Exercise and Rehabilitation in Heart Failure

Editor

ROSS A. ARENA

HEART FAILURE CLINICS

www.heartfailure.theclinics.com

Consulting Editors
MANDEEP R. MEHRA
JAVED BUTLER

January 2015 • Volume 11 • Number 1

ELSEVIER

1600 John F. Kennedy Boulevard • Suite 1800 • Philadelphia, Pennsylvania, 19103-2899

http://www.theclinics.com

HEART FAILURE CLINICS Volume 11, Number 1
January 2015 ISSN 1551-7136, ISBN-13: 978-0-323-34176-9

Editor: Adrianne Brigido
Developmental Editor: Susan Showalter

Heart Failure Clinics (ISSN 1551-7136) is published quarterly by Elsevier Inc., 360 Park Avenue South, New York, NY 10010-1710. Months of publication are January, April, July, and October. Business and editorial offices: 1600 John F. Kennedy Boulevard, Suite 1800, Philadelphia, PA 19103-2899. Periodicals postage paid at New York, NY, and additional mailing offices. Subscription prices are USD 235.00 per year for US individuals, USD 382.00 per year for US institutions, USD 80.00 per year for US students and residents, USD 280.00 per year for Canadian individuals, USD 442.00 per year for Canadian institutions, USD 300.00 per year for international individuals, USD 442.00 per year for international institutions, and USD 100.00 per year for Canadian and foreign students/residents. To receive student and resident rate, orders must be accompanied by name of affiliated institution, date of term, and the *signature* of program/residency coordinator on institution letterhead. Orders will be billed at individual rate until proof of status is received. Foreign air speed delivery is included in all *Clinics* subscription prices. All prices are subject to change without notice. **POSTMASTER:** Send address changes to *Heart Failure Clinics*, Elsevier Health Sciences Division, Subscription Customer Service, 3251 Riverport Lane, Maryland Heights, MO 63043. **Customer Service: 1-800-654-2452 (US and Canada). From outside of the US and Canada, call 314-447-8871. Fax: 314-447-8029. For print support, E-mail: JournalsCustomerService-usa@elsevier.com. For online support, E-mail: JournalsOnlineSupport-usa@elsevier.com.**

Reprints. For copies of 100 or more of articles in this publication, please contact the Commercial Reprints Department, Elsevier Inc., 360 Park Avenue South, New York, NY 10010-1710. Tel.: 212-633-3874; Fax: 212-633-3820; E-mail: reprints@elsevier.com.

Heart Failure Clinics is covered in *MEDLINE/PubMed (Index Medicus)*.

Contributors

CONSULTING EDITORS

MANDEEP R. MEHRA, MD
Professor of Medicine, Harvard Medical School; Co-Director, BWH Heart and Vascular Center; Executive Director, Center for Advanced Heart Disease, Brigham and Women's Hospital, Boston, Massachusetts

JAVED BUTLER, MD, MPH
Professor of Internal Medicine, Stony Brook School of Medicine; Chief of Cardiology, Stony Brook University Medical Center, Stony Brook, New York

EDITOR

ROSS A. ARENA, PhD, PT, FAHA
Integrative Physiology Laboratory, Professor and Head, Department of Physical Therapy, College of Applied Health Sciences, University of Illinois at Chicago, Chicago, Illinois

AUTHORS

ANTONIO ABBATE, MD, PhD
Roberts Professor of Cardiology, VCU Pauley Heart Center, Virginia Commonwealth University, Richmond, Virginia

VOLKER ADAMS, PhD
Department of Internal Medicine/Cardiology, University of Leipzig – Heart Center, Leipzig, Germany

SANDEEP AGGARWAL, MD, FRCPC
Associate Clinical Professor of Medicine, Cardiac Wellness Institute of Calgary; Libin Cardiovascular Institute of Alberta, University of Calgary, Calgary, Alberta, Canada

MARTIN A. ALPERT, MD
Brent M. Parker Professor of Medicine, Division of Cardiovascular Medicine, University of Missouri Health Sciences Center, Columbia, Missouri

ROSS A. ARENA, PhD, PT, FAHA
Integrative Physiology Laboratory, Professor and Head, Department of Physical Therapy, College of Applied Health Sciences, University of Illinois at Chicago, Chicago, Illinois

TRACY BAYNARD, PhD
Integrative Physiology Laboratory, College of Applied Health Sciences; Department of Kinesiology and Nutrition, University of Illinois at Chicago, Chicago, Illinois

GIUSEPPE BIONDI-ZOCCAI, MD
Assistant Professor of Cardiology, Department of Medical-Surgical Sciences and Biotechnologies, Sapienza University of Rome, Latina, Italy

AUDREY BORGHI-SILVA, PhD, PT
Cardiopulmonary Physiotherapy Laboratory, Federal University of Sao Carlos, Sao Carlos, Sao Paulo, Brazil

CLINTON A. BRAWNER, PhD
Division of Cardiovascular Medicine, Henry Ford Hospital, Detroit, Michigan

LAWRENCE P. CAHALIN, PhD, PT, CCS, FAHA
Professor, Department of Physical Therapy, Leonard M. Miller School of Medicine, University of Miami, Miami, Florida

JUSTIN M. CANADA, CEP,
Adjunct Professor, Department of Kinesiology and Health Sciences, College of Humanities and Sciences, Virginia Commonwealth University, Richmond, Virginia

DAVE L. DIXON, PharmD
Assistant Professor of Pharmacotherapy, School of Pharmacy, Virginia Commonwealth University, Richmond, Virginia

DANIEL E. FORMAN, MD
Chair, Geriatric Cardiology Section, University of Pittsburgh Medical Center; Director, Cardiac Rehabilitation, VA Pittsburgh Healthcare System, University of Pittsburgh, Pittsburgh, Pennsylvania

NINA C. FRANKLIN, PhD, MS, LMT
Integrative Physiology Laboratory, Department of Physical Therapy, College of Applied Health Sciences, University of Illinois at Chicago, Chicago, Illinois

MARCO GUAZZI, MD, PhD, FACC
Heart Failure Unit, IRCCS Policlinico San Donato, University of Milano, Milano, Italy

TRINA HAUER, BPAS, MSc
Cardiac Wellness Institute of Calgary, Calgary, Alberta, Canada

MARK HAYKOWSKY, PhD
Professor, Department of Physical Therapy, University of Alberta, Edmonton, Alberta, Canada

MARK J.F. HAYKOWSKY, PhD
Faculty of Rehabilitation Medicine, Alberta Cardiovascular and Stroke Research Centre (ABACUS), Mazankowski Alberta Heart Institute, University of Alberta, Edmonton, Alberta, Canada

LEONARD A. KAMINSKY, PhD, FACSM
Professor and Director, Clinical Exercise Physiology Program, Human Performance Laboratory, Ball State University, Muncie, Indiana

VALENTINA LABATE, MD
Heart Failure Unit, IRCCS Policlinico San Donato, University of Milano, Milano, Italy

CARL J. LAVIE, MD, FACC, FACP, FCCP
Professor of Medicine, Department of Cardiovascular Diseases; Medical Director, Cardiac Rehabilitation; Director, Exercise Laboratories, John Ochsner Heart and Vascular Institute, Ochsner Clinical School, The University of Queensland School of Medicine, New Orleans, Louisiana; Department of Preventive Medicine, Pennington Biomedical Research Center, Louisiana State University System, Baton Rouge, Louisiana

RENATA G. MENDES, PhD, PT
Cardiopulmonary Physiotherapy Laboratory, Federal University of Sao Carlos, Sao Carlos, Sao Paulo, Brazil

JONATHAN MYERS, PhD
Cardiology Division, Palo Alto VA Health Care System, Stanford University, Palo Alto, California

JOSEF NIEBAUER, MD, PhD, MBA
Specialist in Internal Medicine, Cardiology, Sports Medicine; Full Professor of Medicine; Chair of the University Institute of Sports Medicine, Prevention and Rehabilitation, Research Institute of Molecular Sports Medicine and Rehabilitation, Institute of Sports Medicine of the State of Salzburg, Sports Medicine of the Olympic Center Salzburg-Rif, Paracelsus Medical University Salzburg, Salzburg, Austria

SHANE A. PHILLIPS, PhD, PT, FAHA
Department of Physical Therapy; Integrative Physiology Laboratory, College of Applied Health Sciences, University of Illinois at Chicago, Chicago, Illinois

SHERRY O. PINKSTAFF, PhD, PT
Assistant Professor, Physical Therapy Program, Department of Clinical and Applied Movement Sciences, University of North Florida, Jacksonville, Florida

BUNNY POZEHL, PhD, APRN-NP, FAHA, FAAN
Professor of Nursing, Lincoln Division, College of Nursing, University of Nebraska Medical Center, Lincoln, Nebraska

PEDRO V. SCHWARTZMANN, PhD, MD
Rehabilitation Institute Lucy Montoro-Clinical Hospital, Ribeirao Preto School of Medicine, University of Sao Paulo, Ribeirão Preto, Sao Paulo, Brazil

JAMES A. STONE, MD, PhD, FRCPC, FAACVPR, FACC
Clinical Professor of Medicine, Cardiac Wellness Institute of Calgary; Libin Cardiovascular Institute of Alberta, University of Calgary, Calgary, Alberta, Canada

XING-GUO SUN, MD
Distinguished Professor of Medicine, Cardiology, and Anesthesiology; Director of Heart-Lung Functional Testing Center, State Key Laboratory of Cardiovascular Disease, Fuwai Hospital, National Center for Cardiovascular Diseases, Chinese Academy of Medical Sciences, Peking Union Medical College, Beijing, People's Republic of China; Respiratory and Critical Care Physiology and Medicine, Department of Medicine, St. John's Cardiovascular Research Center, Harbor-UCLA Medical Center, Torrance, California

ROD S. TAYLOR, PhD
Graduate School of Education, University of Exeter Medical School, Exeter, United Kingdom; National Institute of Public Health, University of Southern Denmark, Odense M, Denmark

RENATA TRIMER, PhD, PT
Cardiopulmonary Physiotherapy Laboratory, Federal University of Sao Carlos, Sao Carlos, Sao Paulo, Brazil

MARY S. TUTTLE, MS
Clinical Exercise Physiology Program, Human Performance Laboratory, Ball State University, Muncie, Indiana

BENJAMIN W. VAN TASSELL, PharmD
Assistant Professor of Pharmacotherapy, School of Pharmacy, Virginia Commonwealth University, Richmond, Virginia

HECTOR O. VENTURA, MD
Professor of Medicine, Department of Cardiovascular Diseases, John Ochsner Heart and Vascular Institute, Ochsner Clinical School, The University of Queensland School of Medicine, New Orleans, Louisiana

KAREN VUCKOVIC, RN, PhD
Department of Biobehavioral Health Sciences, College of Nursing, University of Illinois at Chicago, Chicago, Illinois

MARK A. WILLIAMS, PhD, MAACVPR, FACSM
Professor of Medicine, Division of Cardiology, Creighton University School of Medicine, Omaha, Nebraska

Contents

> One of the primary hallmarks of patients diagnosed with heart failure (HF) is a reduced tolerance to exercise and compromised functional capacity. This limitation stems from poor pumping capacity but also major changes in functioning of the vasculature, skeletal muscle, and respiratory systems. Advances in the understanding of the central and peripheral mechanisms of exercise intolerance during HF are critical for the future design of therapeutic modalities devised to improve outcomes. The interrelatedness between systems cannot be discounted. This review summarizes the current literature related to the pathophysiology of HF contributing to poor exercise tolerance, and potential mechanisms involved.

> Until the late 1980s, physical exercise training was a contraindication in patients with heart failure. Extensive research has demonstrated that exercise training reverses heart failure–associated pathology at the clinical and molecular levels. Exercise training has emerged as a class I recommendation in all major national and international guidelines for the treatment of chronic heart failure. Knowledge gained in clinical trials and molecular research builds a strong case for exercise training as a key therapeutic component of an evidence-based treatment of chronic heart failure. It is long overdue to provide patients with an infrastructure that enables them to benefit from this class I intervention.

> A hallmark of heart failure (HF) is exercise intolerance, along with fatigue and shortness of breath. Functional assessments provide important clinical information. As the disease progresses, HF patients experience a downward spiral leading to a functional disability. Reduced functional abilities restrict or prevent HF patients from performing occupational tasks, which may result in loss of work and reduced quality of life. Functional assessments provide a measure of functional capacity and information on prognosis, disease severity, degree of disability, and quality of life. Direct and indirect cardiovascular and muscular functional assessments for patients with HF are provided in this review.

heart failure (HF) will lead to expanded application of exercise therapy for eligible HF patients. Nonetheless, US patterns of referral to and enrollment in CR for coronary heart disease have been notoriously poor, and such persistent under-enrollment suggests that there are entrenched obstacles that will impede the use of exercise therapy despite the new CR HF indication. However, application of CR for HF may still grow due to dynamic shifts in contemporary US health care.

More countries around world have begun to use cardiac rehabilitation in patients diagnosed with chronic heart failure (HF). Asia is the largest continent in the world and, depending on its economy, culture, and beliefs, a given Asian country differs from Western countries as well as others in Asia. The cardiac rehabilitation practice patterns for patients with HF are somewhat different in Asia. In addition to the formal pattern of Western practice, it also includes special techniques and skills, such as Taiji, Qigong, and Yoga. This article describes cardiac rehabilitation patterns for patients with HF in most Asian countries and areas.

The recent European Society of Cardiology position paper strongly advises participation of patients with stable heart failure (HF) in structured exercise training (ET) programs, and in most recent years considerable efforts have been put into standardization of exercise prescription. Up to now, 3 ET modalities are proposed for HF populations with variable combinations and extent of effects: (1) endurance aerobic (continuous and interval); (2) strength/resistance; (3) respiratory. Irrespective of ET modalities, most of the studies have clearly demonstrated significant improvements in exercise physiology (ie, oxygen consumption, muscle function, and ventilation), quality of life, and left ventricular function.

Heart failure (HF) is a clinical syndrome of breathlessness, lower extremity swelling, fatigue, and exercise intolerance affecting a large portion of the population worldwide, and associated with premature death. Despite improvement in the management of HF, many patients remain unable to complete activities of daily living without experiencing exertional symptoms. Although prevention of death in patients with HF is imperative, treatment of symptoms and improving functional capacity are equally important goals. This article discusses treatments (medical and surgical) associated with improved functional capacity in HF.

Obesity adversely affects many cardiovascular disease (CVD) risk factors and increases the risk of most CVD, including heart failure (HF). HF is markedly increased in the setting of obesity. However, obese patients with HF have a better prognosis than lean patients with HF, which has been termed the *obesity paradox*. Therefore, the role of weight loss, which generally improves ventricular structure, systolic and diastolic ventricular function, and New York Heart Association functional class in HF, remains controversial. This article discusses the pros and cons of weight loss and differentiates purposeful (healthy) from nonpurposeful (unhealthy) weight loss.

There is a robust trove of scientific studies that support the positive physical and mental health benefits associated with aerobic exercise for healthy individuals. These recommendations suggest that more vigorous exercise can be performed on fewer days for the same benefit. High-intensity intermittent exercise (HIIE) training has begun to show promise. HIIE seems safe and improves physiology, quality of life, and functional capacity. This review defines HIIE, discusses its physiologic benefit for patients with heart failure, outlines the studies that have been conducted to date, and places it in the context of the current clinical environment of exercise training for these patients.

Breathing exercises (BE) and inspiratory muscle training (IMT) have been demonstrated to improve ventilation and ventilation-to-perfusion matching, and to improve exercise, functional performance, and many pathophysiologic manifestations of heart failure (HF). This article provides an extensive review of BE and IMT in patients with HF and identifies several key areas in need of further investigation, including the role of expiratory muscle training, IMT targeted at various locations of inspiration (early, mid, or late inspiration), and alteration of the ratio of inspiratory time to total breath time, all of which have substantial potential to improve many pathophysiologic manifestations of HF.

Regular physical activity is firmly recommended as part of a multifaceted approach to heart failure (HF) self-management. Unfortunately, research indicates that most patients are less likely to engage in and adhere to such activities. The widespread use of information and communication technology tools and resources offers an innovative and potentially beneficial avenue for increasing physical activity levels in HF patients. This article presents specific ways in which advances in information and communication technologies, including Internet- and mobile-based communications, social media platforms, and self-monitoring health devices, can serve as a means to broadly promote increasing levels of physical activity to improve health outcomes in the HF population.

HEART FAILURE CLINICS

HEART FAILURE CLINICS

Foreword
Get a Move on Heart Failure

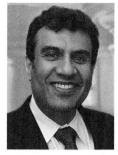 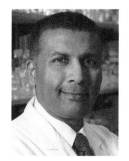

Mandeep R. Mehra, MD   Javed Butler, MD, MPH
Consulting Editors

It was only as recently as 1963 when Burch and colleagues observed the restorative powers of best rest in heart failure. Their observation that prolonged bed rest (combined with digitalis and diuretics) resulted in a return of heart size to normal in half of therapy-compliant patients launched an era of avoidance of exercise in heart failure syndromes. At that time, medical knowledge was largely ignorant of spontaneous recovery in idiopathic cardiomyopathy and did not appreciate the dangers of prolonged inactivity such as venous thromboembolism. Several decades later, the atrophic deconditioning effects of rest and its adverse consequences on the natural history of heart failure became apparent.

As knowledge advanced, the beneficial effects of exercise on functional capacity, quality of life, and skeletal muscle alterations in heart failure became evident. We learned that exercise had effects beyond muscle conditioning, and such lifestyle treatment influenced cellular processes of oxidative stress, resurrected neurohormonal aberrations, and exhibited an impact on the autonomic nervous system, all key arbiters of improved cardiac structure and function in heart failure.

It was only a few years ago that evidentiary support for structured exercise programs in heart failure took root with the demonstration of improved effort tolerance and favorable alteration in the natural history of heart failure, including abrogation of depression symptoms, a key comorbid prognostic marker in this syndrome. The turning tide in favor of rehabilitation using exercise as a lifestyle anchor prompted us to develop this treatise, so ably guest-edited by Dr Ross Arena. We hope that this issue, compiled by an international group of academic stalwarts, will provide a "one-stop shop" for those seeking to understand the fundamentals of exercise and rehabilitation as a key offering in the adjunctive therapeutic armamentarium of all stages of heart failure.

Mandeep R. Mehra, MD
Harvard Medical School
BWH Heart and Vascular Center
Center for Advanced Heart Disease
Brigham and Women's Hospital
75 Francis Street, A Building
3rd Floor, Room AB324
Boston, MA 02115, USA

Javed Butler, MD, MPH
Stony Brook School of Medicine
Stony Brook University Medical Center
101 Nicolls Rd, Stony Brook
NY 11794, USA

E-mail addresses:
MMEHRA@partners.org (M.R. Mehra)
Javed.Butler@stonybrookmedicine.edu (J. Butler)

Heart Failure Clin 11 (2015) xiii
http://dx.doi.org/10.1016/j.hfc.2014.10.002
1551-7136/15/$ – see front matter

heartfailure.theclinics.com

Foreword

Get a Move on Heart Failure

Heart Failure Clin 11 (2015) xvi
http://dx.doi.org/10.1016/j.hfc.2014.10.003
1551-7136/15/ see front matter © 2015 Elsevier Inc. All rights reserved.

Preface
Functional Capacity and Exercise Training Have Earned a Primary Role in the Assessment and Treatment of Patients with Heart Failure

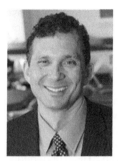

Ross A. Arena, PhD, PT, FAHA
Editor

The importance of functional capacity and lifelong participation in a structured exercise training program to an independent and healthy longevity is no secret. In fact, it has been known and written about for thousands of years,[1–3] and yet, we are only now coming to the realization that functional capacity is a vital sign[4] and "exercise is medicine."[5,6] More importantly, the health care community is also realizing and increasingly acknowledging their importance no matter one's medical status, from the apparently healthy to those diagnosed with a chronic medical condition. No matter, a more appropriate phrase than "better late than never" could not be ascribed to this situation. Universally, successful integration of functional assessment and the prescription of structured exercise training programs into the medical model as well as social and governmental policy/advocacy will undoubtedly result in a healthier global population. We have a long road ahead, but the recent and growing recognition of the importance of physical fitness and activity is a very important first step.

Heart failure (HF) is clearly a global health concern, with an estimated 26 million individuals diagnosed worldwide.[7] Moreover, this chronic condition continues to result in a significant number of hospitalizations around the world[7] and the 5-year survival rate is approximately 50%.[8] The global economic burden (combined direct and indirect costs) is also disconcerting, now estimated to exceed $100 billion.[9] While great strides have been made to improve the prognosis, care, and economic impact of HF,[10] more work is needed, particularly in the realm of effective assessment and treatment strategies; enter quantification of functional capacity and prescription of structured exercise training programs as a clinical indicator of high quality care.

The *Merriam-Webster Dictionary* defines the word "failure" as "omission of occurrence or performance; specifically: a failing to perform a duty or expected action."[11] Given this definition, it would seem counterintuitive to believe assessing function, and participating in exercise training, would be of any benefit. However, nothing could

Heart Failure Clin 11 (2015) xv–xvii
http://dx.doi.org/10.1016/j.hfc.2014.10.001
1551-7136/15/$ – see front matter © 2015 Elsevier Inc. All rights reserved.

be farther from the truth. In this issue of *Heart Failure Clinics*, we take a journey from bench to bedside to clinic to community with respect to all things regarding functional assessment and exercise training. We start at the beginning, understanding why patients with HF oftentimes present with substantial and debilitating functional limitations. The basic-science journey continues with a review of the evidence demonstrating how exercise training actually improves many facets of the pathophysiology brought about by HF, in a sense, helping to reverse and prevent the premise of physiologic "failure." This issue then turns its attention to the bedside and clinic. We start with a comprehensive review on how to assess function; it is not one-size-fits-all and it is also not only about aerobic capacity. While cardiopulmonary exercise testing is the gold standard functional aerobic assessment,[12] it is not feasible in all settings; the important thing is to assess function with resources available, and insights on ways to achieve this in all settings are provided. Moreover, assessing aerobic capacity is oftentimes given more clinical credence than assessing muscular strength and endurance. It is important to remember that both are equally important. The bedside and clinical journey then turns to reasonable functional outcomes associated with exercise training, both aerobic and strength/endurance training, in this case, improving/reversing/preventing the clinical "failure" associated with this condition. The prognostic improvement associated with structured exercise training is another important area and is addressed next. Continuing on the benefits of exercise training in patients with HF, in its purest form, are universal and applicable regardless of where you reside on the planet. However, physical activity promotion and exercise training strategies are not delivered in a universal fashion around the globe. It is therefore important to gain an understanding of these global perspectives, with hopes of working toward a more consistent and optimally effective delivery system. As part of a global health care community, we can all learn from one another; the series of global perspective reviews is presented with that goal in mind. However, the story of functional capacity exercise training related to HF is not that simple or straightforward. Thus, we turn our attention to a series of "special topics" articles: (1) understanding how pharmacologic and surgical interventions improve functional capacity; (2) gaining an appreciation of the obesity paradox and its important interplay with functional capacity and exercise; (3) exploring whether high-intensity interval exercise training is safe and more effective than the traditional moderate intensity continuous exercise approach; (4) discovering the importance of inspiratory muscle weakness and subsequent training strategies in patients with HF; and (5) with the present technologically advanced world in mind and an eye toward the future, we discuss how creative Web-based and mobile platform applications can be used to reach a larger percentage of the HF population, promoting physical activity and providing guidance on exercise training.

It is hoped that this issue of *Heart Failure Clinics* achieves several goals for the readership: (1) to gain an in-depth appreciation of the robust body of literature on the importance of functional assessment and exercise training in the HF population; (2) to be able to describe the physiologic and clinical benefits that can be realized through exercise training in patients with HF; (3) to understand how to assess function and effectively prescribe an exercise training program in patients with HF presenting with a broad array of baseline characteristics and differing degrees of disease severity; (4) to describe the current global perspective of exercise training in patients with HF, understanding strengths and gaps of current practice patterns; and (5) to gain an understanding of an array of unique perspectives associated with (a) changes in functional capacity as it relates to various interventions; (2) the interplay between body habitus, functional capacity, and exercise; (c) forward-thinking models of exercise prescription (eg, high-intensity interval training and inspiratory muscle training); and (d) how technology can be used as an important tool to promote physical activity and guide an exercise training program. As editor of this issue of *Heart Failure Clinics*, I hope this series of review articles will collectively serve as a manifesto that clearly demonstrates the fact that functional capacity assessment and exercise training have earned primary roles in the assessment and treatment of patients with HF. Given the multitude of positive effects gained by leading a physically active lifestyle and participating in a structured exercise training program, perhaps, in the future, we will explore replacing the word "failure" attached to this chronic cardiac condition with a more appropriate term for those who have higher function and lead a healthier lifestyle.

Ross A. Arena, PhD, PT, FAHA
Department of Physical Therapy
College of Applied Health Sciences
University of Illinois Chicago
1919 West Taylor Street (MC 898)
Chicago, IL 60612, USA

E-mail address:
raarena@uic.edu

REFERENCES

1. Tipton CM. Susruta of India, an unrecognized contributor to the history of exercise physiology. J Appl Physiol 2008;104:1553–6.
2. Bhatti SK, O'Keefe JH, Lavie CJ. Of mice and men: atrial fibrillation in veteran endurance runners. J Am Coll Cardiol 2007;63:89.
3. Agarwal SK. Cardiovascular benefits of exercise. Int J Gen Med 2012;5:541–5.
4. Arena R, Myers J, Guazzi M. The future of aerobic exercise testing in clinical practice: is it the ultimate vital sign? Future Cardiol 2010;6:325–42.
5. Coleman KJ, Ngor E, Reynolds K, et al. Initial validation of an exercise "vital sign" in electronic medical records. Med Sci Sports Exerc 2012;44:2071–6.
6. Sallis RE. Exercise is medicine and physicians need to prescribe it! Br J Sports Med 2009;43:3–4.
7. Ambrosy AP, Fonarow GC, Butler J, et al. The global health and economic burden of hospitalizations for heart failure: lessons learned from hospitalized heart failure registries. J Am Coll Cardiol 2014;63:1123–33.
8. Go AS, Mozaffarian D, Roger VL, et al. Heart disease and stroke statistics—2014 update: a report from the American Heart Association. Circulation 2014;129:e28–292.
9. Cook C, Cole G, Asaris P, et al. The annual global economic burden of heart failure. Heart 2014;100:A28–9.
10. Jessup M, Abraham WT, Casey DE, et al. 2009 Focused update: ACCF/AHA guidelines for the diagnosis and management of heart failure in adults: a report of the American College of Cardiology Foundation/American Heart Association Task Force on practice guidelines: developed in collaboration with the International Society for Heart and Lung Transplantation. Circulation 2009;119:1977–2016.
11. Merriam-Webster Dictionary. Available at: http://www.merriam-webster.com/dictionary/failure. Accessed August 10, 2014.
12. Guazzi M, Adams V, Conraads V, et al. EACPR/AHA Scientific Statement. Clinical recommendations for cardiopulmonary exercise testing data assessment in specific patient populations. Circulation 2012;126:2261–74.

Defining the System: Contributors to Exercise Limitations in Heart Failure

Shane A. Phillips, PhD, PT[a,b,*], Karen Vuckovic, RN, PhD[c],
Lawrence P. Cahalin, PhD, PT[d], Tracy Baynard, PhD[b,e]

KEYWORDS

• Exercise • Intolerance • Heart failure • Cardiopulmonary • Vascular • Skeletal muscle

KEY POINTS

• Exercise intolerance is a hallmark symptom of heart failure that severely limits functional capacity, the determinants of which include cardiovascular, skeletal muscle, and respiratory systems.
• Chronotropic incompetence and poor heart-rate reserve in the face of poor pump function further contributes to diminished exercise capacity during heart failure.
• Alterations in the ability of the peripheral and central vasculature to vasodilate at rest and during exercise in heart failure contribute to limit oxygen supply and demand matching.
• The currently identified changes that occur in the skeletal muscles of patients with heart failure are not disease specific, but are similar to those found in aging, deconditioning, and other chronic conditions associated with inflammation.
• The function and compensatory mechanisms of the heart and lungs are intimately related; the primary respiratory factors limiting exercise in patients with heart failure include ventilation, perfusion, and ventilation-perfusion abnormalities.

INTRODUCTION

Chronic heart failure (HF) is marked by severe exercise intolerance with fatigue and dyspnea on exertion. The underlying mechanism of reduced exercise capacity (measured as reduced peak oxygen consumption [Vo_2]) is multifactorial (**Box 1**). Reduced exercise tolerance is a strong prognostic indicator and contributes to poor quality of life.[1] The traditional concepts of exercise limitations have focused on central dysfunction related to poor cardiac pump function, and pulmonary limitations related to congestion of the lungs and dyspnea. However, the mechanisms are not exclusive to the heart and lungs, and the understanding of the pathophysiology of this disease has evolved.[2] The constellation of numerous neurohumoral effects activated by poor pump function can lead to severe changes in the peripheral systems (see **Box 1**). Muscle fatigue and dyspnea are hallmark symptoms of HF that contribute to and exacerbate the symptoms of exercise intolerance (**Fig. 1**). The interrelationships between the

[a] Department of Physical Therapy, College of Applied Health Sciences, University of Illinois at Chicago, 1919 West Taylor Street, MC 898, Chicago, IL 60612, USA; [b] Integrative Physiology Laboratory, College of Applied Health Sciences, University of Illinois at Chicago, 1919 West Taylor Street, Chicago, IL 60612, USA; [c] Department of Biobehavioral Health Sciences, College of Nursing, University of Illinois at Chicago, 845 South Damen Avenue, MC 802, Chicago, IL 60612, USA; [d] Department of Physical Therapy, Leonard M. Miller School of Medicine, University of Miami, 5919 Ponce de Leon Blvd, 5th floor Coral Gables, Miami, FL 33146-2435, USA; [e] Department of Kinesiology and Nutrition, University of Illinois at Chicago, 1919 West Taylor Street, Chicago, IL 60612, USA
* Corresponding author. Department of Physical Therapy, College of Applied Health Sciences, University of Illinois at Chicago, 1919 West Taylor Street, MC 898, Chicago, IL 60612.
E-mail address: shanep@uic.edu

Heart Failure Clin 11 (2015) 1–16
http://dx.doi.org/10.1016/j.hfc.2014.08.009

Box 1
Summary of the system contributors to exercise intolerance in heart failure

1. Cardiac contributors

   ↓ Cardiac reserve

   ↓ End-systolic volume

   ↓ or ↔ End-diastolic volume

   ↑ Left ventricular filling pressures

   Failure of the Starling mechanism

   ↓ Left atrial function

   Left and/or right ventricular remodeling

   ↑ Sympathetic outflow/autonomic dysfunction

   Chronotropic incompetence

   Altered cardiomyocyte physiology/calcium handling

2. Vascular contributors

   ↓ Endothelial function

   ↓ Endothelial nitric oxide synthase protein expression and activity

   ↓ Limb blood flow

   ↑ Arterial stiffness

   ↑ Sympathetic activity

   ↑ Oxidative stress

3. Skeletal muscle contributors

   Muscle atrophy with a shift in muscle fiber type

   ↓ Muscle bulk and fiber cross-sectional area

   ↓ Mitochondria size and function

   ↓ Capillary density

   Increased intracellular acidosis

   ↓ Phosphocreatine and glycogen content

   Impaired calcium homeostasis

   ↓ Insulin-like growth factor 1 expression

4. Respiratory contributors

   Pulmonary edema

   ↓ Elastic recoil of the lungs

   Ascites

   Inspiratory muscle weakness

   ↓ Right ventricular performance

   ↑ Pulmonary artery pressure and vascular resistance

   Ventilation-perfusion mismatch

   Ventricular asynchrony

   Cardiac arrhythmias

   Loss of viable and elastic lung tissue

central hemodynamics and the peripheral systems (vascular, skeletal, and pulmonary) that affect exercise tolerance are poorly understood. However, this review outlines current knowledge about the contribution of these systems to exercise performance and the potential implications of these contributors for the symptoms of HF.

CARDIAC CONTRIBUTORS TO EXERCISE LIMITATIONS IN HEART FAILURE

HF is often defined as the inability to achieve and/or maintain an appropriate cardiac output (Q),[3] and one of the important signs of HF is exercise intolerance, as measured by low peak Vo_2 values. Exercise intolerance in HF patients can be currently explained by numerous inadequacies ranging from peripheral to ventilatory; however, specific cardiac limitations are discussed here, in particular in relation to the cardiac side of the Fick equation ($Vo_2 = Q \times a\text{-}vO_{2diff}$). With Q being composed of both stroke volume and heart rate (HR), HF patients often have diminished capacities on both of these fronts.

Overview of Heart Failure with Preserved Ejection Fraction

HF with preserved ejection fraction (HFpEF) (eg, diastolic HF) has recently been the focus of many investigations intent on understanding the pathophysiology behind low peak aerobic capacities in this population, which warrants discussion here. Despite a normal resting EF, patients with HFpEF exhibit an attenuated change in EF with exercise in comparison with hypertensive patients.[4–7] This change demonstrates that EF may not be the best measure of contractility, owing to the dependence on load and remodeling effects. Nevertheless, this smaller change in EF with exercise does not seem to have one firm culprit, but several contenders, which include either a smaller change in end-diastolic volume (EDV) (eg, less EDV reserve),[6] and/or a smaller end-systolic volume (ESV) reserve.[4,5,8] Of interest, most recent studies have not been able to support the findings of Kitzman and colleagues[6] that demonstrated a lower EDV response with exercise, which would suggest the failure of the Frank-Starling mechanism. Rather, several studies demonstrate similar EDV responses to exercise when comparing HFpEF patients with a control group,[4,5,8,9] suggesting that the left ventricle may fill to an appropriate EDV. However, this does not mean that the Frank-Starling mechanism is fully operational, despite normal EDV reserve.

Evidence suggests indeed that both the static Starling[7] and the novel dynamic Starling

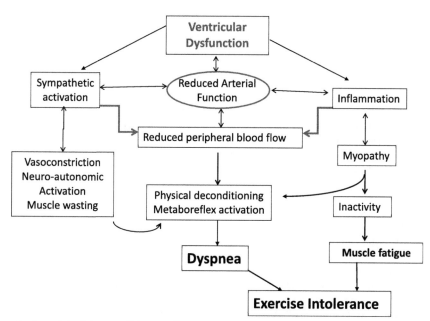

Fig. 1. Conceptual model of the possible contributors to exercise intolerance in heart failure.

mechanisms[10] are compromised in HFpEF either at rest or with exercise,[11] resulting in elevated left ventricular (LV) filling pressures (LVFP). Increased LVFP are often coupled to increased LV elastance and prolonged relaxation,[12,13] and collectively contribute altered filling properties in HFpEF patients.[14] Skaluba and Litwin[15] found that high filling pressures were highly correlated with exercise intolerance in patients with HFpEF. Furthermore, global contractile indices are impaired in HFpEF patients, in that contractile and ventricular-vascular coupling reserve is diminished in HFpEF both at low-level exercise and peak exercise.[8] Contractile dysfunction among patients with HFpEF has also been supported by population-based work.[16]

In addition to the pathophysiologic LV changes and reduced reserves that occur with HFpEF, left atrial (LA) function is also impaired both at rest[17–20] and with exercise,[21,22] which can help explain poor atrial compensation during late diastole and higher LVFP and, thus, poor systolic and diastolic performance in this population. A recent report on individuals without overt HF observed that LA volume index (LA volume/body surface area) was an important predictor for an abnormal exercise LVFP.[23] It is obvious that numerous impairments exist among patients with HFpEF that span across a wide array of both diastolic and systolic-related measurements, all contributing to reduced cardiac performance, with exercise possibly enhancing the lack of cardiac reserve available in patients with HFpEF, thus contributing to exercise intolerance.

Overview of Heart Failure with Reduced Ejection Fraction

HF patients with reduced ejection fraction (HFrEF) (eg, systolic HF) also suffer from severe exercise intolerance, with maximal Q estimated to be approximately less than 50% of that in a healthy control group.[24,25] Earlier work by Sullivan and colleagues[26,27] demonstrated that HFrEF is associated with poor cardiac reserve during exercise, largely because of diminished systolic volume (SV) and maximal HR responses. In many cases of HFrEF the left ventricle is dilated, which corresponds with an inability to appropriately increase LVEDV, because the left ventricle is at or near maximal volume, resulting in the failure of the Starling mechanism and reductions in preload and EF. The higher LVESV and LVEDV collectively contribute to augmented LVFP and pulmonary capillary wedge pressure, which are important contributors to pulmonary hypertension, dyspnea, and right ventricular dysfunction. In the many cases of HFrEF with diastolic dysfunction, resistance to filling exists because of higher ventricular elastance and lower distensibility.

Heart Rate and Chronotropic Incompetence

With Q reserve at less than 50% of that in healthy controls, HF patients must rely on cardioacceleration to substitute for diminished SV during periods of increased physical activity. However, chronotropic incompetence, which is present in approximately 25% to 70% of the HF population,[28] further contributes to diminished exercise capacity and demonstrates the integrated nature of multiple mechanisms contributing to poor exercise tolerance.

Despite several different ways to determine chronotropic incompetence (reviewed by Brubaker and Kitzman[28]), it serves as a strong determinant of exercise intolerance in HF patients. In studies of patients with heart disease (not specifically HF), chronotropic incompetence is strongly related to observed myocardial perfusion abnormalities and increased risk of mortality.[29,30] Specifically in HF patients, HR reserve (difference between peak and resting HR) is attenuated and associated with peak Vo_2. This diminished reserve accounted for 16% of the differences in peak Vo_2 among those defined as either having or not having chronotropic incompetence, which has clinical and functional manifestations when peak aerobic capacities average approximately 15 mL O_2/kg/min in the HF population.[31] In support of this, Witte and colleagues[32] observed that peak aerobic capacity was 14% lower in HF patients with chronotropic incompetence. Of note, this study found similar correlations between peak Vo_2 and the change in HR among HF patients who were either taking or not taking β-blockers ($r = 0.56$ and 0.60), suggesting the importance of chronotropic incompetence.[32] Borlaug and colleagues[9] observed in patients with HFpEF that the HR response and afterload were primarily associated with Q, but that peak Vo_2 was not associated with changes in either SV or EDV with exercise. Again this suggests the importance of HR reserve as a determinant of exercise intolerance.

Chronotropic incompetence coupled with impaired HR recovery (HRR) following exercise suggests autonomic dysfunction, which is known to exist among HF patients as evidenced by heightened sympathetic[33] and altered parasympathetic tone.[34,35] Corroborating this concept, Keller-Ross and colleagues[36] observed that locomotor metaboreflex stimulation using regional circulatory occlusion significantly altered both the arterial baroreflex and HRR following exercise in patients with HFrEF. Again this demonstrates the various levels of impairments throughout the "cardiovascular tree," with autonomic dysfunction possibly playing a central role with regard to cardiac issues at hand for exercise intolerance.

Molecular and Cellular Factors of Ventricular Dysfunction

Many structural and functional changes occur throughout the pathogenesis of HF at the molecular and cellular levels. Remodeling involves changes in cardiomyocyte physiology, factors involved in the intercellular/extracellular matrix, and vessel reorganization, which can lead to increased ventricular stiffness, impaired contractility, or both.[37] It is important to bear in mind that remodeling of one chamber will often result in negative consequences for another chamber (eg, LV failure can lead to right ventricular remodeling because of higher filling pressures).

With respect to cardiomyocytes, volume-overload conditions (ie, HFrEF) can cause increases in length, whereas pressure overload (ie, HFpEF) can increase myocyte thickness.[38] Increased apoptosis and necrosis, combined with lower rates of autophagy, can also contribute to adverse remodeling, especially in situations where infracts are present.[37] Furthermore, the renin-angiotensin system can be activated with wall stress that can lead to cardiac hypertrophy,[39] with concomitant interstitial remodeling stemming from upregulation of aldosterone and angiotensin II, transforming growth factor, and alterations in matrix metalloproteinases (MMP) and tissue inhibitors of MMPs.[37,40–42] Adding further insult, calcium handling becomes impaired with HF, thus limiting excitation-contraction coupling.[43] This process occurs largely through diminished calcium uptake in the sarcoplasmic reticulum and/or elevations in diastolic calcium leak (specifically the ryanodine receptors) of the sarcoplasmic reticulum, or through changes in sodium handling.[43]

Ventricular stiffness can also be attributed to changes in the extracellular matrix, because this matrix is important in preventing overstretch, myocyte slippage, and tissue deformation during filling.[42] Furthermore, the extracellular matrix is also involved with factors of growth and tissue differentiation. For instance, collagen deposition is increased with pressure overload and has been associated with extracellular matrix-related stiffness.[42,44] As many of the aforementioned mechanisms have not been studied specifically in relation to exercise intolerance, it would follow that these factors (and others) provide the molecular and cellular basis for the clinically measured LV dysfunction present in HF, and contribute to poor exercise performance.

VASCULAR CONTRIBUTORS TO EXERCISE LIMITATIONS IN HEART FAILURE

Previous work has found that the often observed major limitations of exercise capacity in HF are related to peripheral abnormalities in the exercising muscle and vasculature.[27,45] Cardiac output increases more than 7-fold during exercise, and a major component of this increase is related to metabolic vasodilation of the exercising muscle.[46,47] In patients with HF, the impaired ability of the circulation to vasodilate and, hence, the restriction of enhanced perfusion in exercising muscle may have severe consequences for exercise tolerance (see **Fig. 1**). The causes of this apparent dysfunction at the level of the circulation during exercise appear to have multiple mechanistic contributors during HF, including (1) increased sympathetic nervous system (SNS) activation, (2) activation of the renin-angiotensin system that enhances vasonconstrictor tone, (3) impaired endothelial-dependent vasodilation, (4) reduced blood vessel density, and (5) increased arterial stiffness, all of which limits tissue perfusion and distribution to the working muscle.[48]

Peripheral Vascular Impairments

Up to 85% of the total Q is used to perfuse the working muscle.[49] During acute exercise in healthy individuals, there is rapid vasodilation of the resistance arteries with concomitant increases in muscle pumping action that serve to supply sufficient oxygen to the working muscles. At very high metabolic demand, the cardiovascular systems' supply of blood to working muscle is excessive.[27] In patients with HF the mechanisms that serve to compensate and preserve cardiac output (ie, activation of the renin-angiotensin-aldosterone system, increased SNS, and sodium and water retention) result in many physiologic imbalances that damage the vasculature and contribute to an earlier mismatch between oxygen supply and demand.[50] The exercise response is hampered by the mechanisms outlined above, resulting in reduced myocardial perfusion, reduced peripheral vasodilation, and increased afterload.

In terms of reduced blood flow to exercising muscle, there are multiple contributing mechanisms. In patients with HF, there is a dramatic shift toward an increase in vasoconstrictor tone that hampers perfusion at rest and during exercise.[51] For example, chronic inhibition of the SNS with clonidine was shown to increase peak vascular conductance during exercise in an HF cohort.[52] Of importance, a high level of SNS activation that occurs during exercise is associated with reduced exercise capacity.[53,54] This exaggerated increase is likely to contribute to the impact of reduced vascular conductance during exercise and exercise capacity.[53]

Role of Endothelial Dysfunction

Physiologic impairment of the endothelium is known as vascular endothelial dysfunction. Reduced endothelial function is a hallmark of cardiovascular disease, and in HF is severely reduced.[55–57] This condition most commonly results from an imbalance between vasodilator and vasoconstrictor substances produced by the endothelium. There is ample evidence demonstrating that the primary mechanism of endothelial dysfunction is a reduction in endothelium-derived nitric oxide (NO) bioavailability. Although the exact mechanism by which this reduction occurs is still under debate, several key mechanisms have been studied, including: disturbances in the NO signaling pathway; reduced bioavailability of the endothelial nitric oxide synthase (eNOS) substrate L-arginine and/or tetrahydrobiopterin (BH$_4$); modified expression and functional activity of eNOS; extracellular scavenging of NO by reactive oxygen species (ROS); and increased production of endothelium-derived vasoconstrictors.[58]

Mechanisms that contribute to reduce NO bioavailability include lower eNOS expression and/or increased quenching of NO by superoxide.[59] Treatment with antioxidants reduces superoxide levels and improves endothelium-dependent vasodilator function, suggesting that ROS are integral to vascular dysfunction.[60] High levels of oxidative stress that overwhelms the vascular antioxidant systems are observed in HF,[61] and superoxide has been linked to peripheral hypoperfusion, peripheral endothelial dysfunction, and exaggerated SNS activity in patients with HF, leading to further to exercise intolerance. Oxidative stress is closely related to peak VO_2 and severity of HF,[61] suggesting that oxidative stress may be a contributor to exercise intolerance.

Endothelial cells are uniquely positioned between circulating blood and the fixed underlying vascular wall, exposing them to shear stress of up to 50 dyn/cm.[62] In the coronary circulation during HF, the endothelium exposed to reduced blood flow and shear stress adapts in a manner that promotes endothelial dysfunction. During physiologic levels of shear stress, there is improved eNOS generation of NO by enzyme phosphorylation[62] and increases in eNOS expression and NO-dependent dilation.[63] Decreased coronary endothelium-dependent dilation can reduce myocardial perfusion, resulting in reduced ventricular function.[64,65] The dysfunctional endothelium contributes to increased vascular stiffness and impaired arterial distensibility, facilitating further myocardial dysfunction. Furthermore, there is emerging evidence that NO itself may have a positive impact on myocardial function, whereas reductions in NO are linked to myocardial necrosis.[66] Improved endothelial function and NO synthase expression are seen after aerobic exercise training[67] in patients with coronary disease and

HF, which is associated with improved exercise tolerance.

Role of Arterial Stiffness

In addition to reduced endothelial function, increased arterial stiffness is associated with cardiovascular mortality and contributes to premature elevations in blood pressure,[7] and is increased in HF. The relationship between the structure of large vessels and arterial stiffness is strong. For example, carotid artery intima-media thickness (another well-known subclinical risk factor for cardiovascular disease) has been associated with pulse pressure and other markers of arterial stiffness.[68] However, in small blood vessels such as the arterioles where tissue blood flow is tightly regulated during exercise, smooth muscle tone can more directly influence arterial stiffness. These changes can occur in such a way that the loss of vasodilators such as NO and the enhancement of vasoconstrictor reactivity in HF enhances arterial stiffness. Increases in arterial stiffness contribute to increased velocity of the reflected pulse waves during the cardiac cycle and reduction of aortic pressure during diastole.[69] These effects can lead to a decrease in myocardial perfusion, leading to a potential mismatch between myocardial oxygen demand and supply, another vicious cycle in HF that leads to further muscle injury. As the artery stiffens during HF, LV afterload (a milestone of HF) also increases. Increased arterial stiffness is associated with diastolic dysfunction[69] and is increased in patients with HFpEF.[70] Although pulse pressure is a crude index of arterial stiffness, higher values predict cardiovascular events and mortality following a myocardial infarction in HF patients.[71] Arterial stiffness is related to walk-time performance during a functional walk test[72] and aortic stiffness was strongly associated with peak V_{O_2} in patients with dilated cardiomyopathy.[73] Finally, Kitzman and colleagues[70] found that carotid arterial stiffness was significantly correlated with peak V_{O_2} and the 6-minute walk distance in patients with HFpEF.

Role of Inflammation on Peripheral Vasculature Contributors to Exercise Intolerance

Both acute and chronic inflammatory conditions have been associated with increased arterial stiffness[74–76] and reduced endothelial function in patients with HF.[77] Concentrations of inflammatory markers such as interleukin (IL)-6 and tumor necrosis factor (TNF)-α have been shown to be greater in patients with HF.[78] There are multiple studies showing a strong relationship between

elevated C-reactive protein (CRP) during cardiovascular disease and HF and increased arterial stiffness.[79–81] High levels of CRP can decrease eNOS activity[82] and increase endothelin (ET)-1,[83] resulting in reduced vasodilation, enhanced vasoconstriction, and increased arterial stiffness. In addition, both IL-6 and TNF-α can induce vascular inflammation, which may be a critical component of the vicious cycle that occurs between inflammation of the vasculature and further cardiac insult during HF.[84–86] ET-1 is a potent vasoconstrictor peptide that is released from endothelium. The biological effects of ET-1 include vasoconstriction, stimulation of vascular smooth muscle proliferation, and enhanced cardiac hypertrophy. ET-1 is increased in patients with HF, and high plasma ET-1 levels are associated with poor prognosis in these patients.[51] The levels of TNF-α, IL-6, and ET-1 seem to be associated with severity of disease, and peak exercise in these patients accentuates the inflammatory response, suggesting that exercise itself may activate the proinflammatory systems that mitigate blood flow responses to exercise. In addition, this viscous cycle further compromises the ability of the working muscle arterioles to vasodilate. Thus, systemic and local inflammation has a dramatic negative effect on arterial function during exercise.

Vascular Dysfunction in Heart Failure with Preserved and Reduced Ejection Fraction

More than half of the patients with HF have preserved LVEF (HFpEF). This population has dramatic reductions in exercise intolerance that can be in part related to changes in peripheral vasculature. For example, peripheral vascular resistance in HFpEF patients is increased and appears to contribute to exercise intolerance (ie, lower peak V_{O_2}).[8,14] Borlaug and colleagues[8] demonstrated that endothelial function measured as the hyperemic response in finger blood flow following upper arm occlusion was reduced in HFpEF patients compared with patients with hypertension. Patients demonstrating endothelial dysfunction had more fatigue and dyspnea during submaximal exercise, suggesting that vasodilator function may be critical for determining exercise capacity in HFpEF.[14] There are data corroborating this hypothesis in a study by Guazzi and colleagues,[87] where treatment of HFrEF patients with sildenafil improved endothelial function, this improvement being closely related to exercise tolerance. In another study, Kitzman and colleagues[88] found that improvements in peak V_{O_2} following 16 weeks of exercise training occurred without improvements in endothelial function or reduction in arterial stiffness, suggesting that exercise training may affect other determinants of exercise capacity in patients with HFpEF. Obviously the timing and sequence of vascular dysfunction and arterial stiffness that occurs during HFpEF and HFrEF, and the implications for exercise intolerance, will require further investigation.

CONTRIBUTIONS OF SKELETAL MUSCLE TO EXERCISE INTOLERANCE

In patients with HF, the inability of the myocardium to meet the demands of skeletal muscle during exercise initiates compensatory mechanisms that include the neuroactivation of the SNS, renin-aldosterone-angiotensin system, vasopressin, and natriuretic peptides. The overactivation of autonomic signals leads to hypoperfusion and tissue hypoxia of skeletal muscle, resulting in progressive structural, metabolic, and functional adaptations in the peripheral musculature, including atrophy. These critical changes contribute to fatigue during exercise, a cardinal symptom of HF (see **Fig. 1**).

The view that significant alterations in the structure (mass), metabolism, and function of skeletal muscle (SM) play an important role in limiting exercise capacity in patients with HF is well accepted. It has been more than 20 years since the SM hypothesis was first proposed.[89] Since then, accumulating evidence supports the view that the complex pathophysiology of HF may begin with reduced cardiac function but ultimately involves peripheral abnormalities in SM. The alterations in SM (locomotor and diaphragm) are an important determinant of exercise capacity, dyspnea, and fatigue, and increase in conjunction with deterioration of symptoms. From a clinical standpoint, improvements in SM alterations can significantly improve functional abilities, to an extent similar to that of age-matched controls for patients with nonadvanced HF.[90]

Alterations in Skeletal Muscle Structure

In patients with HF, reduced levels of physical activity lead to SM atrophy (disuse and loss of mass)[91] and a low-level systemic inflammatory state.[92] Skeletal muscle atrophy leads to a reduction in cross-sectional area of myofibers, and an overall decrease in SM strength and endurance.[93] The underlying mechanisms that mediate SM atrophy are likely related to activation of signaling pathways that regulate protein degradation,[48] decreased protein synthesis, or both.[94,95] Evidence from animal models and human studies indicate that an imbalance between anabolic factors such as growth hormone and insulin-like

growth factor (IGF)-1[96,97] and catabolic factors such as myostatin,[98] TNF-α,[99] and interleukins[99] modulates apoptosis, inflammation, and protein synthesis, and serves to reinforce the loss of SM mass.[95] Apoptosis has been detected in the SM of patients with HF, and its presence has been shown to be negatively correlated with peak Vo_2, length of illness, and SM atrophy.[100] Atrophy is associated with increased SNS activation and increased levels of angiotensin II,[101–103] which lead to vasoconstriction and reduced O_2 delivery. Increased angiotensin II and oxidative stress coupled with reduced IGF-1 concentration mediate SM inflammation.[92] This negative interaction between atrophy and inflammation is not exclusive to HF but is also associated with aging, deconditioning, diabetes, obesity, chronic pulmonary disease, and chronic kidney disease.[92] Thus the progression of changes in the structure of SM may be driven by and related to the presence of 1 of several chronic conditions.

A consistent morphologic SM change identified in muscle biopsies of patients with HF, and later confirmed using ^{31}P magnetic resonance spectroscopy (MRS), is a shift in muscle fiber type from long endurance type I fibers (aerobic, oxidative) toward the easily fatigued type IIb fibers (anaerobic, glycolytic),[90,91,104] and a reduced capillary-to-fiber ratio.[105] Mancini and colleagues[90] and Lipkin and colleagues[104] were among the first to report a significant relationship between fiber type and peak Vo_2, suggesting that a shift in fiber type might promote exercise intolerance. These fiber changes promote fatigue-related processes and incur an O_2 deficit in the working SM, resulting in glycogenolysis and premature acidosis,[106] occurring independently of changes in blood flow. Furthermore, an augmented blood flow does not delay the onset of anaerobic metabolism or increase exercise capacity.[107] Taken together, these data suggest that SM myopathy in HF is metabolic in origin.

Alterations in Skeletal Muscle Metabolism

In addition to structural changes, intrinsic metabolic abnormalities, such as decreased number of functional mitochondria,[105] decreased capillary density,[108] reduced production and release of endothelial-derived vasodilator factors,[109] and decreased oxidative enzymes, affect the oxidative capacity of SM during HF. These changes result in early anaerobic metabolism and muscle fatigue. MRS studies have been used to examine phosphocreatine and adenosine triphosphate metabolism, and showed that during exercise patients with HF deplete their energy stores at a lower O_2 capacity than age-matched controls, and have a lengthened recovery from exercise.[110] Recently, interest has focused on bioenergetics and the effects inflammatory cytokines and ROS as mediators of SM dysfunction and promoters of oxidative stress.[111]

Alterations in Skeletal Muscle Function

Reduced exercise capacity and some degree of muscle wasting is common even in mild HF.[112] Loss of leg SM mass seems to be an early event in the natural history of HF, while alterations in body composition of the arms occurs as disease progresses.[113] The pathologic SM changes in HF are associated with progressive functional limitations such falls, bone fractures,[114] disability, and frailty.[95]

In patients with HF the working SM must compete with the demands of the respiratory muscles for a share of an already diminished Q and overcome amplified SNS, neurohormonal, and reflex-driven vasoconstriction. In addition, mechanosensitive and metabosensitive afferents within the contracting SM increase global sympathetic activation. In turn, lower V_{O_2}, slower O_2 uptake, and microvascular changes produce metabolites that accumulate and stimulate these afferents (**Fig. 2**).[115] SMs sense tension, displacement, and fatigue via tendon organs, muscle spindles, joint receptors, and small nerve endings. It is the sensory function of SM that likely contributes to the symptoms of dyspnea and fatigue via the exercise pressor reflex.[116] It is clear that SM myopathy may be triggered by alterations in central hemodynamics, but becomes an independent phenomenon in HF.[111]

Although most evidence related to SM changes during HF has been established from studies in animal models and clinical studies of patients with HF and a reduced EF, many of the SM abnormalities discussed are not exclusive to HFrEF. Rather, the same derangements occur in the comorbid conditions associated with HFrEF (eg, diabetes). Thus it is likely that patients with HFpEF are subject to the same SM abnormalities. Further investigation of these changes in HFpEF is warranted.

Although physical deconditioning may be a contributor, intrinsic changes in SM induced by

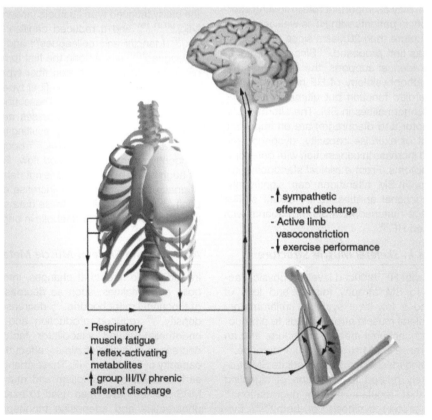

- ↑ sympathetic
  efferent discharge
- Active limb
  vasoconstriction
- ↓ exercise performance

- Respiratory
  muscle fatigue
- ↑ reflex-activating
  metabolites
- ↑ group III/IV phrenic
  afferent discharge

Fig. 2. The respiratory metaboreflex. (*From* Cahalin LP, Arena R, Guazzi M, et al. Inspiratory muscle training in heart disease and heart failure: a review of the literature with a focus on method of training and outcomes. Expert Rev Cardiovasc Ther 2013;11(2):161–77; with permission.)

chronic hypoperfusion are important factors in exercise intolerance. These factors include SM atrophy, poor O_2 utilization, and delayed recovery of SM after submaximal exercise. It may be that the extent of atrophy and inflammation and the corresponding cross-talk among these factors mediate the mechanisms underlying exercise intolerance. However, unlike limb musculature, which is underused, as the HF syndrome progresses the respiratory musculature is exposed to an ever increasing workload as lung compliance decreases.

CONTRIBUTIONS OF THE RESPIRATORY SYSTEM TO EXERCISE INTOLERANCE

Respiratory contributions have been shown to limit exercise in patients with HF. The manner in which the respiratory system limits exercise is due to abnormalities in ventilation, perfusion, or both.[117–121] However, the etiology of these abnormalities seems to be due to impairments in pulmonary function, respiratory muscle strength, and endurance, in addition to impairments in tissue perfusion both centrally and peripherally.[118,119,122–124] The effects of each of these impairments on exercise tolerance are described here within the context of ventilation, perfusion, and ventilation-perfusion abnormalities. Two key pathophysiologic consequences of ventilation-perfusion abnormalities in HF are a steep minute ventilation (VE) to carbon dioxide production (VE/VCo_2) slope and exercise oscillatory ventilation (EOV).[121,122,125,126] The VE/VCo_2 slope is captured during submaximal or maximal exercise, with a slope greater than 30 associated with inefficient ventilation; EOV is usually identified during exercise, but can occur at rest, and is defined as 3 or more oscillatory fluctuations in VE at a minimal average amplitude of 5 L/min persisting for a particular percentage of time during exercise.[121,125,126] The pathophysiologic basis for a steep VE/VCo_2 slope and EOV are discussed because both are key reasons why the respiratory system is a major factor in limiting exercise and functional performance in patients with HF.[121,122,125,126] Furthermore, EOV is used as a conceptual model, highlighting the interrelatedness of cardiorespiratory and neurohormonal activity in the failing heart and providing the mechanisms by which the respiratory system limits exercise in HF.

Ventilation Abnormalities

Abnormalities in ventilation include those listed in **Box 1**. The key factors limiting ventilation in HF include pulmonary edema, loss of elastic recoil of the lungs, ascites, and inspiratory muscle

weakness.[117–119,127] Thus, in view of these key factors the abnormalities in ventilation in HF appear to be mostly restrictive in origin. In fact, the ventilatory response during exercise in HF is more typical of a restrictive lung disorder in view of: (1) decreased tidal volume, end-tidal carbon dioxide, peak Vo_2, and tidal volume (VT) to ventilation ratio (VT/VE); and (2) increased respiratory rate, VE, peak dead space ventilation to tidal volume ratio (VD/VT), ventilation to Vo_2 ratio (VE/Vo_2), and the VE/VCo_2 slope.[123,125,128] In HF, a steep VE/VCo_2 slope (>30) is identified by substantially greater VE for a given level of VCo_2, and thus reflects inefficient ventilation.[125] Nonetheless, pulmonary function tests of patients with HF reveal restrictive, obstructive, and combined restrictive and obstructive patterns.[120,129] It is likely that these pulmonary function patterns reflect lifestyle, the pathophysiologic consequences of HF, and the key factors limiting ventilation.[120,129] Of note is that noninvasive positive pressure ventilation (NIPPV) is a key modality in the management of patients with acute HF exacerbations, highlighting the manner whereby all of the aforementioned factors likely contribute to functional and exercise limitations in HF.[124] In fact, recent research has revealed that NIPPV provided to patients with stable HF during exercise can improve not only ventilation but also cardiovascular performance.[130]

A seminal article investigating the influence of pulmonary edema on exercise tolerance revealed that even subclinical fluid retention can significantly impair exercise ability, but that targeted therapy via diuresis alone can significantly increase exercise tolerance, with improvement in symptoms and cardiorespiratory performance. Diuresis of 4.5 ± 2.2 kg over 4 ± 2 days to a resting right atrial pressure of 6 ± 4 mm Hg and wedge pressure of 19 ± 7 mm Hg increased exercise duration from 9.2 ± 4.2 to 12.5 ± 4.7 minutes, which was associated with significant improvements in ventilation, lactate levels, and dyspnea.[117]

These results support the likelihood of alveolar gas diffusion abnormalities limiting exercise tolerance in HF.[117] Furthermore, important correlations have been found to support the role of alveolar gas diffusion abnormalities in limiting exercise in HF despite a lack of significant arterial oxygen desaturation during exercise, including significant correlations between: (1) baseline diffusion capacity for carbon monoxide (DLCO) and peak Vo_2; (2) alveolar-capillary membrane conductance and the VE/VCo_2; and (3) the improvement in DLCO and peak Vo_2 after enalapril treatment.[118]

The most likely reason for the lack of arterial oxygen desaturation during exercise in patients with

HF is the recruitment of alveolar-capillary membrane conductance areas to compensate for decreased pulmonary perfusion. Such recruitment suggests that the alveolar-capillary membrane is pliable, at least in less advanced HF, and accommodates imposed demands, which is important in regard to therapeutic efforts to improve exercise tolerance in patients with HF. Therapeutic efforts that promote such recruitment may improve arterial oxygenation despite poor pulmonary perfusion.[118]

Inspiratory muscle weakness is another key factor responsible for abnormal ventilation in HF.[119,127] A substantial body of literature has identified the relationship between inspiratory muscle weakness and symptoms, exercise intolerance, inefficient ventilation, and abnormal cardiopulmonary exercise testing (CPX).[119,127] Poor inspiratory muscle endurance is also a key factor responsible for abnormal ventilation in HF but has an even greater potential than inspiratory muscle weakness to limit exercise tolerance, because respiratory muscle fatigue stimulates the respiratory metaboreflex.[127,128,131] The respiratory metaboreflex is stimulated by respiratory muscle fatigue and, as outlined in **Fig. 2**, includes SNS activation and vasoconstriction in resting and exercising limbs to shunt oxygenated blood to fatiguing respiratory muscles, providing exercising limb muscles with less available oxygenated blood and limiting exercise tolerance.[128] It is important that expiratory muscle fatigue also has the capacity to contribute to the respiratory metaboreflex.[128]

A substantial body of literature has also identified the favorable role inspiratory muscle training (IMT) may have in patients with HF who have inspiratory muscle weakness and poor inspiratory muscle endurance.[128] In fact, patients with HF who have maximal inspiratory strength that is 75% or less of the predicted value appear to receive the greatest benefit from IMT, with improvements in exercise and functional performance as well as in many CPX results.[128] The role of expiratory muscle training in HF has drawn limited investigation despite the fact that expiratory muscle strength is poor in HF and is related to dyspnea in HF[119]; however, preliminary findings on improving exercise and functional performance appear promising.[128]

Perfusion Abnormalities

Abnormalities in perfusion include those listed in **Box 1**. The key factors limiting perfusion in HF include poor right ventricular performance and elevated pulmonary artery pressure in addition to pulmonary vascular resistance (PVR).[118,120,121]

An elegant study examined the influence of right ventricular performance, the VE/VCO_2 slope, and PVR on right ventricular oxidative metabolism via positron emission tomography, and found that the VE/VCO_2 slope was significantly correlated with right ventricular oxidative metabolism ($r = 0.61$; $P = .003$).[121] In addition, right ventricular oxidative metabolism was significantly greater in patients with a VE/VCO_2 slope of 34 or greater compared with patients with a VE/VCO_2 slope of less than 34 (0.93 ± 0.16 vs 0.77 ± 0.16; $P = .04$).[121] Thus, PVR appears to be a major determinant of ventilatory inefficiency in patients with HF.[118,121,123,125] Interventions aimed at improving PVR are likely to improve right ventricular performance and metabolism, and the efficiency of ventilation, all of which are likely to improve functional and exercise performance.[118,121,123]

Ventilation-Perfusion Abnormalities

Ventilation-perfusion abnormalities in HF are due to the aforementioned factors in addition to several other key potential factors, including ventricular asynchrony, cardiac arrhythmias, and loss of viable and elastic lung tissue such as in advanced HF. All of these factors contribute to a ventilation-perfusion mismatch of varying degrees.

The influence of cardiac arrhythmias and ventricular asynchrony on ventilation-perfusion matching in patients with HF was keenly investigated via biventricular cardiac resynchronization therapy (CRT).[126] Ventilatory, cardiovascular, metabolic, and symptomatic parameters were studied in a randomized, double-blind, crossover study by turning the CRT modality on and off. Ventilatory, cardiovascular, metabolic, and symptomatic parameters improved significantly when the CRT was turned on rather than off, and was reflected by greater work, peak VO_2, oxygen pulse, and ventilatory threshold, in addition to a less steep VE/VCO_2 slope and decreased operating lung volumes expressed as a percentage of predicted total lung capacity as ventilation increased during incremental CPX.[126]

The restrictive constraints on tidal volume during incremental exercise in HF appear to be significantly reduced by CRT by favorably increasing lung volumes, as shown in **Fig. 3**. **Fig. 3** shows that CRT increases lung volumes from both above (inspiratory reserve volume) and below (inspiratory capacity), and subsequently appears to improve all of the aforementioned CPX measures as well as symptoms throughout incremental exercise.[126] Thus, exercise tolerance can be markedly improved by modalities such as CRT, which

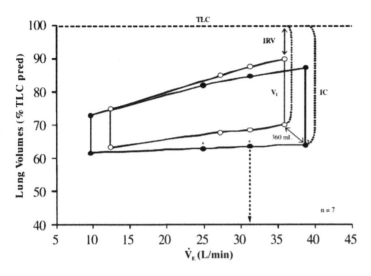

Fig. 3. The effect of cardiac resynchronization therapy (CRT) on lung volumes in heart failure. Lung volumes are expressed as %TLC as V_E increases during cycle exercise in patients with heart failure. CRT is represented by the closed circles. Off CRT is represented by the open circles. **P<0.05, CRT on vs CRT off; IC, inspiratory capacity; IRV, inspiratory reserve volume; TLC, total lung capacity; V_E, minute ventilation; V_T, tidal volume. (*From* Laveneziana P, O'Donnell DE, Ofir D, et al. Effect of biventricular pacing on ventilatory and perceptual responses to exercise in patients with stable chronic heart failure. J Appl Phys 2009;106(5):1579; with permission.)

optimize the relationships between the cardiac and pulmonary systems but also demonstrate the role of the respiratory system in limiting exercise in HF.[126]

Exercise Oscillatory Ventilation

The pathophysiologic mechanisms leading to EOV are not completely understood. In patients with HF, EOV has been hypothetically linked to: (1) instability in the feedback systems that control ventilation, stemming from an increased circulation time; (2) increased chemosensitivity to the partial pressure in CO_2 and O_2 in arterial blood; (3) impaired baroreflex activity; and (4) abnormally increased pulmonary pressures with right ventricle to pulmonary circulation uncoupling.[15] **Fig. 4** is a depiction of EOV highlighting the interrelatedness of the cardiorespiratory and neurohumoral systems, and the method whereby the respiratory system can be a major determinant of exercise and functional performance. This conceptual

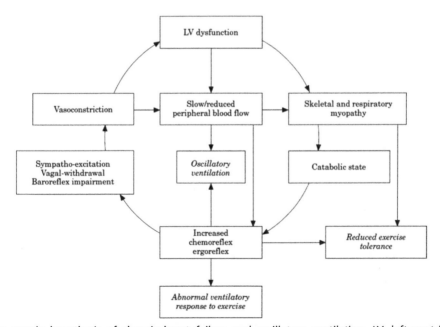

Fig. 4. The muscle hypothesis of chronic heart failure and oscillatory ventilation. LV, left ventricle. (*From* Piepoli MF, Ponikowski PP, Volterrani M, et al. Aetiology and pathophysiological implications of oscillatory ventilation at rest and during exercise in chronic heart failure. Do Cheyne and Stokes have an important message for modern-day patients with heart failure? Eur Heart J 1999;20(13):951; with permission.)

model provides a framework to understand and manage both the factors responsible for EOV and the respiratory limits to exercise.

SUMMARY

The function and compensatory mechanisms of the heart and lungs are intimately related and linked because they both supply oxygen to the body and are coordinated by the autonomic nervous system. Because of the intimate and linked functional and compensatory relationships it is often difficult to identify the primary determinant limiting exercise in HF, but from this review it is apparent that the vascular, SM, and respiratory systems contribute substantially to limitations in exercise and functional performance during HF. Future therapeutic strategies are needed to improve exercise tolerance by targeting the integrated functions of these systems.

REFERENCES

1. Arena R, Guazzi M, Myers J, et al. The prognostic utility of cardiopulmonary exercise testing stands the test of time in patients with heart failure. J Cardiopulm Rehabil Prev 2012;32(4):198–202.
2. Conraads VM, Van Craenenbroeck EM, De Maeyer C, et al. Unraveling new mechanisms of exercise intolerance in chronic heart failure: role of exercise training. Heart Fail Rev 2013;18(1):65–77.
3. Denolin H, Kuhn H, Krayenbuehl HP, et al. The definition of heart failure. Eur Heart J 1983;4(7):445–8.
4. Ennezat PV, Lefetz Y, Marechaux S, et al. Left ventricular abnormal response during dynamic exercise in patients with heart failure and preserved left ventricular ejection fraction at rest. J Card Fail 2008;14(6):475–80.
5. Haykowsky MJ, Brubaker PH, John JM, et al. Determinants of exercise intolerance in elderly heart failure patients with preserved ejection fraction. J Am Coll Cardiol 2011;58(3):265–74.
6. Kitzman DW, Higginbotham MB, Cobb FR, et al. Exercise intolerance in patients with heart failure and preserved left ventricular systolic function: failure of the Frank-Starling mechanism. J Am Coll Cardiol 1991;17(5):1065–72.
7. Abudiab MM, Redfield MM, Melenovsky V, et al. Cardiac output response to exercise in relation to metabolic demand in heart failure with preserved ejection fraction. Eur J Heart Fail 2013;15(7):776–85.
8. Borlaug BA, Olson TP, Lam CS, et al. Global cardiovascular reserve dysfunction in heart failure with preserved ejection fraction. J Am Coll Cardiol 2010;56(11):845–54.
9. Borlaug BA, Melenovsky V, Russell SD, et al. Impaired chronotropic and vasodilator reserves limit exercise capacity in patients with heart failure and a preserved ejection fraction. Circulation 2006;114(20):2138–47.
10. Shibata S, Hastings JL, Prasad A, et al. Congestive heart failure with preserved ejection fraction is associated with severely impaired dynamic Starling mechanism. J Appl Phys 2011;110(4):964–71.
11. Borlaug BA, Nishimura RA, Sorajja P, et al. Exercise hemodynamics enhance diagnosis of early heart failure with preserved ejection fraction. Circ Heart Fail 2010;3(5):588–95.
12. Borlaug BA, Jaber WA, Ommen SR, et al. Diastolic relaxation and compliance reserve during dynamic exercise in heart failure with preserved ejection fraction. Heart 2011;97(12):964–9.
13. Westermann D, Kasner M, Steendijk P, et al. Role of left ventricular stiffness in heart failure with normal ejection fraction. Circulation 2008;117(16):2051–60.
14. Borlaug BA. Mechanisms of exercise intolerance in heart failure with preserved ejection fraction. Circ J 2013;78(1):20–32.
15. Skaluba SJ, Litwin SE. Mechanisms of exercise intolerance: insights from tissue Doppler imaging. Circulation 2004;109(8):972–7.
16. Borlaug BA, Lam CS, Roger VL, et al. Contractility and ventricular systolic stiffening in hypertensive heart disease insights into the pathogenesis of heart failure with preserved ejection fraction. J Am Coll Cardiol 2009;54(5):410–8.
17. Kurt M, Wang J, Torre-Amione G, et al. Left atrial function in diastolic heart failure. Circ Cardiovasc Imaging 2009;2(1):10–5.
18. Pagel PS, Kehl F, Gare M, et al. Mechanical function of the left atrium: new insights based on analysis of pressure-volume relations and Doppler echocardiography. Anesthesiology 2003;98(4):975–94.
19. Patel DA, Lavie CJ, Milani RV, et al. Left atrial volume index predictive of mortality independent of left ventricular geometry in a large clinical cohort with preserved ejection fraction. Mayo Clin Proc 2011;86(8):730–7.
20. Tan YT, Sanderson JE. Forgotten atrial: driver of symptoms in heart failure with normal ejection fraction? Heart 2012;98(17):1261–2.
21. Obokata M, Negishi K, Kurosawa K, et al. Incremental diagnostic value of la strain with leg lifts in heart failure with preserved ejection fraction. JACC Cardiovasc Imaging 2013;6(7):749–58.
22. Phan TT, Abozguia K, Shivu GN, et al. Increased atrial contribution to left ventricular filling compensates for impaired early filling during exercise in heart failure with preserved ejection fraction. J Card Fail 2009;15(10):890–7.

23. Hammoudi N, Achkar M, Laveau F, et al. Left atrial volume predicts abnormal exercise left ventricular filling pressure. Eur J Heart Fail 2014. [Epub ahead of print].

24. Pina IL, Apstein CS, Balady GJ, et al. Exercise and heart failure: a statement from the American Heart Association Committee on exercise, rehabilitation, and prevention. Circulation 2003;107(8):1210–25.

25. Sullivan MJ, Hawthorne MH. Exercise intolerance in patients with chronic heart failure. Prog Cardiovasc Dis 1995;38(1):1–22.

26. Sullivan MJ, Cobb FR. Central hemodynamic response to exercise in patients with chronic heart failure. Chest 1992;101(5 Suppl):340S–6S.

27. Sullivan MJ, Knight JD, Higginbotham MB, et al. Relation between central and peripheral hemodynamics during exercise in patients with chronic heart failure. Muscle blood flow is reduced with maintenance of arterial perfusion pressure. Circulation 1989;80(4):769–81.

28. Brubaker PH, Kitzman DW. Prevalence and management of chronotropic incompetence in heart failure. Curr Cardiol Rep 2007;9(3):229–35.

29. Dresing TJ, Blackstone EH, Pashkow FJ, et al. Usefulness of impaired chronotropic response to exercise as a predictor of mortality, independent of the severity of coronary artery disease. Am J Cardiol 2000;86(6):602–9.

30. Lauer MS, Francis GS, Okin PM, et al. Impaired chronotropic response to exercise stress testing as a predictor of mortality. JAMA 1999;281(6): 524–9.

31. Brubaker PH, Joo KC, Stewart KP, et al. Chronotropic incompetence and its contribution to exercise intolerance in older heart failure patients. J Cardiopulm Rehabil 2006;26(2):86–9.

32. Witte KK, Cleland JG, Clark AL. Chronic heart failure, chronotropic incompetence, and the effects of beta blockade. Heart 2006;92(4):481–6.

33. Floras JS. Sympathetic nervous system activation in human heart failure: clinical implications of an updated model. J Am Coll Cardiol 2009;54(5): 375–85.

34. Kishi T. Heart failure as an autonomic nervous system dysfunction. J Cardiol 2012;59(2):117–22.

35. Zhang DY, Anderson AS. The sympathetic nervous system and heart failure. Cardiol Clin 2014;32(1): 33–45, vii.

36. Keller-Ross ML, Johnson BD, Joyner MJ, et al. Influence of the metaboreflex on arterial blood pressure in heart failure patients. Am Heart J 2014; 167(4):521–8.

37. Heusch G, Libby P, Gersh B, et al. Cardiovascular remodelling in coronary artery disease and heart failure. Lancet 2014;383(9932):1933–43.

38. van Heerebeek L, Borbely A, Niessen HW, et al. Myocardial structure and function differ in systolic and diastolic heart failure. Circulation 2006; 113(16):1966–73.

39. Patel BM, Mehta AA. Aldosterone and angiotensin: role in diabetes and cardiovascular diseases. Eur J Pharmacol 2012;697(1–3):1–12.

40. Spinale FG. Myocardial matrix remodeling and the matrix metalloproteinases: influence on cardiac form and function. Physiol Rev 2007;87(4): 1285–342.

41. van Heerebeek L, Franssen CP, Hamdani N, et al. Molecular and cellular basis for diastolic dysfunction. Curr Heart Fail Rep 2012;9(4):293–302.

42. Weber KT, Sun Y, Tyagi SC, et al. Collagen network of the myocardium: function, structural remodeling and regulatory mechanisms. J Mol Cell Cardiol 1994;26(3):279–92.

43. Neef S, Maier LS. Novel aspects of excitation-contraction coupling in heart failure. Basic Res Cardiol 2013;108(4):360.

44. Berk BC, Fujiwara K, Lehoux S. ECM remodeling in hypertensive heart disease. J Clin Invest 2007; 117(3):568–75.

45. Wilson JR, Martin JL, Ferraro N. Impaired skeletal muscle nutritive flow during exercise in patients with congestive heart failure: role of cardiac pump dysfunction as determined by the effect of dobutamine. Am J Cardiol 1984;53(9):1308–15.

46. Andersen P, Saltin B. Maximal perfusion of skeletal muscle in man. J Physiol 1985;366:233–49.

47. Calbet JA, Gonzalez-Alonso J, Helge JW, et al. Cardiac output and leg and arm blood flow during incremental exercise to exhaustion on the cycle ergometer. J Appl Phys 2007;103(3):969–78.

48. Duscha BD, Schulze PC, Robbins JL, et al. Implications of chronic heart failure on peripheral vasculature and skeletal muscle before and after exercise training. Heart Fail Rev 2008;13(1):21–37.

49. Rowell LB. Blood pressure regulation during exercise. Ann Med 1991;23(3):329–33.

50. Borlaug BA. Heart failure with preserved and reduced ejection fraction: different risk profiles for different diseases. Eur Heart J 2013;34(19): 1393–5.

51. Kinugawa T, Kato M, Ogino K, et al. Plasma endothelin-1 levels and clinical correlates in patients with chronic heart failure. J Card Fail 2003; 9(4):318–24.

52. Lang CC, Rayos GH, Chomsky DB, et al. Effect of sympathoinhibition on exercise performance in patients with heart failure. Circulation 1997;96(1): 238–45.

53. Notarius CF, Ando S, Rongen GA, et al. Resting muscle sympathetic nerve activity and peak oxygen uptake in heart failure and normal subjects. Eur Heart J 1999;20(12):880–7.

54. Notarius CF, Millar PJ, Murai H, et al. Inverse relationship between muscle sympathetic activity

during exercise and peak oxygen uptake in subjects with and without heart failure. J Am Coll Cardiol 2014;63(6):605–6.

55. Drexler H, Hayoz D, Munzel T, et al. Endothelial function in congestive heart failure. Am Heart J 1993;126:761–4.

56. Landmesser U, Spiekermann S, Dikalov S, et al. Vascular oxidative stress and endothelial dysfunction in patients with chronic heart failure: role of xanthine-oxidase and extracellular superoxide dismutase. Circulation 2002;106(24):3073–8.

57. Fichtlscherer S, Breuer S, Zeiher AM. Prognostic value of systemic endothelial dysfunction in patients with acute coronary syndromes: further evidence for the existence of the "vulnerable" patient. Circulation 2004;110(14):1926–32.

58. Vanhoutte PM, Shimokawa H, Tang EH, et al. Endothelial dysfunction and vascular disease. Acta Physiol (Oxf) 2009;196(2):193–222.

59. Laurindo FR, Pedro MA, Barbeiro HV, et al. Vascular free radical release: ex vivo and in vivo evidence for a flow-dependent endothelial mechanism. Circ Res 1994;1994(74):700–9.

60. Taddei S, Virdis A, Ghiadoni L, et al. Vitamin C improves endothelium-dependent vasodilation by restoring nitric oxide activity in essential hypertension. Circulation 1998;97:2222–9.

61. Keith M, Geranmayegan A, Sole MJ, et al. Increased oxidative stress in patients with congestive heart failure. J Am Coll Cardiol 1998;31(6):1352–6.

62. Boo YC, Hwang J, Sykes M, et al. Shear stress stimulates phosphorylation of eNOS at Ser(635) by a protein kinase A-dependent mechanism. Am J Physiol Heart Circ Physiol 2002;283(5):H1819–28.

63. Woodman CR, Price EM, Laughlin MH. Shear stress induces eNOS mRNA expression and improves endothelium-dependent dilation in senescent soleus muscle feed arteries. J Appl Phys 2005;98(3):940–6.

64. Ramsey MW, Goodfellow J, Jones CJ, et al. Endothelial control of arterial distensibility is impaired in chronic heart failure. Circulation 1995;92(11):3212–9.

65. Treasure CB, Vita JA, Cox DA, et al. Endothelium-dependent dilation of the coronary microvasculature is impaired in dilated cardiomyopathy. Circulation 1990;81(3):772–9.

66. Pacher P, Beckman JS, Liaudet L. Nitric oxide and peroxynitrite in health and disease. Physiol Rev 2007;87(1):315–424.

67. Hambrecht R, Adams V, Erbs S, et al. Regular physical activity improves endothelial function in patients with coronary artery disease by increasing phosphorylation of endothelial nitric oxide synthase. Circulation 2003;107(25):3152–8.

68. Morra EA, Zaniqueli D, Rodrigues SL, et al. Long-term intense resistance training in men is associated with preserved cardiac structure/function, decreased aortic stiffness, and lower central augmentation pressure. J Hypertens 2014;32(2):286–93.

69. Mottram PM, Haluska BA, Leano R, et al. Relation of arterial stiffness to diastolic dysfunction in hypertensive heart disease. Heart 2005;91(12):1551–6.

70. Kitzman DW, Herrington DM, Brubaker PH, et al. Carotid arterial stiffness and its relationship to exercise intolerance in older patients with heart failure and preserved ejection fraction. Hypertension 2013;61(1):112–9.

71. Chae CU, Pfeffer MA, Glynn RJ, et al. Increased pulse pressure and risk of heart failure in the elderly. JAMA 1999;281(7):634–9.

72. Lane AD, Wu PT, Kistler B, et al. Arterial stiffness and walk time in patients with end-stage renal disease. Kidney Blood Press Res 2013;37(2–3):142–50.

73. Bonapace S, Rossi A, Cicoira M, et al. Aortic distensibility independently affects exercise tolerance in patients with dilated cardiomyopathy. Circulation 2003;107(12):1603–8.

74. Booth AD, Wallace S, McEniery CM, et al. Inflammation and arterial stiffness in systemic vasculitis: a model of vascular inflammation. Arthritis Rheum 2004;50(2):581–8.

75. Klocke R, Cockcroft JR, Taylor GJ, et al. Arterial stiffness and central blood pressure, as determined by pulse wave analysis, in rheumatoid arthritis. Ann Rheum Dis 2003;62(5):414–8.

76. Vlachopoulos C, Dima I, Aznaouridis K, et al. Acute systemic inflammation increases arterial stiffness and decreases wave reflections in healthy individuals. Circulation 2005;112(14):2193–200.

77. Conraads VM, Bosmans JM, Vrints CJ. Chronic heart failure: an example of a systemic chronic inflammatory disease resulting in cachexia. Int J Cardiol 2002;85(1):33–49.

78. Kinugawa T, Kato M, Ogino K, et al. Interleukin-6 and tumor necrosis factor-alpha levels increase in response to maximal exercise in patients with chronic heart failure. Int J Cardiol 2003;87(1):83–90.

79. Kullo IJ, Seward JB, Bailey KR, et al. C-reactive protein is related to arterial wave reflection and stiffness in asymptomatic subjects from the community. Am J Hypertens 2005;18(8):1123–9.

80. Nagano M, Nakamura M, Sato K, et al. Association between serum C-reactive protein levels and pulse wave velocity: a population-based cross-sectional study in a general population. Atherosclerosis 2005;180(1):189–95.

81. Yasmin, McEniery CM, Wallace S, et al. C-reactive protein is associated with arterial stiffness in

apparently healthy individuals. Arterioscler Thromb Vasc Biol 2004;24(5):969–74.

82. Venugopal SK, Devaraj S, Yuhanna I, et al. Demonstration that C-reactive protein decreases eNOS expression and bioactivity in human aortic endothelial cells. Circulation 2002;106(12):1439–41.

83. Verma S, Li SH, Badiwala MV, et al. Endothelin antagonism and interleukin-6 inhibition attenuate the proatherogenic effects of C-reactive protein. Circulation 2002;105(16):1890–6.

84. Fernandez-Real JM, Ricart W. Insulin resistance and chronic cardiovascular inflammatory syndrome. Endocr Rev 2003;24(3):278–301.

85. Fernandez-Real JM, Broch M, Vendrell J, et al. Smoking, fat mass and activation of the tumor necrosis factor-alpha pathway. Int J Obes Relat Metab Disord 2003;27(12):1552–6.

86. Kalra L, Rambaran C, Chowienczyk P, et al. Ethnic differences in arterial responses and inflammatory markers in Afro-Caribbean and Caucasian subjects. Arterioscler Thromb Vasc Biol 2005;25(11): 2362–7.

87. Guazzi M, Samaja M, Arena R, et al. Long-term use of sildenafil in the therapeutic management of heart failure. J Am Coll Cardiol 2007;50(22):2136–44.

88. Kitzman DW, Brubaker PH, Herrington DM, et al. Effect of endurance exercise training on endothelial function and arterial stiffness in older patients with heart failure and preserved ejection fraction: a randomized, controlled, single-blind trial. J Am Coll Cardiol 2013;62(7):584–92.

89. Coats AJ, Clark AL, Piepoli M, et al. Symptoms and quality of life in heart failure: the muscle hypothesis. Br Heart J 1994;72(2 Suppl):S36–39.

90. Mancini DM, Coyle E, Coggan A, et al. Contribution of intrinsic skeletal muscle changes to ^{31}P NMR skeletal muscle metabolic abnormalities in patients with chronic heart failure. Circulation 1989;80(5): 1338–46.

91. Drexler H, Riede U, Munzel T, et al. Alterations of skeletal muscle in chronic heart failure. Circulation 1992;85(5):1751–9.

92. Anker SD, von Haehling S. Inflammatory mediators in chronic heart failure: an overview. Heart 2004; 90(4):464–70.

93. Fanzani A, Conraads VM, Penna F, et al. Molecular and cellular mechanisms of skeletal muscle atrophy: an update. J Cachexia Sarcopenia Muscle 2012;3(3):163–79.

94. Bonaldo P, Sandri M. Cellular and molecular mechanisms of muscle atrophy. Dis Model Mech 2013; 6(1):25–39.

95. Fulster S, Tacke M, Sandek A, et al. Muscle wasting in patients with chronic heart failure: results from the studies investigating co-morbidities aggravating heart failure (SICA-HF). Eur Heart J 2013; 34(7):512–9.

96. Hambrecht R, Schulze PC, Gielen S, et al. Effects of exercise training on insulin-like growth factor-I expression in the skeletal muscle of non-cachectic patients with chronic heart failure. Eur J Cardiovasc Prev Rehabil 2005;12(4):401–6.

97. Velloso CP. Regulation of muscle mass by growth hormone and IGF-I. Br J Pharmacol 2008;154(3): 557–68.

98. Lenk K, Erbs S, Hollriegel R, et al. Exercise training leads to a reduction of elevated myostatin levels in patients with chronic heart failure. Eur J Prev Cardiol 2012;19(3):404–11.

99. Smart NA, Larsen AI, Le Maitre JP, et al. Effect of exercise training on interleukin-6, tumour necrosis factor alpha and functional capacity in heart failure. Cardiol Res Pract 2011;2011:532620.

100. Vescovo G, Volterrani M, Zennaro R, et al. Apoptosis in the skeletal muscle of patients with heart failure: investigation of clinical and biochemical changes. Heart 2000;84(4):431–7.

101. Cabello-Verrugio C, Córdova G, Salas JD. Angiotensin II: role in skeletal muscle atrophy. Curr Protein Pept Sci 2012;13:560–9.

102. Sukhanov S, Semprun-Prieto L, Yoshida T, et al. Angiotensin II, oxidative stress and skeletal muscle wasting. Am J Med Sci 2011;342:143–7.

103. Tabony AM, Yoshida T, Galvez S, et al. Angiotensin II upregulates protein phosphatase 2C alpha and inhibits AMP-activated protein kinase signaling and energy balance leading to skeletal muscle wasting. Hypertension 2011;58:643–9.

104. Lipkin DP, Jones DA, Round JM, et al. Abnormalities of skeletal muscle in patients with chronic heart failure. Int J Cardiol 1988;18(2):187–95.

105. Massie BM, Simonini A, Sahgal P, et al. Relation of systemic and local muscle exercise capacity to skeletal muscle characteristics in men with congestive heart failure. J Am Coll Cardiol 1996; 27(1):140–5.

106. Poole DC, Hirai DM, Copp SW, et al. Muscle oxygen transport and utilization in heart failure: implications for exercise (in)tolerance. Am J Physiol Heart Circ Physiol 2012;302(5):H1050–1063.

107. von Haehling S, Steinbeck L, Doehner W, et al. Muscle wasting in heart failure: an overview. Int J Biochem Cell Biol 2013;45(10):2257–65.

108. Duscha BD, Kraus WE, Keteyian SJ, et al. Capillary density of skeletal muscle: a contributing mechanism for exercise intolerance in class II-III chronic heart failure independent of other peripheral alterations. J Am Coll Cardiol 1999;33(7):1956–63.

109. Katz SD, Biasucci L, Sabba C, et al. Impaired endothelium-mediated vasodilation in the peripheral vasculature of patients with congestive heart failure. J Am Coll Cardiol 1992;19(5):918–25.

110. Wiener DH, Fink LI, Maris J, et al. Abnormal skeletal muscle bioenergetics during exercise in

patients with heart failure: role of reduced muscle blood flow. Circulation 1986;73(6):1127–36.

111. Rosca MG, Hoppel CL. Mitochondrial dysfunction in heart failure. Heart Fail Rev 2013;18(5):607–22.

112. Mancini DM, Walter G, Reichek N, et al. Contribution of skeletal muscle atrophy to exercise intolerance and altered muscle metabolism in heart failure. Circulation 1992;85(4):1364–73.

113. Anker SD, Ponikowski PP, Clark AL, et al. Cytokines and neurohormones relating to body composition alterations in the wasting syndrome of chronic heart failure. Eur Heart J 1999;20(9):683–93.

114. Majumdar SR, Ezekowitz JA, Lix LM, et al. Heart failure is a clinically and densitometrically independent risk factor for osteoporotic fractures: population-based cohort study of 45,509 subjects. J Clin Endocrinol Metab 2012;97(4):1179–86.

115. Murphy MN, Mizuno M, Mitchell JH, et al. Cardiovascular regulation by skeletal muscle reflexes in health and disease. Am J Physiol Heart Circ Physiol 2011;301(4):H1191–1204.

116. Wang HJ, Zucker IH, Wang W. Muscle reflex in heart failure: the role of exercise training. Front Physiol 2012;3:398.

117. Chomsky DB, Lang CC, Rayos G, et al. Treatment of subclinical fluid retention in patients with symptomatic heart failure: effect on exercise performance. J Heart Lung Transplant 1997; 16(8):846–53.

118. Guazzi M. Alveolar gas diffusion abnormalities in heart failure. J Card Fail 2008;14(8):695–702.

119. McParland C, Resch EF, Krishnan B, et al. Inspiratory muscle weakness in chronic heart failure: role of nutrition and electrolyte status and systemic myopathy. Am J Respir Crit Care Med 1995; 151(4):1101–7.

120. Waxman AB. Pulmonary function test abnormalities in pulmonary vascular disease and chronic heart failure. Clin Chest Med 2001;22(4):751–8.

121. Ukkonen H, Burwash IG, Dafoe W, et al. Is ventilatory efficiency (VE/VCO(2) slope) associated with right ventricular oxidative metabolism in patients with congestive heart failure? Eur J Heart Fail 2008;10(11):1117–22.

122. Dhakal BP, Murphy RM, Lewis GD. Exercise oscillatory ventilation in heart failure. Trends Cardiovasc Med 2012;22(7):185–91.

123. Wasserman K, Zhang YY, Gitt A, et al. Lung function and exercise gas exchange in chronic heart failure. Circulation 1997;96(7):2221–7.

124. Oldenburg O, Bitter T, Lehmann R, et al. Adaptive servoventilation improves cardiac function and respiratory stability. Clin Res Cardiol 2011;100(2): 107–15.

125. Arena RA, Guazzi M, Myers J, et al. The prognostic value of ventilatory efficiency with beta-blocker therapy in heart failure. Med Sci Sports Exerc 2007;39(2):213–9.

126. Laveneziana P, O'Donnell DE, Ofir D, et al. Effect of biventricular pacing on ventilatory and perceptual responses to exercise in patients with stable chronic heart failure. J Appl Phys 2009;106(5): 1574–83.

127. Walsh JT, Andrews R, Johnson P, et al. Inspiratory muscle endurance in patients with chronic heart failure. Heart 1996;76(4):332–6.

128. Cahalin LP, Arena R, Guazzi M, et al. Inspiratory muscle training in heart disease and heart failure: a review of the literature with a focus on method of training and outcomes. Expert Rev Cardiovasc Ther 2013;11(2):161–77.

129. Hawkins NM, Petrie MC, Macdonald MR, et al. Heart failure and chronic obstructive pulmonary disease the quandary of Beta-blockers and Beta-agonists. J Am Coll Cardiol 2011;57(21):2127–38.

130. Borghi-Silva A, Carrascosa C, Oliveira CC, et al. Effects of respiratory muscle unloading on leg muscle oxygenation and blood volume during high-intensity exercise in chronic heart failure. Am J Physiol Heart Circ Physiol 2008;294(6): H2465–2472.

131. Myers J, Oliveira R, Dewey F, et al. Validation of a cardiopulmonary exercise test score in heart failure. Circ Heart Fail 2013;6(2):211–8.

Reversing Heart Failure–Associated Pathophysiology with Exercise
What Actually Improves and by How Much?

Volker Adams, PhD[a], Josef Niebauer, MD, PhD, MBA[b],*

KEYWORDS

- Endothelium • Exercise training • Nitric oxide • Oxidative stress • Skeletal muscle

KEY POINTS

- Improvement in peak oxygen consumption ($\dot{V}O_2$) is due to reverse cardiac remodeling as well as peripheral adaptations in the skeletal muscular and vascular system.
- Central mechanisms include improved myocardial anabolic/catabolic balance, calcium handling, and neurohormonal adaptations; the periphery benefits from less inflammation; and improvement in the catabolic/anabolic balance, energy metabolism, and structural alterations.
- Vascular effects comprise improved endothelial function and regeneration, including positive effects on the nitric oxide (NO) system, microRNA (miRNA), and apoptosis.
- Clinical trials suggest that high-intensity interval training (HIIT) might be superior to other forms of exercise training (ET); underlying molecular mechanisms need to be further elucidated.
- Patients with heart failure with preserved ejection fraction (HFpEF) benefit from ET; molecular mechanisms, however, are only poorly understood.

INTRODUCTION

The first scientific evidence regarding the beneficial effects of work-associated ET was published by Morris and colleagues, in 1953,[1] who examined the incidence of coronary artery disease (CAD) in London bus driver teams. He documented that the incidence of CAD was less in the middle-aged conductors than in the sedentary drivers of the same age. Subsequently, studies in more than 100,000 individuals showed that the higher the level of physical fitness, the less likely an individual would suffer premature cardiovascular (CV) death (reviewed by Lee and colleagues[2]). In a recent meta-analysis, including 883,372 subjects, it became evident that physical activity is associated with a marked risk reduction in CV (risk reduction of 35%) and all-cause mortality (risk reduction of 33%).[3] In addition, exercise capacity or cardiorespiratory fitness is inversely correlated with CV or even all-cause mortality, even after adjustment for confounding factors.[4–6] Based on these studies, all major CV societies made physical activity part of their guidelines for prevention of CV disease (CVD) (class I recommendation), recommending at least 30 minutes of moderate-intensity aerobic activity on 3 to 7 days per week

Disclose: Nothing to disclose.
[a] Department of Internal Medicine/Cardiology, University of Leipzig – Heart Center, Strümpelstraße 39, Leipzig 04289, Germany; [b] University Institute of Sports Medicine, Prevention and Rehabilitation, Research Institut of Molecular Sports Medicine and Rehabilitation, Institute of Sports Medicine of the State of Salzburg, Sports Medicine of the Olympic Center Salzburg-Rif, Paracelsus Medical University Salzburg, Lindhofstrasse 20, Salzburg 5020, Austria
* Corresponding author.
E-mail address: j.niebauer@salk.at

Heart Failure Clin 11 (2015) 17–28
http://dx.doi.org/10.1016/j.hfc.2014.08.001
1551-7136/15/$ – see front matter © 2015 Elsevier Inc. All rights reserved

(ie, greater than 150 min/wk).[7–9] In recent years, molecular biology helped understand the impairment of exercise capacity in patients with chronic heart failure (HF) and the beneficial effects elicited by ET. It also became clear that different organ systems, such as the heart, skeletal muscle, and vascular function, are involved in disease progression and modulation by ET.

This review summarizes current knowledge with respect to molecular changes elicited by ET in HF in different organ systems: the heart, the endothelium, and the skeletal muscle. The last part of the review discusses and summarizes current knowledge on training intensity and if ET is also a potential therapeutic option in patients with HFpEF.

CARDIAC EFFECTS OF EXERCISE TRAINING
Training Effects on Left Ventricular Function and Reverse Remodeling

One of the first small prospective studies, performed by Sullivan and coworkers[10] in HF patients with HF with reduced ejection fraction (HFrEF) (n = 12), demonstrated that 4 to 6 months of training did not worsen left-ventricular ejection fraction (LVEF) and tended to improve maximal cardiac output. The extent of the cardiac changes did not, however, explain the large 23% improvement in peak V̇o$_2$ so that peripheral changes in limb perfusion and oxidative metabolism most likely account for the larger part of the beneficial symptomatic training effects. The first larger prospective randomized study to provide evidence for a training-induced reverse remodeling came from Hambrecht and colleagues,[11] who demonstrated that endurance training led to reverse left ventricular (LV) remodeling, with modest improvements in EF from 30% to 35% as well as reductions of LV end-diastolic diameter. The results of these studies were confirmed in 2 meta-analyses performed in 2007[12] and 2012.[13] In summary, these meta-analyses showed that aerobic training, especially greater than 6 months' duration, significantly reversed LV remodeling, whereas strength training alone or combined with aerobic training had no effect on reverse remodeling.

Mechanisms Explaining Reverse Remodeling in Heart Failure

In the absence of myocardial biopsies for molecular analysis of myocardial changes induced by training, most investigators interpreted this favorable training effect as secondary to afterload reduction with reduced resting blood pressure due to improved endothelial function.[11,14,15] Animal models reveal, however, that there are direct myocardial effects of training that are related to signaling pathways of myocardial hypertrophy and fibrosis.[16,17]

Anabolic/catabolic balance in the myocardium
Animal studies in which a left anterior descending artery ligation model was used demonstrated a significant up-regulation of components of the ubiquitin-proteasome system (UPS) as well as of myostatin.[18,19] Both were significantly reduced by ET over a period of 4 weeks.[18,19]

Calcium handling
Alterations in calcium handling are also associated with pathologic hypertrophy and transition from hypertrophy to failure: sarcoplasmic reticulum CA^{2+} ATPase (SERCA2a) protein levels were reduced in mouse and dog models of HF and were normalized by ET.[20,21] In addition, ET activates Ca^{2+}/calmodulin-dependent protein kinase (CaMK) II, leading to a hyperphosphorylation of phospholamban,[22] which in its phosphorylated form no longer inhibits SERCA2a. In conjunction with an increased expression of Na$^+$-Ca^{2+} exchanger,[23] higher myocardial SERCA-2 and phospholamban lead to improved calcium cycling and thus to better cardiomyocyte function. For more detailed information on exercise-induced improvements on the contractile apparatus and calcium cycling, see the detailed review by Kemi and Wisloff.[24]

Neurohormonal adaptations
An aerobic ET program in patients with HF leads to a reduction in sympathoadrenergic drive. This has also been confirmed for serum catecholamine levels: Coats and colleagues[25] showed a 16% reduction of radiolabeled norepinephrine secretion after 8 weeks of ET. In addition to the reduction in circulating catecholamines, Braith and coworkers[26,27] described a 25% to 30% reduction of angiotensin II, aldosterone, arginine vasopeptide, and atrial natriuretic peptide after 4 months of walking training in patients with HF. In a rat model of ischemic HF, the beneficial training effects on local neurohumoral balance were analyzed in the noninfarcted LV myocardium. Xu and colleagues[28] found a significant reduction of myocardial angiotensin-converting enzyme mRNA expression and angiotensin II, type 1, receptor expression after 8 weeks of treadmill ET. This finding is of special importance given that approximately 90% of angiotensin II is produced locally in the myocardium and implies that local angiotensin II levels are significantly reduced by ET. This reduction also translates into reduced fibrogenesis, as indicated by reduced tissue inhibitor of metalloproteinase-1 expression with unchanged matrix metalloproteinase (MMP)-1

expression and reduced collagen volume fraction in the exercised animals.[28]

VASCULAR EFFECTS OF EXERCISE

Besides the myocardium, the vascular system is significantly impaired in patients with HF,[29] and several studies using ET as a therapeutic intervention during the past decades have proved beneficial effects on this system.[15,30] On a functional level, ET results in better endothelial function and a better compliance of the vessel (reduced stiffness). The following sections focus on molecular changes elicited by ET, especially in the vascular system.

Nitric Oxide System (Nitric Oxide–Reactive Oxygen Species Balance)

One of the most important factors regulating vascular function is NO generated in the endothelial cells (ECs) (reviewed by Feletou and colleagues[31]). In mammals, NO can be generated by 3 different isoforms of NO synthase (NOS), namely endothelial NOS (eNOS), neuronal NOS, and inducible NOS.[32,33] At least in ECs, the most important one for regulating vascular tone is eNOS. NO is responsible for vasodilation, which results in the lowering of peripheral resistance and increase of perfusion. eNOS expression was significantly reduced in animal models of HF, induced by either ventricular pacing or monocrotaline, compared with controls.[34,35] Its activity is up-regulated by an increase in flow-mediated shear stress associated with physical exercise due to a complex pattern of intracellular regulation, such as acetylation,[36] phosphorylation,[37] and translocation to the caveolae.[38] Numerous investigations have documented that exercise or increased shear stress up-regulates eNOS activity in cell culture,[39–41] animal,[42,43] or human studies.[44] With respect to the signal transduction of increased shear stress and eNOS activation, the glycocalyx on the luminar side of the ECs seems to play an important role.[45,46] The deformation of the glycocalyx results in the activation of calcium ion channels, phospholipase activity leading to calcium signaling, prostaglandin I2 release, and cyclic AMP–mediated smooth muscle cell relaxation.[45] In addition, vascular endothelial growth factor receptor 2 is located at the luminal surface and can associate with vascular endothelial cadherin, ß-catenin, and phosphatidylinositol 3 kinase to phosphorylate Akt and induce Akt-mediated eNOS phosphorylation, leading to higher NO production.[47] High-density lipoprotein (HDL) is another factor known to modulate eNOS activity via phosphorylation.[48] This HDL-induced activation is impaired in patients with diabetes,[49] CAD,[50] and HF[51] and an ET program of 12 weeks is able to restore this HDL-mediated eNOS activation.[51]

The bioavailability of NO not only depends on its generation by eNOS but also is influenced by reactive oxygen species (ROS)-mediated breakdown. The low NO bioavailability is partly caused by the reaction of ROS with NO to form peroxynitrite. The application of laminar flow to intact vascular segments has been shown to increase ROS production for a short time period,[52] with NADPH the major source.[53] Extended periods of ET result, however, in a reduced expression of hypoxanthin,[54] NADPH oxidase,[55] and a stimulation of radical scavenging systems that include copper and zinc–containing superoxide dismutase (SOD),[56] extracellular SOD,[57] glutathione peroxidase,[58] and glutathione levels.[59] Another enzyme-generating ROS in the vascular system is eNOS itself. Under several pathologic conditions, the enzymatic reduction of molecular oxygen by eNOS is no longer coupled to L-arginine oxidation, resulting in ROS production.[60–62] NOS uncoupling has been implicated in several pathologies, including atherosclerosis,[63] diabetes,[64] and HF.[65] A critical factor for NOS uncoupling is the bioavailability of tetrahydrobiopterin (BH4), a cofactor for the enzymatic reaction.[66] Cell culture experiments using ECs provide some evidence that elevated blood flow increased BH4 levels.[67–69]

Apoptosis and Endothelial Regeneration

EC senescence and apoptosis are features of numerous human pathologies, including atherosclerosis, diabetic retinopathy, and HF.[70,71] The maintenance of an intact EC layer (repair of damaged or lost ECs) is one important action to counteract endothelial dysfunction. Endothelial progenitor cells (EPCs) or mesenchymal stem cells are mobilized from the bone marrow by specific stimuli and possess the potential to promote angiogenesis and endothelial repair.[72–74] Numerous studies have provided evidence that ET mobilizes EPCs or mononuclear cells (MNCs) from the bone morrow and influences its functional capacity.[75–78] Levels of circulating EPCs correlate inversely with the extent of endothelial dysfunction in humans at various degrees of CV risk.[79] Due to increased shear stress, NO concentration increases in the bone marrow, leading to the activation of MMPs (MMP-2 and MMP-9), leading to the mobilization of stem cells into the circulation.[80,81] This model is supported by the observation that exercise-induced mobilization of EPCs from the bone marrow is impaired in eNOS$^{-/-}$ mice.[82] After mobilization of the cells, the most relevant factor for tissue engraftment is the local concentration of stromal-derived factor 1α and its cell receptor CXCR-4.[83] The expression of CXCR-4 can be up-regulated by either ET[84] or adiponectin,[85] both known to have an impact on EPC migration.[86]

MicroRNA

The coordinated regulation of angiogenesis and maintenance of the EC layer is essential for proper vascular function and prevention of endothelial dysfunction. In recent years miRNAs were identified as critical regulator of gene expression, due to their ability to suppress protein synthesis by inhibiting the translation of protein from mRNA or by promoting mRNA degradation.[87,88] With respect to miRNA and the impact of ET in HF to maintain proper endothelial function, 3 different miRNAs received closer attention: miRNA-21, miRNA-95a, and miRNA-126. miRNA-92a could be identified as an endogenous repressor of the angiogenic program in ECs.[89] In addition, large-scale miRNA profiling of human umbilical vein ECs exposed to different shear stress conditions identified miRNA-92a as an miRNA that is up-regulated by low shear stress.[90] A study of LDLR$^{-/-}$ mice fed a high-fat diet documented that the up-regulation of miRNA-92a by oxidized low-density lipoprotein (LDL) in atheroprone areas (areas of low shear stress) promoted endothelial activation and the development of atherosclerotic lesions.[91] A mechanistic explanation may be that an elevation of miRNA-92a by low or oscillatory shear stress leads to a down-regulation of Krüppel-like factor 2, resulting in a reduced expression of eNOS.[92] Another miRNA up-regulated by elevated shear stress is miRNA-21.[93] Transfection and inhibitions studies documented that an elevation of miRNA-21 led to enhanced NO production via Akt and eNOS phosphorylation.[93] MiRNA-126 is highly enriched in the vascular endothelium and was shown to play distinct roles in angiogenesis, vasculogenesis, and endothelial inflammation. Swim training in rats resulted in an increased expression of miRNA-126 in the myocardium and is related to exercise-induced cardiac angiogenesis, by indirect regulation of the vascular endothelial growth factor receptor pathway.[94] This essential role of miRNA-126 is further supported by the observation that antagomir-mediated silencing of miRNA-126 impairs ischemia-induced angiogenesis in a mouse model.[95]

MUSCULAR EFFECTS OF EXERCISE

Early fatigue and exercise intolerance are hallmarks for the diagnosis of chronic HF in patients. Investigations from the early 1990s documented that exercise intolerance cannot be predicted by LVEF. Based on these observations, the muscle hypothesis of HF was born: that alterations in the peripheral skeletal muscle are a main predictor for exercise intolerance and that these alterations are influenced by ET.[96,97]

Inflammation

During the development of HF, a derangement in inflammatory factors is evident.[98,99] The prototype of inflammatory cytokines elevated in HF is tumor necrosis factor α (TNF-α).[100,101] Besides TNF-α, other inflammatory cytokines, such as interleukin (IL)-6 and IL-1ß, have been described as elevated in patients with HF.[102,103] The elevation of inflammatory cytokines is not restricted to HFrEF but is also evident in HFpEF patients.[104] With respect to the origin of the circulating inflammatory cytokines, at least 3 different hypothesis are discussed: (1) production and secretion by circulating MNCs, like macrophages[105]; (2) secretion by injured cardiomyocytes or by cells from peripheral tissue, mainly skeletal muscle[106,107]; and (3) increased edema of the bowel wall and thereby an induction of TNF-α by lipopolysaccharides.[108–111]

Inflammatory cytokines, especially TNF-α, are able to induce muscle wasting, a phenomenon often observed in patients with end-stage HF, via the activation of the UPS by mitogen-activated protein kinases (MAPKs) and nuclear factor κB.[112] With respect to ET and the level of inflammatory cytokines, several investigators have demonstrated that depending on the severity of chronic heart failure (CHF), elevated baseline cytokine levels did not increase further[113] and in 2 studies even decreased in response to ET, both in the serum[114,115] and in the skeletal muscle.[116,117]

Catabolic/Anabolic Balance

Muscle weakness and muscle atrophy are hallmark characteristics in patients with end-stage HF. An imbalance between anabolic and catabolic factors is responsible for loss of muscle mass. Fortunately, this imbalance can be influenced by ET. With respect to anabolic factors, growth hormone, androgens (testosterone), insulin, and insulinlike growth factor 1 (IGF-1) play an important role, with IGF-1 in a central position due to its ability to regulate muscle cell proliferation and differentiation and muscle regeneration.[118–120] In support of this pivotal role of IGF-1, the transgenic overexpression of IGF-1 in the skeletal muscle is associated with muscle hypertrophy, increased muscle strength, and improved muscle regeneration.[119,120] Mechanistically, an overexpression of

IGF-1 seems to prevent muscle atrophy by inhibiting protein degradation pathways, like the UPS, in the skeletal muscle.[121] Analyzing skeletal muscles from animal models or patients with HF, a significant reduction of IGF-1 was evident,[122–124] which could be reversed by an ET program.[125]

On the catabolic site, the activation of the UPS in the skeletal muscle of HF[126] and the up-regulation of myostatin[19] could be documented. A relation between the inflammation and the activation of the UPS could be identified. TNF-α seems to activate the UPS, and this activation is essential for the TNF-α–induced loss of muscle function.[127] Performing regular ET counteracts this dysregulation of the UPS[126,128] and myostatin.[19]

Energy Metabolism

HF is associated with an augmented energy demand and a diminished energy metabolism, resulting in an energetic imbalance.[129,130] The phosphocreatine (PCr) shuttle, in particular, transporting energy from the mitochondria to the cytosolic ATPases, and the recovery of the PCr after exercise are impaired.[131,132] Creatine kinase (CK) and mitochondrial CK expression is altered in the skeletal muscle of experimental HF[129] and in muscle biopsies obtained from HF patients.[132,133] When performing prolonged exercise, skeletal muscle metabolism adapts very fast by quantitative and qualitative changes in mitochondria and the capillary supply.[134,135] For all these adaptive responses, peroxisome proliferator-activated receptor γ coactivator 1α (PGC-1α) plays an important and central role. It regulates mitochondrial biogenesis, as shown in animals overexpressing PGC-1α.[136] Besides PGC-1α, other signaling molecules, such as MAPKs, CaMKs, and AMP-activated protein kinase, are activated during exercise and are relevant for the exercise-induced changes observed in the skeletal muscle (for review Ventura-Clapier and colleagues[137] and Russell and colleagues[138]).

Structural Alterations

In skeletal muscle biopsies of patients with HF, a shift in fiber-type composition is evident compared with healthy controls. Patients with HF exhibit a relative increase in less aerobic type II and a relative decrease in aerobic type I fibers.[139,140] Recently, also in patients with HFpEF, the percentage of type I fibers, the type I-to–type II fiber ratio, and capillary-to-fiber ratio were reduced, whereas the percentage of type II fibers was greater.[141] Using ET as a therapeutic intervention in patients with HF resulted in a reversal of the changes observed in fiber-type composition and the reduced capillary-to-fiber ratio.[140,142] On the molecular level, PGC-1α seems to be an important regulator of fiber-type composition. This important role is supported by studies using transgenic animals[136] and by the positive correlation between PGC-1α expression and fiber type composition.[143]

EXERCISE TRAINING INTENSITY—INTERVAL VERSUS MODERATE CONTINUOUS TRAINING

Applying the knowledge obtained in sports medicine using HIIT, Wisloff and coworkers[144] demonstrated a superior CV effect of aerobic HIIT compared with moderate continuous training (MCT) in HF patients. From the molecular standpoint, it seems that HIIT improves endothelial function much better than MCT due to greater bioavailability of NO (increase of the antioxidant status in the plasma) and reduced oxidized LDL. In addition, the activation of PGC-1α in the skeletal muscle is more pronounced after HIIT. It is speculated that higher shear stress during the on phase of HIIT triggers larger responses at the cellular and molecular level compared with MCT. In myocytes, HIIT partly reversed contractile dysfunction and impaired Ca^{2+} handling in rats with postinfarction HF.[145] In recent years, several studies were performed to confirm the result of Wisloff and colleagues,[144] with mixed results. Performing a meta-analysis on 7 randomized trails comparing HIIT with MCT,[146–152] the investigators came to the conclusion that in clinically stable HF patients, HIIT is more effective than MCT in improving peak $\dot{V}o_2$, but no difference is obvious with respect to altering LV remodeling.[146] Nevertheless, all these results have to be taken with care, because this meta-analysis is only based on 180 patients in total, with all studies using a single-center design. Therefore, results of larger, multicenter trials comparing the different training intensities in HF or CAD, such as SmartEx[153] or SAINTEX-CAD,[154] currently underway, must be awaited.

EXERCISE AND HEART FAILURE WITH PRESERVED EJECTION FRACTION

HFpEF is the only CVD with increasing prevalence and incidence and a mortality rate similar to HFrEF.[155] The poor clinical outcome in patients with HFpEF is not explained by age, gender, or the high prevalence of CV risk factors and comorbidities.[156] Thus, the underlying mechanisms and, therefore, treatment options are incompletely understood. The pharmacologic therapy of HFpEF to improve outcome and symptoms has been particularly disappointing. Several large clinical trials using established pharmacologic strategies in HFpEF, such as angiotensin-converting enzyme inhibitors (PEP-CHF),[157] angiotensin II receptor blockers (PARAMOUNT,[158] CHARM-Preserved,[159] and I-Preserve[160]), or spironolactone (Aldo-DHF[161]), have failed to convincingly demonstrate substantially improved symptoms, morbidity, or mortality. Currently, no pharmacologic agent has shown to improve symptoms, exercise capacity, or prognosis in this severely debilitated patient population. From a pathophysiologic point of view, ET could be one possible therapeutic option to improve symptoms in this patient population. Small randomized trials in HFpEF patients showed improvements in peak $\dot{V}O_2$ of approximately 20%.[162–164] With respect to the molecular basis for these beneficial training effects, not much is known so far. A recent study analyzing the training effects in heart and diaphragmatic muscles in a mouse model of HFpEF revealed alterations in the titin isoform composition.[165] With respect to endothelial function and arterial stiffness, no impact of a 16-week ET program in older HFpEF patients could be documented.[163] More studies investigating the molecular basis for the beneficial effects of ET in HFpEF are warranted.

SUMMARY

The evidence discussed in this article from clinical and bench-type studies has demonstrated that ET does reverse the HF-associated pathology at the clinical and molecular levels. There are clinically relevant exercise-induced changes of LV function and reverse remodeling, of the vascular system, of the skeletal muscle, and even in HFpEF. Even though this debilitated patient population refers to patients with CHF has resulted in a class I recommendation for ET in chronic HF in all major national and international guidelines, further research is warranted to investigate molecular changes induced by ET in patients with preserved ejection fraction. Furthermore, mechanisms underlying the supposedly superior effects of HIIT need to be further elucidated.

REFERENCES

1. Morris J, Heady JA, Raffle PA, et al. Coronary artery disease and physical activity of work. Lancet 1953; 265:1053–7.
2. Lee DC, Artero EG, Xuemei S, et al. Review: mortality trends in the general population: the importance of cardiorespiratory fitness. J Psychopharmacol 2010;24:27–35.
3. Nocon M, Hiemann T, Müller-Riemenschneider F, et al. Association of physical activity with all-cause and cardiovascular mortality: a systematic review and meta-analysis. Eur J Cardiovasc Prev Rehabil 2008;15:239–46.
4. Myers J, Prakash M, Froelicher V, et al. Exercise capacity and mortality among men referred for exercise testing. N Engl J Med 2002;346:793–801.
5. Kokkinos P, Myers J, Faselis C, et al. Exercise capacity and mortality in older men: a 20-year follow-up study. Circulation 2010;122:790–7.
6. Kokkinos P, Doumas M, Myers J, et al. A graded association of exercise capacity and all-cause mortality in males with high-normal blood pressure. Blood Press 2009;18:261–7.
7. Haskell WL, Lee IM, Pate RR, et al. Physical activity and public health: updated recommendation for adults from the american college of sports medicine and the american heart association. Circulation 2007;116:1081–93.
8. Graham I, Atar D, Borch-Johnsen K, et al. European guidelines on cardiovascular disease prevention in clinical practice: executive summary. Eur Heart J 2007;28:2375–414.
9. Smith SC, Benjamin EJ, Bonow RO, et al. AHA/ACCF secondary prevention and risk reduction therapy for patients with coronary and other atherosclerotic vascular disease: 2011 update. Circulation 2011;124:2458–73.
10. Sullivan MJ, Higginbotham MB, Cobb FR. Exercise training in patients with severe left ventricular dysfunction: hemodynamic and metabolic effects. Circulation 1988;78:506–15.
11. Hambrecht R, Gielen S, Linke A, et al. Effects of exercise training on left ventricular function and peripheral resistance in patients with chronic heart failure. A randomised trial. JAMA 2000; 283:3095–101.
12. Haykowsky MJ, Liang Y, Pechter D, et al. A meta-analysis of the effect of exercise training on left ventricular remodeling in heart failure patients: the benefit depends on the type of training performed. J Am Coll Cardiol 2007;49:2329–36.
13. Chen YM, Li ZB, Zhu M, et al. Effects of exercise training on left ventricular remodelling in heart failure patients: an updated meta-analysis of randomized trails. Int J Clin Pract 2012;66:782–91.
14. Giannuzzi P, Temporelli PL, Corra U, et al. Antiremodeling effect of long-term exercise training in patients with stable chronic heart failure: results of the Exercise in Left Ventricular Dysfunction and Chronic Heart Failure (ELVD-CHF) Trial. Circulation 2003;108:554–9.
15. Hambrecht R, Fiehn E, Weigl C, et al. Regular physical exercise corrects endothelial dysfunction and improves exercise capacity in patients with chronic heart failure. Circulation 1998;98:2709–15.
16. Emter CA, Baines CP. Low-intensity aerobic interval training attenuates pathological left ventricular

remodeling and mitochondrial dysfunction in aortic-banded miniature swine. Am J Physiol Heart Circ Physiol 2010;299:H1348–56.

17. Miyachi M, Yazawa H, Furukawa M, et al. Exercise training alters left ventricular geometry and attenuates heart failure in dahl salt-sensitive hypertensive rats. Hypertension 2009;53:701–7.

18. Adams V, Link A, Gielen S, et al. Modulation of Murf-1 and MAFbx expression in the myocardium by physical exercise training. Eur J Cardiovasc Prev Rehabil 2008;15:293–9.

19. Lenk K, Schur R, Linke A, et al. Impact of exercise training on myostatin expression in the myocardium and skeletal muscle in a chronic heart failure model. Eur J Heart Fail 2009;11:342–8.

20. Rolim NP, Medeiros A, Rosa KT, et al. Exercise training improves the net balance of cardiac Ca2+ handling protein expression in heart failure. Physiol Genomics 2007;29:246–52.

21. Lu L, Mei DF, Gu AG, et al. Exercise training normalizes altered calcium-handling proteins during development of heart failure. J Appl Physiol (1985) 2002;92:1524–30.

22. Kemi OJ, Ellingsen O, Ceci M, et al. Aerobic interval training enhances cardiomyocyte contractility and Ca2+ cycling by phosphorylation of CaMKII and Thr-17 of phospholamban. J Mol Cell Cardiol 2007;43:354–61.

23. Wisloff U, Loennechen JP, Falck G, et al. Increased contractility and calcium sensitivity in cardiac myocytes isolated from endurance trained rats. Cardiovasc Res 2001;50:495–508.

24. Kemi OJ, Wisloff U. Mechanisms of exercise-induced improvements in the contractile apparatus of the mammalian myocardium. Acta Physiol (Oxf) 2010;199:425–39.

25. Coats AJ, Adamopoulos S, Radaelli A, et al. Controlled trial of physical training in chronic heart failure: exercise performance, hemodynamics, ventilation, and autonomic function. Circulation 1992;85:2119–31.

26. Braith R, Welsch M, Feigenbaum M, et al. Neuroendocrine activation in heart failure is modified by endurance training. J Am Coll Cardiol 1999;34: 1170–5.

27. Braith RW, Edwards DG. Neurohormonal abnormalities in heart failure: impact of exercise training. Congest Heart Fail 2003;9:70–6.

28. Xu X, Wan W, Powers AS, et al. Effects of exercise training on cardiac function and myocardial remodeling in post myocardial infarction rats. J Mol Cell Cardiol 2008;44:114–22.

29. Kubo SH, Rector TS, Williams RE, et al. Endothelium dependent vasodilitation is attenuated in patients with heart failure. Circulation 1994;84:1589–96.

30. Belardinelli R, Capestro F, Misiani A, et al. Moderate exercise training improves functional capacity,

quality of life, and endothelium-dependent vasodilation in chronic heart failure patients with implantable cardioverter defibrillators and cardiac resynchronization therapy. Eur J Cardiovasc Prev Rehabil 2006;13:818–25.

31. Feletou M, Köhler R, Vanhoutte PM. Nitric oxide: orchestrator of endothelium-dependent responses. Ann Med 2012;44:694–716.

32. Förstermann U, Sessa WC. Nitric oxide synthases: regulation and function. Eur Heart J 2012;33:829–37.

33. Balligand JL, Feron O, Dessy C. eNOS activation by physical forces: from short-term regulation of contraction to chronic remodeling of cardiovascular tissues. Physiol Rev 2009;89:481–534.

34. Comini L, Bachetti T, Gaia G, et al. Aorta and skeletal muscle NO synthase expression in experimental heart failure. J Mol Cell Cardiol 1996;28:2241–8.

35. Smith CJ, Sun D, Hoegler C, et al. Reduced gene expression of vascular endothelial no synthase and cyclooxygenase-1 in heart failure. Circ Res 1996;78:58–64.

36. Busconi L, Michel T. Endothelial nitric oxide synthase; N-terminal myristoylation determines subcellular localization. J Biol Chem 1993;268:8410–3.

37. Kolluru GK, Siamwala JH, Chatterjee S. eNOS phosphorylation in health and disease. Biochimie 2010;92:1186–98.

38. Ortiz PA, Garvin JL. Trafficking and activation of eNOS in epithelial cells. Acta Physiol Scand 2003;179:107–14.

39. Boo YC, Sorescu G, Boyd N, et al. Shear stress stimulates phosphorylation of endothelial nitric-oxide synthase at Ser1179 by Akt-independent mechanisms: role of protein kinase A. J Biol Chem 2002; 277:3388–96.

40. Uzarski JS, Scott EW, McFetridge PS. Adaptation of endothelial cells to physiologically-modeled, variable shear stress. PLoS One 2013;8:e57004.

41. Niebauer J, Dulak J, Chan JR, et al. Gene transfer of nitric oxide synthase: effects on endothelial biology. J Am Coll Cardiol 1999;34:1201–7.

42. Woodman CR, Muller JM, Laughlin MH, et al. Induction of nitric oxide synthase mRNA in coronary resistance arteries isolated from exercise-trained pigs. Am J Physiol 1997;273:H2575–9.

43. Touati S, Meziri F, Devaux S, et al. Exercise reverses metabolic syndrome in high-fat diet-induced obese rats. Med Sci Sports Exerc 2011;43:398–407.

44. Hambrecht R, Adams V, Erbs S, et al. Regular physical activity improves endothelial function in patients with coronary artery disease by increasing phosphorylation of endothelial nitric oxide synthase. Circulation 2003;107:3152–8.

45. Pahakis MY, Kosky JR, Dull RO, et al. The role of endothelial glycocalyx components in mechanotransduction of fluid shear stress. Biochem Biophys Res Commun 2007;355:228–33.

46. Zeng Y, Tarbell JM. The adaptive remodeling of endothelial glycocalyx in response to fluid shear stress. PLoS One 2014;9:e86249.

47. Jin ZG, Ueba H, Tanimoto T, et al. Ligand-independent activation of vascular endothelial growth factor receptor 2 by fluid shear stress regulates activation of endothelial nitric oxide synthase. Circ Res 2003; 93:354–63.

48. Yuhanna IS, Zhu Y, Cox BE, et al. High-density lipoprotein binding to scavenger receptor-BI activates endothelial nitric oxide synthase. Nat Med 2001;7: 853–7.

49. Sorrentino SA, Besler C, Rohrer L, et al. Endothelial-vasoprotective effects of high-density lipoprotein are impaired in patients with type 2 diabetes mellitus but are improved after extended-release Niacin therapy. Circulation 2010;121:110–22.

50. Besler C, Heinrich K, Rohrer L, et al. Mechanisms underlying adverse effects of HDL on eNOS-activating pathways in patients with coronary artery disease. J Clin Invest 2011;121:2693–708.

51. Adams V, Besler C, Fischer T, et al. Exercise training in patients with chronic heart failure promotes restoration of HDL functional properties. Circ Res 2013;113:1345–55.

52. Laurindo FR, Pedro Mde A, Barbeiro HV, et al. Vascular free radical release. Ex vivo and in vivo evidence for a flow-dependent endothelial mechanism. Circ Res 1994;74:700–9.

53. De Keulenaer GW, Chappell DC, Ishizaka N, et al. Oscillatory and steady laminar shear stress differentially affect human endothelial redox state. Role of a superoxide-producing NADH-Oxidase. Circ Res 1998;82:1094–101.

54. Niebauer J, Clark AL, Webb-Peploe KM, et al. Home-based exercise training modulates pro-oxidant substrates in patients with chronic heart failure. Eur J Heart Fail 2005;7:183–8.

55. Adams V, Linke A, Kränkel N, et al. Impact of regular physical activity on the NAD(P)H oxidase and angiotensin receptor system in patients with coronary artery disease. Circulation 2005;111: 555–62.

56. Inoue N, Ramasamy S, Fukai T, et al. Shear stress modulates expression of Cu/Zn superoxide dismutase in human aortic endothelial cells. Circ Res 1996;79:32–7.

57. Fukai T, Siegfried MR, Ushio-Fukai M, et al. Regulation of the vascular extracellular superoxide dismutase by nitric oxide and exercise training. J Clin Invest 2000;105:1631–9.

58. Takeshita S, Inoue N, Ueyama T, et al. Shear stress enhances glutathione peroxidase expression in endothelial cells. Biochem Biophys Res Commun 2000;273:66–71.

59. Mueller CF, Widder JD, McNally JS, et al. The role of the multidrug resistance preotein-1 in modulation of

60. Vasquez-Vivar J, Kalyanaraman B, Martasek P, et al. Superoxide generation by endothelial nitric oxide synthase: the influence of cofactors. Proc Natl Acad Sci U S A 1998;95:9220–5.

61. Xia Y, Tsai AL, Berka V, et al. Superoxide generation from endothelial nitric-oxide synthase. A Ca2+/calmodulin-dependent and tetrahydrobiopterin regulatory process. J Biol Chem 1998;273:25804–8.

62. Pou S, Pou WS, Bredt DS, et al. Generation of superoxide by purified brain nitric oxide synthase. J Biol Chern 1992;267:24173–6.

63. Hattori Y, Hattori S, Wang X, et al. Oral administration of tetrahydrobiopterin slows the progression of atherosclerosis in apolipoprotein E-knockout mice. Arterioscler Thromb Vasc Biol 2007;27:865–70.

64. Landmesser U, Dikalov S, Price SR, et al. Oxidation of tetrahydrobiopterin leads to uncoupling of endothelial cell nitric oxide synthase in hypertension. J Clin Invest 2003;111:1201–9.

65. Yamamoto E, Kataoka K, Shintaku H, et al. Novel mechanism and role of angiotensin II induced vascular endothelial injury in hypertensive diastolic heart failure. Arterioscler Thromb Vasc Biol 2007; 27:2569–75.

66. Alkaitis M, Crabtree M. Recoupling the cardiac nitric oxide synthases: tetrahydrobiopterin synthesis and recycling. Curr Heart Fail Rep 2012;9:200–10.

67. Widder JD, Chen W, Li L, et al. Regulation of tetrahydrobiopterin biosynthesis by shear stress. Circ Res 2007;101:830–8.

68. Lam CF, Peterson TE, Richardson DM. Increased blood flow causes coordinated upregulation of arterial eNOS and biosynthesis of tetrahydrobiopterin. Am J Physiol Heart Circ Physiol 2006;290: H786–93.

69. Rössig L, Hoffmann J, Hugel B, et al. Vitamin C inhibits endothelial cell apoptosis in congestive heart failure. Circulation 2001;104:2182–7.

70. Rössig L, Dimmeler S, Zeiher AM. Apoptosis in the vascular wall and atherosclerosis. Basic Res Cardiol 2001;96:11–22.

71. Rössig L, Haendeler J, Mallat Z, et al. Congestive heart failure induces endothelial cell apoptosis: protective role of carvedilol. J Am Coll Cardiol 2000;36:2081–9.

72. HUang NF, Li S. Mesenchymal stem cells for vascular regeneration. Regen Med 2008;3:877–92.

73. Becher MU, Nickenig G, Werner N. Regeneration of the vascular compartment. Herz 2010; 35:342–51.

74. Kirton JP, Xu Q. Endothelial precursors in vascular repair. Microvasc Res 2010;79:193–9.

75. Lenk K, Uhlemann M, Schuler G, et al. Role of endothelial progenitor cells in the beneficial effects of physical exercise on atherosclerosis and coronary

artery disease. J Appl Physiol (1985) 2011;111: 321–8.

76. Adams V, Lenk K, Linke A, et al. Increase of circulating endothelial progenitor cells in patients with coronary artery disease after exercise-induced ischemia. Arterioscler Thromb Vasc Biol 2004;24: 684–90.

77. Van Craenenbroeck EM, Beckers PJ, Possemiers NM, et al. Exercise acutely reverses dysfunction of circulating angiogenic cells in chronic heart failure. Eur Heart J 2010;31(15): 1924–34.

78. Van Craenenbroeck E, Hoymans V, Beckers P, et al. Exercise training improves function of circulating angiogenic cells in patients with chronic heart failure. Basic Res Cardiol 2010;105:665–76.

79. Hill JM, Zalos G, Halcox JP, et al. Circulating endothelial progenitor cells, vascular function, and cardiovascular risk. N Engl J Med 2003; 348:593–600.

80. Aicher A, Heeschen C, Mildner-Rihm C, et al. Essential role of endothelial nitric oxide synthase for mobilization of stem and progenitor cells. Nat Med 2003;9:1370–6.

81. Iwakura A, Shastry S, Luedemann C, et al. Estradiol enhances recovery after myocardial infarction by augmenting incorporation of bone marrow-derived endothelial progenitor cells into sites of ischemia-induced neovascularization via endothelial nitric oxide synthase-mediated activation of matrix metalloproteinase-9. Circulation 2006;113:1605–14.

82. Laufs U, Werner N, Link A, et al. Physical training increases endothelial progenitor cells, inhibition of neointima formation, and enhances angiogenesis. Circulation 2004;109:220–6.

83. Askari AT, Unzek S, Popovic ZB, et al. Effect of stromal-cell-derived factor 1 on stem-cell homing and tissue regeneration in ischaemic cardiomyopathy. Lancet 2003;362:697–703.

84. Sandri M, Adams V, Gielen S, et al. Effects of exercise and ischemia on mobilization and functional activation of blood-derived progenitor cells in patients with ischemic syndromes: results of 3 randomized studies. Circulation 2005;111:3391–9.

85. Adams V, Heiker JT, Höllriegel R, et al. Adiponectin promotes the migration of circulating angiogenic cells through p38-mediated induction of the CXCR4 receptor. Int J Cardiol 2012;167:2039–46.

86. Shibata R, Skurk C, Ouchi N, et al. Adiponectin promotes endothelial progenitor cell number and function. FEBS Lett 2008;582:1607–12.

87. Aghabozorg Afjeh SS, Ghaderian SM. The role of microRNAs in cardiovascular disease. Int J Mol Cell Med 2013;2:50–7.

88. Vickers KC, Rye KA, Tabet F. MicroRNAs in the onset and development of cardiovascular disease. Clin Sci 2014;126:183–94.

89. Bonauer A, Carmona G, Iwasaki M, et al. MicroRNA-92a controls angiogenesis and functional recovery of ischemic tissues in mice. Science 2009; 324:1710–3.

90. Fogelman AM. When good cholesterol goes bad. Nat Med 2004;10:902–3.

91. Loyer X, Potteaux S, Vion AC, et al. Inhibition of microrna-92a prevents endothelial dysfunction and atherosclerosis in mice. Circ Res 2014;114: 434–43.

92. Marin T, Gongol B, Chen Z, et al. Mechanosensitive MicroRNAs—role in endothelial responses to shear stress and redox state. Free Radic Biol Med 2013; 64:61–8.

93. Weber M, Baker MB, Moore JP, et al. MiR-21 is induced in endothelial cells by shear stress and modulates apoptosis and eNOS activity. Biochem Biophys Res Commun 2010;393:643–8.

94. Da Silva ND, Fernandes T, Soci UP, et al. Swimming training in rats increases cardiac MicroRNA-126 expression and angiogenesis. Med Sci Sports Exerc 2012;44:1453–62.

95. Van Solingen C, Seghers L, Bijkerk R, et al. Antagomir-mediated silencing of endothelial cell specific microRNA-126 impairs ischemia-induced angiogenesis. J Cell Mol Med 2009;13:1577–85.

96. Clark AL, Poole-Wilson PA, Coats AJ. Exercise limitation in chronic heart failure: central role of the periphery. J Am Coll Cardiol 1996;28: 1092–102.

97. Coats AJ. The muscle hypothesis of chronic heart failure. J Mol Cell Cardiol 1996;28:2255–62.

98. Yndestad A, Damas JK, Oie E, et al. Role of inflammation in the progression of heart failure. Curr Cardiol Rep 2007;9:236–41.

99. Niebauer J. Inflammatory mediators in heart failure. Int J Cardiol 2000;72:209–13.

100. Gullestad L, Ueland T, Vinge LE, et al. Inflammatory cytokines in heart failure: mediators and markers. Cardiology 2012;122:23–35.

101. von Haehling S, Schefold JC, Lainscak M, et al. Inflammatory biomarkers in heart failure revisited: much more than innocent bystanders. Heart Fail Clin 2009;5:549–60.

102. Deswal A, Petersen NJ, Feldman AM, et al. Cytokines and cytokine receptors in advanced heart failure: an analysis of the cytokine database from the Vesnarinone Trial (VEST). Circulation 2001; 103:2055–9.

103. Cappuzzello C, Di Vito L, Melchionna R, et al. Increase of plasma IL-9 and decrease of plasma IL-5, IL-7, and IFN-gamma in patients with chronic heart failure. J Transl Med 2011;9:28–34.

104. Niethammer M, Sieber M, von Haehling S, et al. Inflammatory pathways in patients with heart failure and preserved ejection fraction. Int J Cardiol 2008;129:111–7.

105. Batista J, Santos RV, Cunha LM, et al. Changes in the pro-inflammatory cytokine production and peritoneal macrophage function in rats with chronic heart failure. Cytokine 2006;34:284–90.

106. Panaro MA, Gagliardi N, Saponaro C, et al. Toll-like receptor 4 mediates LPS-induced release of nitric oxide and tumor necrosis factor-alpha by embryonal cardiomyocytes: biological significance and clinical implications in human pathology. Curr Pharm Des 2010;16:766–74.

107. Meador BM, Krzyszton CP, Johnson RW, et al. Effects of IL-10 and age on IL-6, IL-1beta, and TNF-α responses in mouse skeletal and cardiac muscle to an acute inflammatory insult. J Appl Physiol (1985) 2008;104:991–7.

108. Sandek A, Rauchhaus M, Anker SD, et al. The emerging role of the gut in chronic heart failure. Curr Opin Clin Nutr Metab Care 2008;11:632–9.

109. Peschel T, Schönauer M, Thiele H, et al. Invasive assessment of bacterial endotoxin and inflammatory cytokines in patients with acute heart failure. Eur J Heart Fail 2003;5:609–14.

110. Sandek A, Bjarnason I, Volk HD, et al. Studies on bacterial endotoxin and intestinal absorption function in patients with chronic heart failure. Int J Cardiol 2012;157:80–5.

111. Niebauer J, Volk HD, Kemp M, et al. Endotoxin and immune activation in chronic heart failure: a prospective cohort study. Lancet 1999;353:1838–42.

112. Li YP, Reid MB. NF-kB mediates the protein loss induced by TNF-α in differentiated skeletal muscle. Am J Physiol 2000;279:R1165–70.

113. Niebauer J, Clark AL, Webb-Peploe KM, et al. Exercise training in chronic heart failure: effects on pro-inflammatory markers. Eur J Heart Fail 2005;7:189–93.

114. Adamopoulos S, Parissis J, Kroupis C, et al. Physical training reduces peripheral markers of inflammation in patients with chronic heart failure. Eur Heart J 2001;22:791–7.

115. Smart NA, Larsen AI, Le Maitre JP, et al. Effect of exercise training on interleukin-6, tumour necrosis factor alpha and functional capacity in heart failure. Cardiol Res Pract 2011;2011:532620.

116. Gielen S, Adams V, Möbius-Winkler S, et al. Anti-inflammatory effects of exercise training in the skeletal muscle of patients with chronic heart failure. J Am Coll Cardiol 2003;42:861–8.

117. Batista J, Rosa JC, Lopes RD, et al. Exercise training changes IL-10/TNF-[alpha] ratio in the skeletal muscle of post-MI rats. Cytokine 2010;49:102–8.

118. Florini JR, Ewton DZ, Magri KA. Hormones, growth factors and myogenic differentiation. Annu Rev Physiol 1991;53:201–16.

119. Coleman ME, DeMayo F, Yin KC, et al. Myogenic vector expression of insulin-like growth factor I stimulates muscle cell differentiation and myofiber hypertrophy in transgenic mice. J Biol Chem 1995;270:12109–16.

120. Musaro A, McCullagh K, Paul A, et al. Localized Igf-1 transgene expression sustains hypertrophy and regeneration in senescent skeletal muscle. Nat Genet 2001;27:195–200.

121. Schulze PC, Fang J, Kassik KA, et al. Transgenic overexpression of locally acting insulin-like growth factor-1 inhibits ubiquitin-mediated muscle atrophy in chronic left ventricular dysfunction. Circ Res 2005;97:418–26.

122. Hambrecht R, Schulze PC, Gielen S, et al. Reduction of insulin-like growth factor-I expression in the skeletal muscle of noncachectic patients with chronic heart failure. J Am Coll Cardiol 2002;39:1175–81.

123. Niebauer J, Pflaum CD, Clark AL, et al. Deficient insulin-like growth factor 1 in chronic heart failure predicts altered body composition, anabolic deficiency, cytokine and neurohormonal activation. J Am Coll Cardiol 1998;32:393–7.

124. Kackstein K, Teren A, Matsumoto Y, et al. Impact of angiotensin II on skeletal muscle metabolism and function in mice: contribution of IGF-1, Sirtuin-1 and PGC-1a. Acta Histochem 2013;115:363–70.

125. Hambrecht R, Schulze PC, Gielen S, et al. Effects of exercise training on insulin-like growth factor-I expression in the skeletal muscle of non-cachectic patients with chronic heart failure. Eur J Cardiovasc Prev Rehabil 2005;12:401–16.

126. Gielen S, Sandri M, Kozarez I, et al. Exercise training attenuates MuRF-1 expression in the skeletal muscle of patients with chronic heart failure independent of age: the randomized Leipzig Exercise Intervention in Chronic Heart Failure and Aging (LEICA) catabolism study. Circulation 2012;125:2716–27.

127. Adams V, Mangner N, Gasch A, et al. Induction of MuRF1 Is essential for TNF-[alpha]-induced loss of muscle function in mice. J Mol Biol 2008;384:48–59.

128. Höllriegel R, Beck EB, Linke A, et al. Anabolic effects of exercise training in patients with advanced chronic heart failure (NYHA IIIb): impact on ubiquitin–protein ligases expression and skeletal muscle size. Int J Cardiol 2013;167(3):975–80.

129. De Sousa E, Veksler V, Bigard X, et al. Heart failure affects mitochondrial but not myofibrillar intrinsic properties of skeletal muscle. Ciculation 2000;102:1847–53.

130. Quigley AF, Kapsa RM, Esmore D, et al. Mitochondrial respiratory chain activity in idiopathic dilated cardiomyopathy. J Card Fail 2000;6:47–55.

131. Massie BM, Conway M, Yonge R, et al. 31P nuclear magnetic resonance evidence of abnormal skeletal muscle metabolism in patients with congestive heart failure. Am J Cardiol 1987;60:309–15.

132. Hambrecht R, Adams V, Gielen S, et al. Exercise intolerance in patients with chronic heart failure and increased expression of inducible nitric oxide synthase in the skeletal muscle. J Am Coll Cardiol 1999;33:174–9.

133. Garnier A, Fortin D, Zoll J, et al. Coordinated changes in mitochondrial function and biogenesis in healthy and diseased human skeletal muscle. FASEB J 2005;19:43–52.

134. Flück M, Hoppeler H. Molecular basis of skeletal muscle plasticity-from gene to form and function. Rev Physiol Biochem Pharmacol 2003;146: 159–216.

135. Hood DA, Irrcher I, Ljubicic V, et al. Coordination of metabolic plasticity in skeletal muscle. J Exp Biol 2006;209:2265–75.

136. Lin J, Wu H, Tarr PT, et al. Transcriptional co-activator PGC-1[alpha] drives the formation of slow-twitch muscle fibres. Nature 2002;418: 797–801.

137. Ventura-Clapier R, Mettauer B, Bigard X. Beneficial effects of endurance training on cardiac and skeletal muscle energy metabolism in heart failure. Cardiovasc Res 2007;73:10–8.

138. Russell AP, Foletta VC, Snow RJ, et al. Skeletal muscle mitochondria: a major player in exercise, health and disease. Biochim Biophys Acta 2014; 1840:1276–84.

139. Larsen AI, Lindal S, Aukrust P, et al. Effect of exercise training on skeletal muscle fibre characteristics in men with chronic heart failure. Correlation between skeletal muscle alterations, cytokines and exercise capacity. Int J Cardiol 2002;83:25–32.

140. Hambrecht R, Fiehn E, Yu J, et al. Effects of endurance training on mitochondrial ultrastructure and fiber type distribution in skeletal muscle of patients with stable chronic heart failure. J Am Coll Cardiol 1997;29:1067–73.

141. Kitzman DW, Nicklas B, Kraus WE, et al. Skeletal muscle abnormalities and exercise intolerance in older patients with heart failure and preserved ejection fraction. Am J Physiol Heart Circ Physiol 2014;306:H1364–70.

142. Erbs S, Höllriegel R, Linke A, et al. Exercise training in patients with advanced chronic heart failure (NYHAIIIb) promotes restoration of peripheral vasomotor function, induction of endogenous regeneration, and improvement of left ventricular function. Circ Heart Fail 2010;3:486–94.

143. Krämer DK, Ahlsen M, Norrbom J, et al. Human skeletal muscle fibre type variations correlate with PPAR alpha, PPAR delta and PGC-1 alpha mRNA. Acta Physiol (Oxf) 2006;188:207–16.

144. Wisloff U, Stoylen A, Loennechen JP, et al. Superior cardiovascular effect of aerobic interval training versus moderate continuous training in heart failure patients. Circulation 2007;115:3086–94.

145. Johnsen AB, Hoydal M, Rosbjorgen R, et al. Aerobic interval training partly reverse contractile dysfunction and impaired Ca2+ handling in atrial myocytes from rats with post infarction heart failure. PLoS One 2013;8:e66288.

146. Haykowsky MJ, Timmons MP, Kruger C, et al. Meta-analysis of aerobic interval training on exercise capacity and systolic function in patients with heart failure and reduced ejection fractions. Am J Cardiol 2013;111:1466–9.

147. Smart NA, Steele M. A comparison of 16 weeks of continuous vs intermittent exercise training in chronic heart failure patients. Congest Heart Fail 2012;18:205–11.

148. Iellamo F, Manzi V, Caminiti G, et al. Matched dose interval and continuous exercise training induce similar cardiorespiratory and metabolic adaptations in patients with heart failure. Int J Cardiol 2013;167:2561–5.

149. Dimopoulos S, nastasiou-Nana M, Sakellariou D, et al. Effects of exercise rehabilitation program on heart rate recovery in patients with chronic heart failure. Eur J Prev Cardiol 2006;13:67–73.

150. Nechwatal RM, Duck C, Gruber G. Physical training as interval or continuous training in chronic heart failure for improving functional capacity, hemodynamics and quality of life–a controlled study. Z Kardiol 2002;91:328–37.

151. Fu TC, Wang CH, Lin PS, et al. Aerobic interval training improves oxygen uptake efficiency by enhancing cerebral and muscular hemodynamics in patients with heart failure. Int J Cardiol 2013; 167:41–50.

152. Freyssin C, Verkindt C, Prieur F, et al. Cardiac rehabilitation in chronic heart failure: effect of an 8-week, high-intensity interval training versus continuous training. Arch Phys Med Rehabil 2012; 93:1359–64.

153. Stoylen A, Conraads V, Halle M, et al. Controlled study of myocardial recovery after interval training in heart failure: SMARTEX-HF–rationale and design. Eur J Prev Cardiol 2012;19:813–21.

154. Conraads VM, Van Craenenbroeck EM, Pattyn N, et al. Rationale and design of a randomized trial on the effectiveness of aerobic interval training in patients with coronary artery disease: the SAINTEX-CAD study. Int J Cardiol 2013;168: 3532–6.

155. Owan TE, Hodge DO, Herges RM, et al. Trends in prevalence and outcome of heart failure with preserved ejection fraction. N Engl J Med 2006;355: 251–9.

156. Campbell RT, Jhund PS, Castagno D, et al. What have we learned about patients with heart failure and preserved ejection fraction from DIG-PEF, CHARM-preserved, and I-PRESERVE? J Am Coll Cardiol 2012;60:2349–56.

157. Cleland JG, Tendera M, Adamus J, et al. The peri-ndopril in elderly people with chronic heart failure (PEP-CHF) study. Eur Heart J 2006;27:2338–45.

158. Solomon SD, Zile M, Pieske B, et al. The angiotensin receptor neprilysin inhibitor LCZ696 in heart failure with preserved ejection fraction: a phase 2 double-blind randomised controlled trial. Lancet 2012;380:1387–95.

159. Yusuf S, Pfeffer MA, Swedberg K, et al. Effects of candesartan in patients with chronic heart failure and preserved left-ventricular ejection fraction: the CHARM-Preserved Trial. Lancet 2003;362:777–81.

160. Zile MR, Gaasch WH, Anand IS, et al. Mode of death in patients with heart failure and a preserved ejection fraction: results from the Irbesartan in heart failure with preserved ejection fraction study (I-Preserve) trial. Circulation 2010;121:1393–405.

161. Edelmann F, Wachter R, Schmidt AG, et al. Effect of spironolactone on diastolic function and exercise capacity in patients with heart failure with preserved ejection fraction: the Aldo-DHF randomized controlled trial. JAMA 2013;309:781–91.

162. Edelmann F, Gelbrich G, Düngen HD, et al. Exercise training improves exercise capacity and diastolic function in patients with heart failure with preserved ejection fraction: results of the Ex-DHF (Exercise training in Diastolic Heart Failure) pilot study. J Am Coll Cardiol 2011;58:1780–91.

163. Kitzman DW, Brubaker PH, Morgan TM, et al. Exercise training in older patients with heart failure and preserved ejection fraction: a randomized, controlled, single-blind trial. Circ Heart Fail 2010;3:659–67.

164. Smart NA, Haluska B, Jeffriess L, et al. Exercise training in heart failure with preserved systolic function: a randomized controlled trial of the effects on cardiac function and functional capacity. Congest Heart Fail 2012;18:295–301.

165. Hidalgo C, Saripalli C, Granzier HL. Effect of exercise training on post-translational and post-transcriptional regulation of titin stiffness in striated muscle of wild type and IG KO mice. Arch Biochem Biophys 2014;552–553:100–7.

Functional Assessment of Heart Failure Patients

Leonard A. Kaminsky, PhD*, Mary S. Tuttle, MS

KEYWORDS

- Functional capacity • Peak oxygen consumption • Six-minute walk test • Muscular strength
- Handgrip

KEY POINTS

- The gold standard measurement of cardiovascular functional capacity is peak oxygen consumption obtained from a cardiopulmonary exercise test.
- The 6-minute walk test provides an indirect measure of cardiovascular functional capacity.
- Muscular functional capacity is assessed using either a 1-repetition maximum test of the upper and lower body or other methods, such as handgrip measurement.
- The short physical performance battery may provide a helpful, indirect indication of muscular functional capacity.

INTRODUCTION

Heart failure (HF) is the condition characterized by the inability of the heart to pump sufficient blood to meet the demands of the body. It has been well established that both the prevalence and incidence of HF is increasing.[1] There are 2 primary types of HF, categorized by ejection fraction: Reduced ejection fraction and preserved ejection fraction.[2] Additionally, HF is commonly classified into stages from mild to severe using a symptom-based scale related to functional limitations.

One of the hallmark features of HF is exercise intolerance, which is accompanied by symptoms of fatigue and shortness of breath.[3] As the disease progresses, patients experience a downward spiral as these symptoms typically result in reduced physical activity, which leads to progressively worsening exercise intolerance. Typically, patients with HF are faced with what can be termed a functional disability. Often, their reduced functional abilities restrict or may even prevent them from performing occupational tasks, which may result in loss of work. Additionally, it is well known that patients with HF experience impairment in the ability to carry out activities of daily living and suffer from reduced quality of life.

The objective of this paper was to provide an overview of assessments of functional ability of patients with HF. Two categories of assessment are reviewed: Cardiovascular function and muscular function. The review includes procedural guidance on how to administer the assessments and information related to the advantages and disadvantages of each method. Because both HF types (reduced ejection fraction and preserved ejection fraction) are characterized by exercise intolerance, the procedures can be used effectively with either type of HF.

CARDIOVASCULAR FUNCTION

The gold standard method for assessing cardiovascular functional capacity is measurement of oxygen consumption (Vo_2) during a maximal exercise test. This procedure is known as cardiopulmonary exercise testing (CPX). The principle outcome variable is maximal or peak oxygen Vo_2 (Vo_{2max} or Vo_{2peak}). Weber and colleagues[4] established a classification system based on peak Vo_2

Clinical Exercise Physiology Program, Human Performance Laboratory, Ball State University, Muncie, IN 47306 USA
* Corresponding author.
E-mail address: kaminskyla@bsu.edu

Heart Failure Clin 11 (2015) 29–36
http://dx.doi.org/10.1016/j.hfc.2014.08.002
1551-7136/15/$ – see front matter © 2015 Elsevier Inc. All rights reserved.

for patients with HF (**Table 1**). Although exercise testing guidelines have existed for more than 40 years,[5] there is not a uniformly accepted standard for assessing cardiovascular functional capacity in terms of Vo_2. Review of the scientific and clinical literature reveals that both Vo_{2max} and peak Vo_2 are routinely reported. As reviewed by Arena and colleagues,[6] historically Vo_{2max} is used when the measurement methodology includes determination of a plateau in Vo_2 measurement values during the last 2 work rates of the exercise test. However, not all studies that report the variable in terms of Vo_{2max} used that as a criterion and this method is not typically suitable for use with ramp-style protocols. Alternatively, peak Vo_2 is used when the method determines the highest Vo_2 value, expressed as milliliters of oxygen per kilogram of body weight per minute (mL $O_2 \bullet kg^{-1} \bullet min^{-1}$) during the exercise test. Another challenge in interpretation is that different studies have used various measurement sampling intervals to determine Vo_2. A recent scientific statement from the American Heart Association recommends using a rolling average of three 10-s sampling intervals during the exercise test to help standardize this important outcome measurement.[7] For the purposes of this paper, the term peak Vo_2 is used to indicate cardiovascular functional capacity for patients with HF.

As mentioned, guidelines for exercise testing have been available for more than 40 years. However, in the past 10 years as the evidence base has grown, establishing the clinical importance of CPX measures, there have been a number of scientific statements released.[7–10] Although the focus of this paper is on the assessment of cardiovascular functional capacity, it is important to recognize that CPX is clearly recognized as a valuable component in the diagnosis and prognosis of HF patients. Indeed, the joint report from the European Society of Cardiology/European Association for Cardiovascular Prevention and Rehabilitation and the American Heart Association provides a stratification approach for diagnosis and prognosis of patients with HF.[9] The key CPX measurements, all clearly defined in the report, included in the stratification are the slope of minute ventilation (VE) relative to carbon dioxide production (VCo_2; VE/VCo_2 slope); peak Vo_2; exercise oscillatory ventilation; and the change in the partial pressure of carbon. The stratification also includes consideration of the blood pressure and electrocardiographic response during the exercise test, the rate of decline in heart rate after 1 minute of recovery and the reason for test termination.

Assessing Peak Oxygen Consumption from Exercise Tests

Recent guidelines and scientific statements are available that provide comprehensive recommendations for procedures for clinical exercise testing. A brief overview of some of the important methodologic points is reviewed in this section for obtaining the gold standard assessment of peak Vo_2.

Exercise testing can be performed with various exercise modes; however, the 2 most common choices are cycle ergometers and treadmills. The advantages and disadvantages to both modes of testing are listed in **Table 2**. There are 2 types of cycle ergometers; Mechanically braked and electrically braked. Work rates on mechanically braked cycle ergometers can be varied by both the rate of pedaling and the resistance to pedaling. This requires a fixed pedal rate of typically 50 or 60 rpm to achieve the desired fixed work rate. Electrically braked cycle ergometers are designed to automatically change the resistance on the pedal as the pedal rate varies to maintain a desired fixed work rate.

Exercise tests are administered according to specified protocols with multiple variations possible. The duration of an exercise test should require at least 6 minutes but no more than 15 minutes, with an ideal time of 10 minutes. The first decision in selecting a protocol is between a fixed incremental or ramp style. A fixed incremental protocol uses a specific work rate either in watts on a cycle ergometer or by a combination of speed and elevation on a treadmill for a set period of time (stage) of 1, 2, or 3 minutes. One of the most desirable features of fixed incremental protocols is that the Vo_2 of each stage can be estimated (standard error of estimate [SEE] $\pm$ 7%) using equations provided by the American College of Sports

Table 1
Classification of heart failure patients based on functional status

Peak Vo_2 (mL $O_2 \bullet kg^{-1} \bullet min^{-1}$)	Classification
>20	A. Normal
16–20	B. Mild to moderate impairment
10–15.9	C. Moderate to severe impairment
<10	D. Severe impairment

Abbreviation: Vo_2, oxygen consumption.
Data from Weber KT, Janicki JS, Ward DM, et al. Measurement and interpretation of maximal oxygen uptake in patients with chronic cardiac or circulatory failure. J Clin Monit 1987;3:31–7.

Table 2
Advantages and disadvantages of cycle and treadmill modes of exercise testing

Mode	Advantages	Disadvantages
Cycle	Smaller, portable	Less familiar activity for patients
	Less expensive	Leg fatigue may cause early termination
	Ausculatory blood pressure measurement is easier	Electrically braked ergometers are difficult to calibrate
	Electrocardiogram tracings have fewer artifacts	Lack of standardized testing protocols
Treadmill	Walking is a more common activity for patients	Balance issues, risk of falling
	Typically higher peak Vo_2 values are achieved	Handrail use will impact prediction of peak Vo_2
	Work rates can be increased by elevation at a fixed speed	Blood pressure and electrocardiogram measures are more difficult

Abbreviation: Vo_2, oxygen consumption.

Medicine.[5] There are many standardized incremental treadmill protocols. The Bruce protocol was commonly used in routine cardiac diagnostic assessments; however, the relatively high first work rate of approximately 5 metabolic equivalents (METs; 1 MET = 3.5 mL $O_2 \bullet kg^{-1} \bullet min^{-1}$) and the large stage increments of 2 to 3 METs makes it unsuitable for patients with HF. Preferred options for this population are either the modified Naughton or a modified Balke protocol. For cycle testing, few standardized protocols exist because the maximal watt level varies directly with the total body weight (muscle mass) of the patient. Certainly, some clinics use a number of standardized incremental protocol options for cycle testing to achieve different expected maximal watt levels. Alternatively, both standardized and individualized ramp-style protocols can be used. Unfortunately, there are no standardized ramp protocols suitable for HF patients. Individualized ramp protocols can be derived using software options with metabolic systems, which require setting a starting and maximal speed of walking (or fixed speed) and an estimate of the functional capacity of the patient in METs. The software then generates the increments in speed and elevation to obtain the estimated MET level in a targeted test time (usually 10 minutes). A similar process is used for cycle testing, setting a starting and expected watt level and then computing the rate of increase in watts to be obtained in a linear fashion over a 10-minute period of time.

Determination of peak Vo_2 during a CPX requires collecting ventilatory expired gases during the test. The 3 primary variables measured during the test are the total ventilation and the fractional concentrations of expired oxygen and carbon dioxide. As mentioned, additional CPX variables can also be measured, which have prognostic and diagnostic utility. CPX measurements require specialized equipment and trained personnel, which can be a limiting factor, because these resources may not be readily available. However, as more academic programs have developed for training individuals to administer these tests and the costs of the equipment are relatively fixed (ie, the primary cost is the purchase of the equipment, the costs per test are minimal) the opportunities for obtaining a measured peak Vo_2 are growing.

The next best option for assessing cardiovascular functional capacity is from a maximal exercise test, performed without ventilatory expired gas measurements. This option is commonly available in cardiology clinics and practices. These tests are primarily performed for diagnostic purposes with routine monitoring of the exercise electrocardiogram, along with blood pressure, heart rate, and signs and symptoms. These tests also require specifically trained personnel. Cardiovascular functional capacity can be estimated from either a prediction equation using maximal test time with standardized protocols or from the maximal work rate obtained during the test. With use of any prediction equation, there is some degree of error associated with the estimation. Prediction equations using test time typically have reported error ranges of approximately ± 3 to 5 mL $O_2 \bullet kg^{-1} \bullet min^{-1}$. Estimations from maximal work rate are derived using the American College of Sports Medicine equations. However, it is important to recognize that this creates some issues, because these equations were developed for steady-state submaximal work rates (not maximal). Thus, the estimates may result in greater error ranges than those reported for the submaximal level (ie, more than $\pm 7\%$).

A third option for assessing cardiovascular functional capacity is from a submaximal exercise test. These procedures rely on having a reasonable estimation of maximal heart rate, commonly estimated using age. A heart rate to Vo_2 (predicted from work rate) relationship is established at 2 submaximal levels and then a linear line is extrapolated to derive an estimated maximal value. Advantages of submaximal testing are that it requires less training from staff, takes less time, and because the patient's effort is submaximal has lower associated risks. However, because many patients with HF are prescribed β-blocker medications,[2] prediction of maximal heart rate is compromised. Thus, this method may not be viable for many patients with HF. A summary of the advantages and disadvantages of 3 exercise testing methods is provided in **Table 3**.

Assessing Cardiovascular Functional Capacity Without Exercise Tests

Exercise testing has inherent limitations (expense [equipment and personnel], time, and risks associated with maximal exercise effort); thus, it is not feasible in all settings. However, because understanding an HF patient's exercise intolerance is important for guiding therapy, alternative methods of assessing cardiovascular functional capacity have been developed.

Field tests for estimating aerobic fitness were originally used with apparently healthy populations and most often involved running 1.5 miles or 12 minutes.[5] Variations of this approach were explored with clinical populations using fixed distance or time while walking. More than 30 years ago, Butland and colleagues[11] reported that walking for 6 minutes may provide useful information in patient populations with functional limitations. Since that time, the 6-minute walk test (6MWT) has gained acceptance in the clinical community as a feasible option to obtain an estimate of cardiovascular functional capacity in disease-based populations known to experience exercise intolerance. Although it is beyond the scope of this paper to provide a thorough review of the clinical uses and limitations of the 6MWT, it is important to recognize that the 6MWT does not accurately predict peak Vo_2.[12] Some reports have suggested that failure to achieve a certain distance, such as 300 m[13] or 450 m,[14] on the 6MWT has prognostic value. Additionally, some have proposed that measures other than total distance achieved, such as total work performed[15] or heart rate after 1 minute of recovery[16] may provide useful information from the 6MWT. However, there are no well-accepted normative values available to interpret 6MWT results.

The 6MWT is considered simple in concept in terms of the patient directions; however, there are important methodologic requirements. These are briefly reviewed here, with more detailed information available in the guideline statement from the American Thoracic Society (ATS).[17] The first consideration is the location. Ideally, this should be in a semiprivate area free from distractions and potential obstacles. In most clinical settings, this can be done in a hallway that is at least 30 m long. However, it should be mentioned that the length and type (oval vs back-and-forth) may result

Table 3
Advantages and disadvantages of 3 exercise testing methods for assessing cardiovascular functional capacity

Mode	Advantages	Disadvantages
Maximal CPX	Gold standard method Same diagnostic measures from maximal exercise test Additional measures have prognostic value	Expense of equipment Specialized training required for technicians Additional time required for results processing
Maximal without CPX	More widely available in clinical settings Less expense (equipment and personnel)	Prediction errors in estimating functional capacity Important prognostic indicators not available
Submaximal	Lower risk because test effort is submaximal Less expense (equipment and personnel)	Maximal heart rate predictions not accurate for those on β-blockers Prediction errors in estimating functional capacity

Abbreviation: CPX, cardiopulmonary exercise test.

in slight differences in performance. Attempts to perform this test on a treadmill have not been found to be successful.[18]

Although there are few pretest requirements for the patient, it is important to provide a clear set of instructions pertaining to the objective (walk as far as possible), the requirement to walk, not jog, and the ability to stop and rest if needed. The ATS guidelines provide a brief script that can easily be read before each test. During the test, the amount and type of verbal encouragement should be consistent, because this can influence test performance.[19] The ATS guidelines also provide recommendations for standardizing the communication with the patient during the test.

One of the most important issues with 6MWT administration is a learning effect. The ATS guidelines suggest that "a practice test is not needed in most clinical settings"; however, the guidelines acknowledged that test performance is improved on a second trail. In clinical programs where the 6MWT will be used to influence therapeutic options and in research settings, the validity of the measurement is paramount. Thus, having patients perform at least 1 practice trial is important. Interestingly, Hanson and colleagues[20] reported that 6MWT distance continued to improve over 3 trials (regardless if performed on the same day or over 3 different days) in patients in a cardiac rehabilitation program. Similarly, Wu and colleagues[21] found improvement over 3 consecutive trials both at baseline and after 2 months. In patients with more severe exercise tolerance limitations, such as advanced HF, it was shown that a repeated trial did not result in improvement in 6MWT distance.[22]

Key methodologic considerations for the 6MWT are listed in **Box 1**. The importance of using standardized procedures cannot be overemphasized.

Although the 6MWT is the most commonly used nonexercise test indicator of cardiovascular functional capacity, other assessments have been studied. Some investigators have determined the ability of a shuttle walk test (SWT) to evaluate chronic disease patient populations.[14,23,24] This test requires patients to walk back and forth around 2 markers on a 10-m course (each 10 m = 1 shuttle) at a pace dictated by audio signals recorded on a cassette tape or CD. The speed is initially set at 0.5 m/s and increased by 0.17 m/s every minute. The test is terminated when the patient cannot complete a shuttle in the required time interval. As with the 6MWT, it is recommended that only standardized comments (no encouragement) be provided and that the SWT is repeated at least twice to account for a learning effect.

The major distinguishing characteristic between the 6MWT and SWT is the incremental nature of

---

> **Box 1**
> **Important methodologic considerations for the 6-minute walk test**
>
> Standardized location is needed; free from distractions/obstacles; distance between turn around point of ~30 m.
>
> Clear, standardized instructions should be read to the patient before each test.
>
> Clear, standardized feedback should be given to the patient during each test.
>
> Although not required, assessments of heart rate, blood pressure, and rating of perceived exertion are desirable.
>
> To eliminate a learning effect impacting test results, a minimum of 2 trials should be performed (either with a short rest period or on a separate day).

---

the SWT. Proponents of the SWT suggest this should result in a greater level of effort, compared with the self-pace nature of the 6MWT, and thus provide a better indicator of cardiovascular functional capacity. Although this test may have merit, to date, the research evidence base is lacking to recommend it be used in place of the 6MWT.

Finally, there have been other attempts to improve on the limitations of the 6MWT by evaluating shorter distances. Studies have investigated the utility of a 100-m walk test in patients with pulmonary disease,[25] 200-m fast walking in patients in cardiac rehabilitation,[26] and a 400-m walk test in patients with HF.[27] All of these tests showed some utility in evaluating patient populations; however, additional research is needed before recommending their use as an assessment of cardiovascular functional capacity.

MUSCULAR FUNCTION

One of the most frequent misconceptions of HF is that the limitations are solely related to the heart. Evidence has existed for some time that one of significant factors associated with exercise intolerance in patients with HF is skeletal muscle deconditioning.[28] Recent studies have identified mechanisms underlying the weakness observed in the skeletal muscles or patients with HF.[29,30] Thus, is it now well accepted that functional assessments of patients with HF should include measures of muscular performance. In general, tests of muscular performance are not as common as cardiovascular function in healthy adult populations. Even less has been done with disease-based populations to evaluate muscular function.

Thus, the review of muscular function assessments provided herein is primarily based on work with healthy adults. However, the procedures for assessing patients with HF would not vary significantly, only the interpretation of the results.

The gold standard method to assess muscular strength is the 1-repetition maximum test (1-RM). The procedures for this assessment are described in **Box 2**. The resistance for the lifting can be either free weights or resistance exercise machines. Although a 1-RM can be obtained from any weight lifting exercise, the 2 most common lifts are the bench press (for upper body strength) and the leg press (for lower body strength). The American College of Sports Medicine guidelines provide a set of normative values derived from an adult population that was free from chronic disease.[5] Unfortunately, there are no definitive standards for interpreting 1-RM performance in patients with HF. One of the major issues with performing 1-RM assessments is the time requirement, especially if patients need to be familiarized with using the free weights or machines. Other issues are the need for specialized equipment and trained personnel and the risks associated with maximal effort.

Box 2
Important methodologic considerations for the 1 repetition maximum

To eliminate a learning effect impacting test results, patient should be familiarized with the equipment used for the assessment (ideally on a separate day).

Clear instructions regarding proper breathing (no breath holding) needs to be explained before each test.

A warm up of ~5 repetitions of each movement (bench press or leg press) with no weight is important.

Select a weight that is submaximal (estimated to be ~75% of the patient's capacity) and have the patient complete 1 repetition.

Based on feedback from the patient, select a higher weight that should be able to be lifted 1 time and after a 3-minute rest period attempt 1 repetition. If successful, have the patient attempt 1 more lift of the next highest weight increment. If not successful, lower the weight by 1 increment and have the patient attempt to complete 1 repetition.

Because different muscle groups are involved, both the chest press and leg press tests should be able to be completed at the same testing session.

A second option for performing muscular function assessments is to use a handgrip dynamometer. This test has been used for many years as a physical fitness measure in school-aged children. It does require a handgrip dynamometer; however, these devices are relatively inexpensive (<$400) and are durable. The procedure is simple, only requiring the patient to squeeze the handle of the dynamometer as hard as they can for 3 seconds. After a short rest, the test is repeated 2 more times, with each hand being tested. Although normative values specific for patients with HF do not exist, large population standards are available.[31] These tests are starting to be administered in the HF population and seem to have some merit.[32,33]

There are also indirect measures of muscular strength that can be used as indicators of muscular functional ability. The origins for many of these evaluations came from work with geriatric populations. The method that seems to be gaining the most acceptance is the Short Physical Performance Battery.[34] This functional test includes assessments of gait speed (4 m), strength (sit to stand, repeated 5 times), and balance (standing position). A composite score is formulated, with higher scores indicating better functional ability. A recent study reported that the Short Physical Performance Battery was reduced in patients with HF with preserved ejection fraction compared with age-matched controls and also correlated with total and leg lean mass.[35]

There are other assessments used in geriatric populations that may have utility in assessing the muscular performance of patients with HF. These include both the instrumental activities of daily living[36] and the timed up and go test.[37]

Finally, there are some questionnaire-based methods that have been used in the HF population. Myers and colleagues[38] evaluated the Duke Activity Status Index, the Kansas City Cardiomyopathy Questionnaire, and the Veterans Specific Activity Questionnaire. They compared these questionnaires with results from CPX and the 6MWT in a group of patients with HF. Their findings revealed that these different methods did not correlate well with each other and concluded that they should not be used as surrogate indicators of functional status in this population.

SUMMARY

Functional assessments of patients with HF provide important clinical information. Cardiovascular functional capacity measures have been utilized for many years. The gold standard method is measuring peak Vo_2 from a CPX, which has added value by providing measurements with prognostic utility. Peak V_{O_2} can also be estimated from diagnostic maximal exercise tests, commonly used in cardiac care and from submaximal exercise tests. Indirect indicators of cardiovascular functional capacity can also be obtained, the most common of which is the 6MWT. When performed with standardized procedures, the 6MWT can provide useful information when measurements of peak V_{O_2} are not available or are not feasible.

The importance of skeletal muscle as a limiting factor for patients with HF is now well understood. This has led to increased interest in evaluating muscular functional capacity in patients with HF. Efforts are beginning to utilize measures that have been commonly applied to evaluate the muscular fitness of adults, the most common of which are the 1-RM and handgrip. Interpretation of results with normative standards for patients with HF with these 2 assessments is lacking at this time. Work is also beginning to utilize indirect indicators of muscular functional capacity that have been established in geriatric populations. The assessment that may have the most promise for patients with HF is the Short Physical Performance Battery.

REFERENCES

1. Go AS, Mozaffarian D, Roger VL, et al. Heart disease and stroke statistics—2014 update: a report from the American Heart Association. Circulation 2014;129(3):399–410.
2. Yancy CW, Jessup M, Bozkurt B, et al. 2013 ACCF/AHA guideline for the management of heart failure: a report of the American College of Cardiology Foundation/American Heart Association Task Force on Practice Guidelines. Circulation 2013;128(16):e240–327.
3. Watson RD, Gibbs CR, Lip GY. ABC of heart failure. Clinical features and complications. BMJ 2000; 320(7229):236–9.
4. Weber KT, Janicki JS, Ward DM, et al. Measurement and interpretation of maximal oxygen uptake in patients with chronic cardiac or circulatory failure. J Clin Monit 1987;3:31–7.
5. Pescatello LS, editor. ACSM's guidelines for exercise testing and prescription. 9th edition. Philadelphia: Wolters Kluwer/Lippincott Williams & Wilkins Health; 2014.
6. Arena R, Myers J, Williams MA, et al. Assessment of functional capacity in clinical and research settings: a scientific statement from the American Heart Association Committee on Exercise, Rehabilitation, and Prevention of the Council on Clinical Cardiology and the Council on Cardiovascular Nursing. Circulation 2007;116(3):329–43.
7. Myers J, Arena R, Franklin B, et al. Recommendations for clinical exercise laboratories: a scientific statement from the American Heart Association. Circulation 2009;119(24):3144–61.
8. Balady GJ, Arena R, Sietsema K, et al. Clinician's guide to cardiopulmonary exercise testing in adults: a scientific statement from the American Heart Association. Circulation 2010;122(2):191–225.
9. Guazzi M, Adams V, Conraads V, et al. Clinical recommendations for cardiopulmonary exercise testing data assessment in specific patient populations. Circulation 2012;126(18):2261–74.
10. Palange P, Ward SA, Carlsen KH, et al. Recommendations on the use of exercise testing in clinical practice. Eur Respir J 2007;29(1):185–209.
11. Butland R, Pang J, Gross ER, et al. Two-, six-, and 12-minute walking tests in respiratory disease. Br Med J (Clin Res Ed) 1982;284(6329):1607–8.
12. Lucas C, Stevenson LW, Johnson W, et al. The 6-min walk and peak oxygen consumption in advanced heart failure: aerobic capacity and survival. Am Heart J 1999;138:618–24.
13. Cahalin LP, Mathier MA, Semigran MJ, et al. The six-minute walk test predicts peak oxygen uptake and survival in patients with advanced heart failure. Chest 1996;110(2):325–32.
14. Lewis ME, Newall C, Townend JN, et al. Incremental shuttle walk test in the assessment of patients for heart transplantation. Heart 2001;86:183–7.
15. Hendrican MC, McKelvie RS, Smith T, et al. Functional capacity in patients with congestive heart failure. J Card Fail 2000;6(3):214–9.
16. Cahalin LP, Arena R, Guazzi M. Comparison of heart rate recovery after the six-minute walk test to cardiopulmonary exercise testing in patients with heart failure and reduced and preserved ejection fraction. Am J Cardiol 2012;110(3):467–8.
17. American Thoracic Society, ATS Committee on Proficiency Standards for Clinical Pulmonary Function Laboratories. ATS statement: guidelines for the six-minute walk test. Am J Respir Crit Care Med 2002;166:111–7.
18. Lenssen AF, Wijnen LC, Vankan DG, et al. Six-minute walking test done in a hallway or on a treadmill: how close do the two methods agree? Eur J Cardiovasc Prev Rehabil 2010;17(6):713–7.
19. Guyatt GH, Pugsley SO, Sullivan MJ, et al. Effect of encouragement on walking test performance. Thorax 1984;39:818–22.
20. Hanson LC, McBurney H, Taylor NF. The retest reliability of the six-minute walk test in patients referred to a cardiac rehabilitation programme. Physiother Res Int 2012;17:55–61.
21. Wu G, Sanderson B, Bittner V. The 6-minute walk test: how important is the learning effect? Am Heart J 2003;146(1):129–33.
22. Adsett J, Mullins R, Hwang R, et al. Repeat six-minute walk tests in patients with chronic heart failure: are they clinically necessary? Eur J Cardiovasc Prev Rehabil 2011;18(4):601–6.

23. Morales FJ, Martinez A, Mendez M, et al. A shuttle walk test for assessment of functional capacity in chronic heart failure. Am Heart J 1999;138(2 Pt 1): 291–8.

24. Singh SJ, Morgan MD, Scott S, et al. Development of a shuttle walking test of disability in patients with chronic airways obstruction. Thorax 1992;47:1019–24.

25. Morice A, Smithies T. The 100 m walk: a simple and reproducible exercise test. Br J Dis Chest 1984; 78(4):392–4.

26. Gremeaux V, Hannequin A, Laroche D, et al. Reproducibility, validity and responsiveness of the 200-metre fast walk test in patients undergoing cardiac rehabilitation. Clin Rehabil 2012;26(8):733–40.

27. Zdrenghea D, Beudean M, Pop D, et al. Four hundred meters walking test in the evaluation of heart failure patients. Rom J Intern Med 2010;48(1):33–8.

28. Wilson JR, Mancini DM. Factors contributing to the exercise limitation of heart failure. J Am Coll Cardiol 1993;22(4 Suppl A):93A–8A.

29. von Haehling S, Steinbeck L, Doehner W, et al. Muscle wasting in heart failure: an overview. Int J Biochem Cell Biol 2013;45(10):2257–65.

30. Miller MS, Vanburen P, Lewinter MM, et al. Mechanisms underlying skeletal muscle weakness in human heart failure: alterations in single fiber myosin protein content and function. Heart Fail 2009;2:700–6.

31. Spruit MA, Sillen MJ, Groenen MT, et al. New normative values for handgrip strength: results from the UK Biobank. J Am Med Dir Assoc 2013; 14:775.e5–11.

32. Izawa KP, Watanabe S, Osada N, et al. Handgrip strength as a predictor of prognosis in Japanese patients with congestive heart failure. Eur J Cardiovasc Prev Rehabil 2009;16:21–7.

33. Sunnerhagen KS, Cider A, Schaufelberger M, et al. Muscular performance in heart failure. J Card Fail 1998;4(2):97–104.

34. Guralnik JM, Simonsick EM, Ferrucci L, et al. A short physical performance battery assessing lower extremity function: association with self-reported disability and prediction of mortality and nursing home admission. J Gerontol 1994;49(2):M85–94.

35. Haykowsky MJ, Brubaker PH, Morgan TM, et al. Impaired aerobic capacity and physical functional performance in older heart failure patients with preserved ejection fraction: role of lean body mass. J Gerontol A Biol Sci Med Sci 2013;68(8): 968–75.

36. Lawton MP, Brody EM. Assessment of older people: self-maintaining and instrumental activities of daily living. Gerontologist 1969;9(3):179–86.

37. Podsiadlo D, Richardson S. The timed "Up & Go": a test of basic functional mobility for frail elderly persons. J Am Geriatr Soc 1991;39(2):142–8.

38. Myers J, Zaheer N, Quaglietti S, et al. Association of functional and health status measures in heart failure. J Card Fail 2006;12(6):439–45.

Reasonable Expectations
How Much Aerobic Capacity, Muscle Strength, and Quality of Life Can Improve with Exercise Training in Heart Failure

Mark A. Williams, PhD, MAACVPR, FACSM[a],*, Bunny Pozehl, PhD, APRN-NP, FAHA, FAAN[b]

KEYWORDS

- Exercise training • Functional capacity • Health-related quality of life
- Reduced ejection fraction (HFrEF) • Preserved ejection fraction (HFpEF)

KEY POINTS

- Despite variability in regimens, aerobic exercise training, which may include resistance training, provides for significant increases in functional capacity in patients with heart failure.
- Using moderate-intensity exercise training, benefits seem to be similar in patients with reduced ejection fraction (HFrEF) as well as those with preserved ejection fraction (HFpEF).
- Although some inconsistencies exist, overall, exercise training in HFrEF results in positive effects on health-related quality of life (HRQoL).
- Despite small sample sizes and underpowered trials, findings also suggest a positive impact on HRQoL of exercise training in HFpEF.

INTRODUCTION

Over the previous 25 years, the use of exercise training in patients with diagnoses of heart failure (HF) has been shown to improve exercise capacity, functional disability, and overall clinical outcomes, including quality of life (QoL).[1–8] Patients included within these investigations of exercise training have generally been those with a diagnosis of HF with reduced ejection fraction (HFrEF) (ie, <35%–40%). More recently, determining the impact of exercise training in patients with HF with preserved ejection fraction (HFpEF), which is greater than 50%, has received increasing attention.

The purpose of this article is to provide an overview of the magnitude of changes in functional capacity as determined by measurement of peak oxygen consumption (Vo_2), as well as the impact on QoL using a variety of tools. This discussion also describes reported comparisons between the impact of exercise training in patients with HFrEF versus HFpEF. In addition, exercise training methodology is discussed in relation to these patient groups within the population with HF.

MAGNITUDE OF FUNCTIONAL GAINS AFTER EXERCISE TRAINING

Since the early days of investigation and discussion of its potential impact,[1,9,10] the role of exercise training in patients with HF, using traditional moderate-intensity aerobic exercise, and in some instances resistance training, has been associated with significant improvement in the physiologic

[a] Division of Cardiology, Creighton University School of Medicine, 3006 Webster Street, Omaha, NE 68131, USA; [b] University of Nebraska Medical Center, College of Nursing, Lincoln Division, 1230 "O" Street, Suite 131, P.O. Box 880220, Lincoln, NE 68588-0220, USA
* Corresponding author.
E-mail address: MarkWilliams@creighton.edu

Heart Failure Clin 11 (2015) 37–57
http://dx.doi.org/10.1016/j.hfc.2014.08.003
1551-7136/15/$ – see front matter © 2015 Elsevier Inc. All rights reserved.

heartfailure.theclinics.com

indices of functional capacity and specifically, peak Vo_2. However, perhaps at least as important as increased levels of the peak values of these parameters is the benefit of decreased myocardial work during submaximal effort, as shown by decreased submaximal heart rates, lower systolic blood pressures (reduced rate pressure product [ie, heart rate x systolic blood pressure], which is associated with lower myocardial oxygen demand), and the corresponding patient descriptions of lessened perceived effort. Consequently, as a result of exercise training, patients become less symptomatic during usual daily activities (eg, decreased dyspnea and fatigue), and may be able to increase the intensity of activities, which heretofore had not been possible.

Exercise Training in Patients with Reduced Ejection Fraction

Findings from an extensive review by Smart and Marwick[2] in 2004 (81 studies in patients, ejection fraction <40% [HFrEF], mean 27% $\pm$ 7%, **Table 1**) showed important results. In those studies, which directly assessed peak Vo_2 (n = 57) before and after exercise training (including aerobic, resistance, combinations of the 2, and inspiratory training), there was an associated overall increase of 15.3% $\pm$ 8.1% (range: 0%–39%) in peak Vo_2, from a baseline of 16.5 mL/kg/min to 19.0 mL/kg/min. When findings were separated by training regimen, aerobic training alone was associated with a 17% increase in peak Vo_2, the largest improvement within the 4 training regimen groups. Although the components of the exercise prescriptions used in the training regimens varied, overall, studies included within this review generally used moderate-intensity exercise, as characterized by targets of 60%, 70%, and 65% of peak Vo_2, maximal heart rate, and heart rate reserve, respectively.

More recent individual trials (**Table 2**) indicated similar findings to those described earlier.[3,11–14] Klocek and colleagues[11] used constant, progressively increasing workloads versus interval training, showing that the progressive protocol was associated with a 26% increase in peak Vo_2 compared with only a 7.1% increase for the interval protocol versus a 9.6% decrease in the no training control group. The constant, progressively increasing workload group also showed overall improved QoL and sexual life (P<.01) compared with the other 2 groups. Passino and colleagues[12] and Mueller and colleagues[13] reported improvements of 13.2% and 18.8%, respectively, in peak Vo_2 compared with control groups. O'Connor and colleagues,[3] reporting on data from the Heart Failure-A Controlled Trial Investigating Outcomes

of Exercise Training (HF-ACTION) trial, reported smaller increases in peak Vo_2 with exercise training. However, the magnitude of the trial (more than 2300 patients from 82 centers) and including analyses of both 3-month and 12-month data, indicated significant increases in peak Vo_2 compared with controls, as well as modest significant reductions in (1) all-cause mortality or hospitalization and (2) cardiovascular mortality or HF hospitalization. Certainly, even modest reductions in mortality and hospitalizations have tremendous implications for the use of cardiac rehabilitation.

Exercise Training in Women with Heart Failure and Reduced Ejection Fraction

Historically, the inclusion of women within studies of exercise training in HF has generally been limited. Thus, there continues to be less evidence regarding the value of exercise training in women with HF, when compared with that of men. In the Smart and Marwick meta-analysis,[2] only approximately 21% of patients studied were women, although women are more likely to have HF after myocardial infarction or revascularization.[14] In addition, it is suggested that women are less likely to be referred, and to participate if referred, in cardiac rehabilitation exercise programs.[14–16] Reviewing findings from HF-ACTION, Pina and colleagues[14] in 2014 suggested that there is no significant difference between women and men in the effect of exercise training on peak Vo_2.

The Exercise Training Regimen

Although the dose of exercise training described within the Smart and Marwick[2] review ranged widely for some parameters, in general, it is similar to that described in the 2014 Cochrane review,[17] identified as exercise session duration of 15 to 120 minutes, 1 to 7 sessions per week, at an exercise intensity of 40% to 80% of maximal heart rate or 50% to 85% of peak Vo_2, along with a Borg rating of 12 to 18, and carried out over a period of 15 to 120 weeks.

Although the focus here is to generally describe the impact of moderate-intensity exercise training on functional capacity, use of higher-intensity exercise training is increasing, not only in standard cardiac rehabilitation programs but within studies of patients with HF. The review by Smart and Marwick[2] suggests that this is not a new concept, in that the studies reported, and the ranges within the exercise intensity parameters, indicate some use of higher intensities, at least within the research environment (eg, 85%, 95%, and 80% peak Vo_2), maximal heart rate, and heart rate reserve, respectively. In the meta-analysis of the

Table 1
Meta-analyses of the impact of exercise training programming on functional capacity as measured by peak oxygen in patients with HFrPF and HFpPF

		Baseline		Exercise Training						
Study	Patients	Ejection Fraction (%)	Peak V_{O_2}[a] (mL/kg/min)	Session Duration (min)	Sessions per wk	Duration (wk)	Intensity (%max V_{O_2})	Intensity (%max HR)	Intensity HR Reserve (%)	Change in Peak V_{O_2} after Training (%)
Smart & Marwick,[2] 2004, 81 studies	N = 2387 59 ± 7 y 79% men	27 ± 7 (<40)	16.5 ± 6.9	43 ± 21.2 R: 15–120	3.9 ± 1.3 R: 1–7	17.1 ± 16.1 R: 1–104	60.6 ± 10.1 R: 40–85	71 ± 6.5 R: 45–95	66.7 ± 8.5 R: 40–80	Overall: ↑15.3 ± 8 R: 0–39 Aerobic: ↑17 Strength: ↑9 Combined: ↑15 Inspiratory training: 16
Taylor et al,[6] 2012, 5 studies	N = 228 57 y 59% men	≥45	Not reported	30–60	3	12–24	40–80	—	—	Compared with control, ExTr group had 3.0 mL/kg/min greater increase in peak V_{O_2}, $P<.0001$[b]

Abbreviations: ↑, increase; ExTr, exercise training; R, range.
[a] Reported in 57 studies.
[b] Reported in 4 studies.
Data from Refs.[2,6]

Table 2
Additional individuals trials of the impact of exercise training on functional capacity as measured by peak oxygen in patients with HFrEF

Study	Subjects	Baseline		Exercise Training				Change in Peak VO$_2$ After Training
		Ejection Fraction (%)	Peak VO$_2$ (mL/kg/min)	Session Duration (min)	Sessions per wk	Duration	Intensity	
Klocek et al,[11] 2005	100% men ET (C): n = 14, age 54 ± 7 y ET (P): n = 14, age 57 ± 8 y Con: n = 14, age 55 ± 9 y	ET (C): 33.6 ± 3.6 ET (P): 34.2 ± 4.2 Con: 33.2 ± 3.8	ET (C): 15.4 ET (P): 15.3 Con: 15.7	ET (Int): 25 ET (P): 25 C: no training	3	6 mo	ET (Int): 4 min interval/ 1 min recovery; 60% age pred maximum HR ET (P): increasing workload every 5 min (10–25 W) limited by exercise tolerance/75% age pred maximum HR	ET (Int): ↑7.1%, 16.5 mL/kg/min, P<.05 ET (P): ↑26.1%, 19.3 mL/kg/min, P<.01 Con: ↓9.6%, 14.2 mL/kg/min
Passino et al,[12] 2006	84.2% men ET: n = 44, age 60 ± 2 y Con: n = 41, age 61 ± 2 y	ET: 35.3 ± 1.6 Con: 32.3 ± 2.2	ET: 15.1 Con: 14.1	ET: 30 Con: usual care	3	9 mo	65% of peak VO$_2$ HR	ET: ↑13.2%, 17 ± 1 mL/kg/min P<.001 vs baseline and group Con: ↓7.1%, 13 ± 1 mL/kg/min
Mueller et al,[13] 2007	100% men, age <40 55 ± 10 y ET: n = 25 Con: n = 25	ET: Con:	ET: 20.7 ± 3.7 Con: 19.1 ± 3.5	ET: 30 min cycling and 45 cycling twice daily Con: usual care	5 d cycling 7 d walking	1 mo	60%–80% HRR and RPE of 12–14	ET: ↑18.8%, 24.5 ± 5.1 mL/kg/min P<.01 Con: ↑ 3.7%, 20.4 ± 3.6 mL/kg/min
O'Connor et al,[3] 2009	72% men ET: n = 1159 59.2 y Con: n = 1172, age 59.3 y	ET: 24.6 Con: 24.9	ET: 14.4 Con: 14.5	ET: 15–40 Con: usual care	3–5	Initial 36 supervised sessions followed by home-based training for up to 4 y, mean 30.1 mo	60%–70% HRR	ET: 3 mo ↑4.3%, P<.001 vs Con 12 mo ↑4.9%, P<.001 vs Con Con: 3 mo ↑1.4% 12 mo ↑.7%
Pina et al,[14] 2014	72% men Women: n = 661, age, 57 y Men: 1,670, age 60 y	Women: 25 Men: 25	Women: 13.4 Men: 14.9	30	3–5	Initial 36 supervised sessions	60%–70% HRR	ET women (n = 290) - ↑6.2%, 14.3 mL/kg/ min P = .42 vs men ET men (n = 682) ↑5.2%, 15.7 mL/kg/min

Abbreviations: ↑, increase; ↓, decrease; Con, control; ET, exercise training; HR, heart rate; HRR, heart rate reserve; Int, constant workload; interval group; P, progressive workload; pred, predicted; RPE, rating of perceived exertion.
Data from Refs.[3,11–14]

impact of aerobic interval training on exercise capacity in patients with HFrEF, Haykowsky and colleagues[7] in 2013 also found that vigorous aerobic interval exercise training (eg, short periods 80%–120% of peak power output or 90%–95% of peak heart rate followed by periods of reduced exercise intensity), was more effective in increasing peak Vo_2. Wisloff and colleagues[18] in 2007 also reported that exercise intensity was an important factor for reversing left ventricular (LV) remodeling as well as improving aerobic capacity, endothelial function, and QoL. In that study, the high-intensity arm of the exercise interval protocol was performed at 95% of peak heart rate. These findings are supported by the systematic review and meta-analysis of Ismail and colleagues[19] in 2013, which found that as exercise training intensity increased, the magnitude of improvement in functional capacity also increased. Conversely, data from HF-ACTION reported by Keteyian and colleagues[20] in 2012 suggested that a moderate level of exercise, 3 to 7 metabolic equivalent of task (MET) hours per week, is sufficient to provide clinical benefit.

Although not the focus here, beyond the impact on peak Vo_2 and the response of the body to submaximal exercise, several reviews and meta-analyses have also described the positive impact of exercise training on mortality and morbidity,[2] LV remodeling,[21] and in patients with reduced and preserved ejection fraction.[6,7,17] Within each of these analyses are provided identification of the impact of the exercise training program on functional capacity, including changes in peak Vo_2 and the methods of exercise prescription.

Exercise Training in Patients with Preserved Ejection Fraction

HF with HFpEF is a more recently recognized disorder than HFrEF, but the incidence of the diagnosis is rapidly increasing, and it is occurring more frequently in older patients, especially in women, with the primary symptom in patients with HFpEF being chronic exercise intolerance.[22] Consequently, and not surprisingly, interest in studying the role and use of exercise training in this patient group is also on the increase. The systematic review and meta-analysis of Taylor and colleagues[6] in 2012 provides evidence of the use of exercise training to enhance exercise capacity in patients with HFpEF (see **Table 1**). In patients with ejection fractions 45% or greater, findings indicated that exercise training was associated with a 3.0 mL/kg/min greater increase in exercise capacity compared with a control group (*P*<.0001), a finding similar to those studies of

exercise training in patients with HFrEF. Training parameters used within the studies of HFpEF were also similar to those described by described in Smart and Marwick[2] and the 2014 Cochrane analyses for HFrEF,[17] 30 to 60 minutes per session, 3 sessions per week over 12 to 24 weeks, and at an intensity of 40% to 80% of peak Vo_2.

Table 3 summarizes the findings of several trials in patients diagnosed with HFpEF.[5,8,23–25] Patients in these studies were older, the range of mean ages was approximately 63 to 70 years, and the range of mean ejection fractions was approximately 56% to 68%. The exercise training groups in all 5 studies of HFpEF reported improved peak Vo_2 after the intervention period, ranging from a low of 8%[25] to a high of 22.9%,[24] although the 8% improvement was not measured using a direct assessment of Vo_2. If these data are removed, the range in improvement is 11.3%[8] to 29.9%.[24] Thus, it seems that the expected magnitude of improvement in functional capacity after exercise training in patients with HFpEF may be similar to that achieved in patients with HFrEF, that is, an increase of 15.3%[2] for overall training programs and an increase of 17% for aerobic-only training programs (see **Table 1**).[2,17]

Adaptation to Exercise Training

The enhancements to skeletal muscle function and cardiovascular adaption, which occur as a result of aerobic exercise training, are significant to the increased ability of the patient with HF to increase the level of daily activity, and these findings have been shown in patients with both HFrEF and HFpEF. Improved arterial-venous oxygen difference is likely a major contributor to the improved postexercise exercise tolerance. The mechanisms for this improvement may include enhanced microcirculation of the skeletal muscle, which has undergone exercise training, such as increased capillaries/muscle fiber ratio, improved metabolic capacity of the muscle tissue resulting from increased size and number of mitochondria, as well as enzymatic changes.[26] The cardiovascular outcomes of these adaptations to exercise include decreased heart rate and systolic blood pressure at submaximal levels of exertion.

Resistance Training

Resistance training is a useful adjunct in attaining additional benefits from the overall exercise training program, particularly in increasing endurance and physical function and increasing the level of activities of daily living. In the Smart and Marwick 2004 study,[2] 21 of 81 (26%) reports identified the use of some form of resistance training, most

Table 3
Controlled group exercise intervention trials in patients with HFpEF

Study	Subjects	Baseline — Ejection Fraction (%)	Peak Vo2 (mL/kg/min)	Exercise Training — Mode	Session Duration (min)	Sessions per wk	Duration (wk)	Intensity (%)	Change in Vo2 After Training
Kitzman et al,[23] 2010	24% men ET: n = 26, age 70 y CG: n = 27, age 69 y	ET: 61% ± 5 CG: 60% ± 10	ET: 13.8 ± 2.5 CG: 12.8 ± 2.6	ET: walking, cycle CG: —	60	3	16	40–70 HRR	ET group: ↑16.7%, 16.1 mL/kg/min Control group: ↓2.3%, 12.5 ± 3.4 mL/kg/min P = .0001 between groups
Edelmann et al,[5] 2011	44% men ET: n = 44, age 64 ± 8 y CG: n = 20 age 65 ± 6 y	ET: 68% ± 7 CG: 67% ± 7	ET: 16.1 ± 4.9 CG: 16.7 ± 4.7	ET: cycle CG: RT	ET: 20–40 CG: 15 reps	ET: 2–3 CG: 2	ET: 12 CG: 5–12	ET: 50–70 HRR CG: 60–65 1RM	ET group: ↑16.1%, 18.7 mL/kg/min Control group: ↓4.2%, 16.0 mL/kg/min P = .001 between groups
Smart et al,[24] 2012	52% men ET: n = 12, age 67 ± 6 y CG: n = 13, age 62 ± 7 y	ET: 58.9 ± 11.9 CG: 56.7 ± 7.7	ET: 12.2 ± 3.6 CG: 14.0 ± 4.1	ET: cycle CG: usual activity	30	3	16	60–70 Vo2	ET group: ↑22.9%, 15.0 ± 4.9 mL/kg/min Control group: ↑5.7%, 14.8 ± 4.6 mL/kg/min P = .06 between groups
Alves et al,[25] 2012[a]	74% men M-SHF: n = 34, age 62.0 ± 9.9 y Mild HF: n = 33, age 63.6 ± 10.9 y HFpEF: 62.9 ± 10.2 y	M-SHF: 37.3 ± 7.9 Mild HF: 49.3 ± 1.9 HFpEF: 56.3 ± 2.5	ET group: M-SHF: 3.86 estMETs Mild HF: 4.34 estMETs HFpEF: 3.62 estMETs	ET: treadmill, cycle	INT: Progress to 7 5-min intervals with 1-min active recovery between intervals	3	6 mo	70–75 maximum HR with 45–55 during recovery intervals	ET group: M-SHF: ↑12.4%, 4.34 estMETs P<.001 Mild HF: ↑15.9%, 5.03 estMETs P<.001 HFpEF: ↑8.0%, 3.91 estMETs P<.046 Control group: No significant change from baseline in any of the 3 control groups
Kitzman et al,[8] 2013	24% men ET: n = 32, age 70 ± 7 y CG: n = 27, age 70 ± 7 y	ET: 58 ± 6 CG: 56 ± 5	ET: 14.2 ± 2.2 CG: 14.0 ± 3.2	ET: walking, cycle CG: —	60	3	16	40–70 HRR	ET group: ↑11.3%, 15.8 mL/kg/min Control group: ↓1.4%, 13.8 mL/kg/min P = .0001 between groups

Abbreviations: ↑, increase; ↓, decrease; 1RM, 1 repetition maximum; CG, control group; estMETs, metabolic equivalents estimated from symptoms-limited treadmill testing using guidelines from the American College of Sports Medicine; ET, exercise training; HRR, heart rate reserve; INT, interval training; M-SHF, moderate to severe HF; RT, resistance training.

[a] Functional capacity was measured by using American College of Sports Medicine equations for estimating METs metabolic equivalents for various treadmill workloads.

Data from Refs.5,8,23–25

often included along with aerobic training. In data reported within the Cochrane analysis of 2014,[17] findings indicated a similar but slightly greater percentage of studies published since 2004, identifying the use of resistance training within the exercise regimen as 31% (8 of 22 programs). However, as mentioned earlier, resistance training was primarily used in addition to aerobic training.

Table 4 identifies 4 reports, 2 of which are from the same study population, in which resistance training was the primary exercise training modality used in patients with HF.[27–30] Patients in these trials were generally older, mean age ranging from 56 to 74 years, primarily men, and primarily consisting of patients with HFrEF, although Savage and colleagues[30] did include 3 patients with HFpEF, with ejection fractions of greater than 40%, mean 50 ± 3% (HFpEF). Mean peak V_{O_2} ranged from 14.4 to 15.3 mL/kg/min across the trials. The resistance training programs were similar, with 1 program, Selig and colleagues',[27] using a gradually increasing intensity approach to resistance intensity, whereas Levinger and colleagues[28,29] and Savage and colleagues[30] using percentages of 1 repetition maximum (RM) (ranging from 40% to 80%), repetitions ranging from 10 to 20, and 1 to 3 sets. All studies used a 3 day per week training regimen. Each study reported a significant improvement in strength, with no episodes of untoward events.

Selig and colleagues[27] reported an improvement of 10.5% in peak V_{O_2} to 16.9 ± 3.8 mL/kg/min from 15.3 ± 3.7 mL/kg/min, whereas the control group decreased by 10.8%. Forearm blood flow and heart rate variability were also improved. Along with increases in strength, Levinger and colleagues[28,29] reported improved QoL, measured by the Living with Heart Failure Questionnaire. Savage and colleagues[30] reported a 7% increase in peak V_{O_2}; however, there was no associated training effect on the self-reported physical function and QoL questionnaire Medical Outcomes Study Short-Form (SF). Findings from these trials suggest that resistance training is a viable and effective component of the overall exercise training program, to be used separately or in conjunction with the aerobic portion of the program.

Exercise Programming

The following sections address specific components of association with moderate-intensity exercise for both aerobic and resistance training for patients with HF. This section is based on experiences of those investigations described earlier in the article as well as from guidelines from both the American College of Sports Medicine and the American Heart Association. The components are intended to provide guidance in developing an exercise program for patients with HFrEF or HFpEF.

Aerobic exercise

The components of traditional, moderate-intensity, aerobic exercise training programs include descriptions of exercise intensity, duration of a session, frequency of sessions per week, and exercise modality(s) (see **Table 1**).[31]

Exercise intensity Exercise intensity, or the level of a patient's effort during activity, can be expressed using a variety of parameters, commonly involving a percentage of peak levels of heart rate (60%–85%) or heart rate reserve (50%–80%), or peak V_{O_2} (50%–80%), but may include other measures, such as rating of perceived exertion (11–14 on the 6–20 scale[20]). In addition, as mentioned earlier, Keteyian and colleagues[20] showed that the volume of exercise undertaken by participants with HF was associated with reduced risk for clinical events and moderate levels (3–7 MET hours per week) of exercise was needed to observe a clinical benefit.

Exercise duration Exercise duration is generally used to describe the total number of minutes of exercise, which might comprise either continuous or intermittent work, generally 20 to 40 minutes in total. However, with intermittent exercise (ie, brief, higher-intensity exercise immediately followed by a period of lower-intensity effort or rest), the duration of the various exercise/rest intervals is also described. As an example, a higher-intensity exercise interval of 3 to 4 minutes followed by 3 to 4 minutes of low intensity exercise could be used. Thus, the duration designation may also be identified along with the intensity with this approach.

Exercise frequency Exercise frequency generally refers to number of exercise days per week, generally 3 to 5 sessions per week.

Exercise modality (mode) Exercise modality describes the various pieces of exercise equipment that may be used, such as treadmill or cycle ergometers.

Resistance exercise

The components of a resistance training program should include an initial consideration of the various potential types of resistance training equipment available to patients, be preceded by an assessment of baseline strength levels and training technique, and the development of an individualized routine of resistance-type training protocol, including education and demonstration.[32] Many

Table 4
Studies using primarily resistance training as the mode of exercise for patients with HF

Study	Baseline			Training Program	
	Subjects	Ejection Fraction (%)	Peak Vo$_2$ (mL/kg/min)	Training Program	Results (Vo$_2$ and Muscle Strength)
Selig et al,[27] 2004	86% men Ex: n = 19, age 65 ± 13 Con: n = 20, age 64 ± 9	Ex: 27 ± 7 Con: 28 ± 6	Ex: 15.3 ± 3.7 Con: 17.0 ± 4.5	Ex: 3 sessions/wk for 3 mo Alternating upper and lower body exercises: leg cycle, arm cycle, and multistation hydraulic RT system: Knee: flex and exten, Elbow: flex and exten, and shoulder press Con: usual care	Ex: peak Vo$_2$ ↑10.5%, 16.9 ± 3.8 mL/kg/min $P<.01$ Sig ↑ knee flex and elbow/knee flex Con: peak Vo$_2$ ↓10.8%, 14.9 ± 4.0 mL/kg/min $P<.01$ between groups No significant change in any strength exercise
Levinger et al,[28] 2005 Levinger et al,[29] 2005	100% men Ex: n = 8, age 57.3 ± 11.1 Con: n = 7, age 56.7 ± 10.0	Ex: 35.4 ± 6.3 Con: 34.0 ± 8.8	Ex: 14.4 ± 2.8 Con: 14.9 ± 1.8	Ex: 3 sessions/wk, 2 d between sessions, for 8 wk 9 exercises of major muscle groups, 40%–60% of maximal strength, 15–20 reps, 1–3 sets Con: nontraining	Ex: total weight lifted (kg): ↑21.3% Pre-ex: 394.4 ± 100.6 kg; post-ex: 478.4 ± 98.2 kg $P<.001$ Con: ↓1.7% Pre-ex: 353.5 ± 123.6 kg; post-ex: 347 ± 124.7 P = not significant
Savage et al,[30] 2011	61.9% men Ex: n = 10, age 73.4 ± 2.4 Con: healthy volunteers: n = 11, age 72.1 ± 2.1	Ex: n = 7, 32 ± 2% (HFrEF); n = 3, >40%, 50 ± 3% (HFpEF) Con: 62.3 ± 1.2	Ex: 14.6 ± 1.4 Con: 23.4 ± 1.3	Ex: 3 sessions/wk, 2 d between sessions, for 8 wk 7 exercises of major muscle groups, 50%–80% of 1RM assessed every 2 wk, 8–10 reps, 1–3 sets	Ex: total weight lifted (kg): ↑34.3% Pre-ex: 248 ± 46 kg; post-ex: 333 ± 58 kg, $P<.001$; Peak Vo$_2$ ↑7% Con: pre-ex: 272 ± 35 kg; post-ex: 362 ± 40, $P<.001$ Peak Vo$_2$ ↑.9%, 23.6 ± 1.0 mL/kg/min

Abbreviations: ↑, increase; ↓, decrease; 1RM, one repetition maximum; Con, control; Ex, exercise; exten, extension; flex, flexion; HFpEF, heart failure with preserved ejection fraction; HFrEF, heart failure with reduced ejection fraction; reps, repetitions; RT, resistance training; Sig, significant.
Data from Refs.[27–30]

patients may have limited or no experience with resistance-type training.

Modality/education/technique For each type of resistance exercise modality (eg, weight machines, free weights, bands, and other equipment), a session of education regarding use and safety should be provided. The techniques of resistance training should include an evaluation of technique. Resistance training should be performed: (1) in a rhythmic manner at a moderate to slow controlled speed; (2) through a full range of motion; and (3) avoiding breath-holding and straining (Valsalva maneuver) by exhaling during the contraction or exertion phase of the exercise (eg, the push, pull, raise, lower), and inhaling during the relaxation phase.

Assessment of baseline strength levels Baseline strength is frequently described using a measurement of RM, which is quantified as the most weight (resistance) that can be lifted, pushed, pulled, and so forth, a single time (1 RM). From this, a percentage of the 1 RM (40%–70%) is used as the initial resistance level for training. In stable HF, typically patients begin at the lower end of this intensity range.

Development of the training protocol The initial resistance or weight load for each exercise should: (1) allow for and be limited to 8 to 12 repetitions at a low level of resistance, for example, 40% of 1 RM; (2) be limited to a single set performed 2 d/wk, increasing to 2 sets as appropriate; (3) involve the major muscle groups of the upper and lower extremities (eg, chest press, shoulder press, triceps extension, biceps curl, pull-down [upper back], lower-back extension, abdominal crunch/curl-up, quadriceps extension or leg press, leg curls [hamstrings], and calf raise); and (4) alternate between upper body and lower body work to allow for adequate rest between exercises, 2 upper body and 2 lower body initially, adding exercise as appropriate.

Summary

Exercise training, both aerobic and resistance, is used in patients with stable HF, and various research protocols suggest its efficacy in both patients with HFrEF as well as those with HFpEF. Aerobic training positively affects peak V_{O_2} and exercise capacity in both groups of patients, leading to improved responses to daily activity, including reduce myocardial work and perceived effort. Thus, daily activities are performed with less dyspnea and fatigue. Although training protocols vary, most HF trials use moderate-intensity

exercise, which has been shown to be safe and effective in these patient groups.

Quality of Life in Exercise Training Trials for Heart Failure

Health-related QoL (HRQoL) gains from exercise training trials in patients with HF have generally been positive; however, there is a great deal of variability in the magnitude of these gains, and in some instances, there has been no effect on HRQoL. In most clinical trials, HRQoL has been evaluated as a secondary end point, so the clinical trials may not be appropriately powered to detect statistically significant differences. The Minnesota Living with Heart Failure Questionnaire (MLwHF) and the Kansas City Cardiomyopathy Questionnaire (KCCQ) have been the 2 most commonly used measures to assess HRQoL. These disease-specific measures have well-documented reliability and validity, and each has a 5-point magnitude of change for clinical meaningfulness. A few studies have used generic QoL measures (eg, Medical Outcomes Study SF-36, EuroQol 5D, and Patient Health Questionnaire 9), which have less documentation of reliability and validity in HF. As mentioned in the exercise training section, training programs vary widely (ie, setting, type of training, frequency, duration, and intensity), and these differences may be a contributing factor to variability in HRQoL results. The following sections of this review summarize the magnitude of effect on HRQoL from moderate-intensity aerobic exercise training trials in patients with both HFrEF and HFpEF. Consideration is given to sustained effects on QoL in exercise trials with follow-up of 12 months or greater.

The 2014 Cochrane review of exercise-based rehabilitation for heart failure by Taylor and colleagues[17] provides an update from the systematic Cochrane review published in 2010.[33] The 2014 review included randomized clinical trials with a parallel group or cross-over design and at least 6 month follow-up or longer. It resulted in a meta-analysis of 33 trials, and of these trials, 19 reported QoL outcomes. The MLwHF questionnaire was the most common measure used and resulted in a significant improvement with exercise (random effects mean difference, −5.8; 95% confidence interval [CI], −9.2 to −2.4; $P = .0007$).[17] A significant improvement in HRQoL was also seen when pooled across all studies regardless of the measure that was used (random effects model standardized mean difference [SMD], −0.46; 95% CI, −0.66 to −0.26; $P<.0001$). Examination of individual studies in the 2014 Cochrane review shows that 11 of the 19 trials had superior HRQoL in the exercise trained group compared with control (**Table 5**).[4,12,34–42]

Table 5
Exercise training and HRQoL in patients with HFrEF

Author, Year	Exercise Training Intervention		QoL		
			Exercise Training	Control	Between Group
			Mean (CI) or Mean ± Standard Deviation	Mean (CI) or Mean ± Standard Deviation	P value
Austin et al,[34] 2005	Supervised facility based (cardiac rehab) Aerobic only 8 wk–2 times per week for 2.5 h 16 wk–1 time per week for 1 h Exercise (n = 85) Attention Control (n = 94)	**MLwHF** *Total* Baseline	41.0 (36.0–46.0)	44.3 (39.5–49.1)	Within group testing only; no between group testing
		8 wk	25.8 (22.3–29.4) **Base to 8 wk P<.001**	38.8 (33.8–43.8) **Base to 8 wk P<.05**	
		24 wk	22.9 (19.5–26.4) **Base to 24 wk P<.01**	36.9 (32.2–41.6) **Base to 24 wk P<.05**	
		5 y	35.5 ± 21.7 **Base to 5 y P = .28**	37.1 ± 24.9 **Base to 5 y P = .15**	
Austin et al,[51] 2008		*Emotional* Baseline	8.6 (7.1–10.1)	9.9 (8.3–11.5)	
		8 wk	5.7 (4.6–6.8) **Base to 8 wk P<.001**	9.1 (7.6–10.6) **Base to 8 wk NS**	
		24 wk	4.4 (3.4–5.3) **Base to 24 wk P<.01**	8.0 (6.6–9.4) **Base to 24 wk P<.05**	
		5 y	7.4 ± 6.5 **Base to 5 y P = .26**	7.6 ± 7.1 **Base to 5 y P = .17**	
		Physical Baseline	21.5 (19.1–23.9)	24.2 (21.8–26.6)	
		8 wk	13.7 (11.8–15.6) **Base to 8 wk P<.001**	20.4 (17.9–23.0) **Base to 8 wk P<.01**	
		24 wk	12.6 (10.7–14.5) **Base to 24 wk P<.001** **8–24 wk P<.01**	20.4 (17.8–23.0) **8–24 wk P<.01**	
		5 y	18.3 ± 11.2 **Base to 5 y P = .26**	19.3 ± 12.5 **Base to 5 y P = .02**	
		EuroQol Baseline	0.67 (0.62–0.72)	0.65 (0.61–0.70)	
		24 wk	0.78 (0.75–0.81) **Base to 24 wk P<.001**	0.65 (0.59–0.71) **Base to 24 wk NS**	
		5 y	0.61 ± 0.32 **Base to 5 y P = .02**	0.60 ± 0.34 **Base to 5 y P = .25**	

Study	Intervention	Outcome	Timepoint	Exercise	Control	Significance
Belardinelli et al,[35] 1999	Supervised facility based (aerobic only) 8 wk – 3 times per week, 60% peak Vo₂ 12 mo – 2 times per week Exercise (n = 50) and control (n = 49)	MLwHF *Total*	Baseline	52 ± 22	50 ± 21	P<.001
			2 mo	40 ± 19	51 ± 22	
			14 mo	39 ± 20	52 ± 20	
			26 mo	44 ± 21	54 ± 22	
Belardinelli et al,[52] 2012	Exercise (n = 63) and control (n = 60) 10 y–2 times per week	MLwHF	10 y	43 ± 12	58 ± 14	P<.05
Bocalini et al,[41] 2008	Supervised facility based aerobic and resistance 6 mo, 90-min sessions (20–40 min aerobic), 3 times per wk, 50% maximum HR Exercise (n = 22) and control (n = 20)	**WHOQoL** Physical		23 ± 4% improvement	2 ± 1% improvement	Between group
		Psychological		20 ± 2% improvement	1 ± 1% improvement	differences for all
		Social		16 ± 1% improvement	3 ± 2% improvement	subscales
		Environmental		15 ± 2% improvement	2 ± 1% improvement	P<.001
Zwisler et al,[45] 2008 (DANREHAB)	Supervised cardiac rehab 6 wk of counseling, education and 12 aerobic exercise sessions (twice weekly) Follow-up at 12 mo Exercise (n = 380) and control (n = 390)	**SF-36** *Physical Component*	Baseline	41 ± 10	42 ± 10	NS
			12 mo	46 ± 10	45 ± 10	
		Mental Component	Baseline	44 ± 12	46 ± 12	NS
			12 mo	48 ± 12.3	50 ± 11	
Davidson et al,[36] 2010	Supervised cardiac rehab (aerobic and resistance) 12 wk of counseling, education and individualized exercise sessions Follow-up at 3 and 12 mo Exercise (n = 53) and attention control (n = 52)	MLwHF *Total*	Baseline	44.11 ± 23.70	52.37 ± 26.38	Significance of intervention group as predictor
			3 mo	27.92 ± 12.46	36.89 ± 16.22	P = .01
			12 mo	52.90 ± 15.68	56.43 ± 18.28	P = .37

(continued on next page)

Table 5
(Continued)

Author, Year	Exercise Training Intervention		QoL		
			Exercise Training	Control	
			Mean (CI) or Mean ± Standard Deviation	Mean (CI) or Mean ± Standard Deviation	Between Group *P* value
Dracup et al,[43] 2007	Home-based walking Aerobic and resistance 10–45 min sessions, 40%–60% maximum HR; 4 times weekly for walking, 3 times weekly resistance Follow-up at 3 and 6 mo Exercise (n = 86) Attention control (n = 87)	**MlwHF** *Total* Baseline 3 mo 6 mo *Mental* Baseline 3 mo 6 mo *Physical* Baseline 3 mo 6 mo			Group x time effects
		Baseline	46.7 ± 23.8	49.2 ± 22.4	*P* = .819
		3 mo	37.5 ± 23.9	46.7 ± 26.5	*P* = .819
		6 mo	35.7 ± 23.7	43.2 ± 27.3	*P* = .819
		Baseline	10.3 ± 7.1	12.0 ± 6.9	*P* = .670
		3 mo	9.0 ± 6.8	10.9 ± 8.4	*P* = .670
		6 mo	7.8 ± 6.6	10.5 ± 7.4	*P* = .670
		Baseline	19.7 ± 10.1	20.5 ± 10.8	*P* = .592
		3 mo	15.7 ± 10.0	21.1 ± 11.5	*P* = .592
		6 mo	16.1 ± 10.0	19.4 ± 11.3	*P* = .592
Gary et al,[44] 2010	Home-based exercise Aerobic and resistance 3 walking sessions per wk; 5 min progressing to 60 min duration 12 weekly home visits for supervision Follow-up at 3 and 6 mo Exercise (n = 20) and control (n = 17)	**MlwHF** *Total* Baseline 12 wk 24 wk			
		Baseline	32.4 ± 22.4	28.1 ± 17.3	NS
		12 wk	29.2 ± 18.1	26.4 ± 23.7	NS
		24 wk	25.6 ± 19.7	28.9 ± 29.9	NS

Study	Intervention	Measure	Exercise	Control	P value
Flynn et al,[4] 2009 (HF-ACTION)	Supervised facility based for 12 wk – 3 times weekly; 60%–70% HRR Home based 5 d per week for up to 4 y Aerobic only Exercise (n = 1159) Control (n = 1172)	**KCCQ** *BL to 3 mo*			
		Overall summary	5.21 (4.42–6.00)	3.28 (2.48–4.09)	P<.001
		Physical limitations	3.55 (2.62–4.48)	1.25 (0.30–2.20)	P<.001
		Social limitations	6.28 (5.13–7.44)	4.50 (3.32–5.67)	P = .02
		Symptoms	3.58 (2.74–4.42)	2.06 (1.21–2.92)	P = .008
		QoL	7.36 (6.35–8.38)	5.73 (4.7–6.77)	P = .02
		3 mo to end			
		Overall summary	0.00 (−0.04 to 0.03)	−0.01 (−0.05 to 0.03)	P = .85
		Physical limitations	−0.05 (−0.10 to −0.01)	−0.06 (−0.10 to −0.02)	P = .84
		Social limitations	0.02 (−0.03 to 0.07)	−0.04 (−0.09 to 0.01)	P = .12
		Symptoms	−0.03 (−0.07 to 0.01)	−0.03 (−0.07 to 0.01)	P = .91
		QoL	0.09 (0.05–0.14)	0.08 (0.03–0.12)	P = .61
Jolly et al,[37] 2009	3 Supervised sessions; 70% peak Vo_2 Home-based walking for 20–30 min 5 d per week Aerobic and resistance Exercise (n = 85) Attention control (n = 85)	**MLwHF** *Total*			
		Base to 6 mo	36.26 ± 24.08	34.49 ± 23.98	P = .30
		Base to 12 mo	37.61 ± 20.97	34.91 ± 24.80	P = .80
		EQ-5D			
		Base to 6 mo	0.663 ± 0.242	0.617 ± 0.319	P = .004
		Base to 12 mo	0.679 ± 0.21	0.691 ± 0.28	P = .07
Jonsdottir et al,[47] 2006	Supervised facility based Aerobic and resistance plus education Twice weekly for 15 min aerobic (starting at 50% peak Vo_2 and progressing) 20 min resistance Exercise (n = 21) and control (n = 22)	**Icelandic QoL**			
		Before	44.50 (10.5)	42.50 (13.7)	NS
		After	47.55 (8.7)	44.10 (14.04)	NS

(continued on next page)

Table 5
(Continued)

Author, Year	Exercise Training Intervention	QoL				
			Exercise Training Mean (CI) or Mean ± Standard Deviation		Control Mean (CI) or Mean ± Standard Deviation	Between Group P value
			Constant workload	Progressive workload		
Klocek et al,[11] 2005	Supervised facility based Aerobic only Constant workload – 25 min; 60% maximum HR; 3 times weekly for 6 mo Progressive workload: 25 min; started at RPM 60 kpm/min for 5 min; every 5 min increased 25 W Constant workload exercise (n = 14) Progressive workload exercise (n = 14) Control (n = 14)	Psychological General Well-being Baseline 6 mo	68.3 99.0	72.6 109.0	63.5 71.7	P<.01 P<.01
Koukouvou et al,[38] 2004	Supervised facility based Aerobic and resistance plus education 60 min sessions; 3–4 times weekly; 50%–70% peak Vo₂ Exercise (n = 16) Control (n = 10)	MLwHF	Base to 6 mo P<.05		Base to 6 mo	Within group testing only; no between group testing
			45.5 (17.1) 34.1 (13.0)		45.1 (9.9) - NS 45.2 (9.0)	
		QLI - Spitzer Index Baseline 6 mo	Base to 6 mo P<.05 7.8 (1.1) 9.1 (1.1)		Base to 6 mo 7.1 (1.0) - NS 7.1 (1.1)	
		LSI - Scale of Life Satisfaction Baseline 6 mo	Base to 6 mo P<.05 50.1 (3.9) 55.0 (3.4)		Base to 6 mo 49.0 (3.1) - NS 48.7 (2.8)	
McKelvie et al,[48] 2002	3 mo supervised facility based 9 mo home based Aerobic and resistance plus education 30 min sessions; 3 times weekly; 60%–70% maximum HR Exercise (n = 90) and control (n = 91)	MLwHF Total Change at 3 mo Change at 12 mo	−3.9 ± 1.9 −3.4 ± 2.4		−1.2 ± 1.5 −3.3 ± 1.7	P = .28 P = .98
Nilsson et al,[39] 2008	Group-based aerobic dancing and counseling 2 d per week for 4 mo 50 min sessions Exercise (n = 40) and control (n = 40)	MLwHF Total Baseline 4 mo 12 mo	33 ± 18 22 ± 12 23 ± 14		22 ± 17 23 ± 20 28 ± 20	Baseline to 12 mo P = .003

Study	Intervention	Measure / Timepoint			P value
Norman et al,[42] 2012	Supervised facility based Aerobic and resistance plus education (12 wk) Aerobic sessions 30 min; 3X (40%–70% HRR) Resistance 2 d per week Exercise (n = 22) and attention control (n = 20)	**KCCQ Overall Summary** Baseline 3 mo 6 mo	69.7 ± 20.2 78.1 ± 18.1 81.0 ± 18.2	72.8 ± 15.6 76.0 ± 17.0 77.9 ± 11.6	Time effect P<.01 Group x time effect P = .20
Passino et al,[12] 2006	Supervised facility based Aerobic only 9-mo training; 3 per week; 65% peak Vo₂ Exercise (n = 44) and control (n = 41)	**MLwHF** *Total* Baseline 9 mo	54 ± 5 32 ± 4 Base to 9 mo P<.01	52 ± 6 53 ± 5 NS	
Willenheimer et al,[58] 2001	Supervised facility based Aerobic only (group based) 4-mo training; 15 min 2 times per week increased to 45 min 3 times per week; 80% peak Vo₂ Exercise (n=17) and control (n=20)	**Patient Global Assessment of Change in QoL** Baseline 4 mo 10 mo	0 ± 0 1.3 ± 1.3 0.7 ± 0.9	0 ± 0 0.4 ± 1.4 0.0 ± 1.0	P = .064 P = .023
Witham et al,[49] 2005	Supervised facility based for 3 mo; twice weekly; group-based exercise Home based for 3 mo; 2–3 times weekly with video Aerobic and resistance Exercise (n = 41) and control (n = 41)	**Guyatt Chronic Heart Failure Questionnaire** Baseline 3 mo 6 mo	67 ± 13 68 ± 11 65 ± 10	70 ± 12 69 ± 12 69 ± 13	P = .11 P = .48
Yeh et al,[40] 2011	Supervised group based Tai chi; 1 h session; 2× for 12 wk plus encouraged to do at home 3× with video Exercise (n = 41) + attention control (n = 41)	**MLwHF** *Total* **Median (Q1, Q3)** Baseline 12 wk	28 (12, 47) 9 (2, 25)	21 (11, 52) 22 (4, 43)	P = .07 adjusted for Baseline P = .02

Abbreviations: BL, baseline; HR, heart rate; KCCQ, Kansas City Cardiomyopathy Questionnaire; MLwHF, Minnesota Living with Heart Failure; NS, not significant; QoL, quality of life; QLI, Quality of Life Index; rehab, rehabilitation; SF-36, Short Form 36 Health Survey; WHOQOL, World Health Organization Quality of Life.
Data from Refs. [4,11,12,34–45,47–51,58]

Table 6
Exercise training and HRQoL in patients with HFpEF

Author, Year	Exercise Training Intervention		QoL Exercise Training (Mean ± Standard Deviation)		Control (Mean ± Standard Deviation)		Between Group P value
Gary,[53] 2006	Control (n = 16) and exercise (n = 16) 12 wk walking program, 3 times weekly 100% women	**MLwHF** Total	Baseline 41.90 ± 24.1	12 wk 24.10 ± 18.0	Baseline 24.2 ± 18.2	12 wk 27.85 ± 21.9	P = .002
Gary et al,[55] 2004	Same study as Gary (2006); additional time point of 24 wk		24 wk 19 ± 18		24 wk 32 ± 27		P = .014
Kitzman et al,[23] 2010	Supervised facility based Endurance only 48 sessions over 16 wk (3 times per week) Exercise (n = 26) Attention control (n = 27) Older, mean age 70 ± 6 y 87% women	**MLwHF**	Baseline	16 wk	Baseline	16 wk	
		Emotional	5 ± 4	3 ± 5	3 ± 5	4 ± 5	P = .35
		Physical	16 ± 10	11 ± 11	12 ± 11	12 ± 9	P = .03
		Total	32 ± 20	25 ± 24	25 ± 22	27 ± 19	P = .11
		SF-36					
		Physical	50 ± 20	54 ± 19	48 ± 23	46 ± 21	P = .53
		General health	42 ± 16	41 ± 14	46 ± 17	51 ± 14	P = .47
		Social role	40 ± 14	41 ± 13	44 ± 14	43 ± 14	P = .74
		Role: Physical	35 ± 34	52 ± 35	38 ± 34	47 ± 35	P = .30
		Role: Emotional	60 ± 38	67 ± 40	55 ± 39	63 ± 42	P = .95
		Pain	46 ± 18	51 ± 19	40 ± 19	42 ± 21	P = .50
		Mental	58 ± 10	57 ± 10	55 ± 12	53 ± 10	P = .76
		Vitality	42 ± 12	48 ± 12	45 ± 14	40 ± 13	P = .20
Edelmann et al,[5] 2011	32 sessions (endurance and resistance) Weeks 1–4 (2×) and weeks 5–12 (3×) Exercise (n = 46) and control (n = 21) 56% women	**MLwHF** Total	Mean Change −8 (−12 to −4)		Mean Change −2 (−6 to 1)		P = .07
		SF-36 Physical functioning	14 (8–19)		−4 (−11 to 4)		P = .001

Study	Measure	Mean Change	Mean Change	P
Nolte,[56] 2014	**MLwHF**			
Same study as Edelmann (2011): additional subscales reported. Both studies are supervised facility based	Physical limitation	−5 (−7 to −3)	−2 (−4 to 0)	P = .04
	Emotional limitation	−1 (−2 to 1)	−1 (−2 to 0)	P = .566
	Total	−8 (−12 to 4)	−2 (−6 to 1)	P = .07
	SF-36			
	Physical functioning	14 (8–19)	−4 (−11 to 4)	P = .001
	Physical problems	10 (−3 to 23)	−7 (−18 to 5)	P = .219
	Bodily pain	8 (0–16)	0 (−7 to 7)	P = .178
	General health perception	12 (8–17)	3 (0–7)	P = .016
	Vitality	9 (3–15)	3 (−2 to 9)	P = .242
	Social functioning	13 (6–19)	8 (−4 to 19)	P = .852
	Emotional problems	6 (−4 to 16)	0 (−5 to 5)	P = .997
	General mental health	7 (3–11)	1 (−5 to 7)	P = .203
	Physical component	5 (3–7)	−1 (−3 to 1)	P = .001
	Mental component	3 (0–5)	3 (0–5)	P = .462
Smart et al,[24] 2012	**MLwHF**			
16 wk program. 30 patients with HFpEF. Mean age 64 ± 8 y. 48% women	Total	34.5 ± 22.9	31.7 ± 28.2	P = .79
	Physical	12.5 ± 9.7	15.1 ± 15.2	P = .62
	Emotion	8.1 ± 6.7	5.6 ± 6.8	P = .37

Study	Measure	Baseline	16 wk	Baseline	16 wk	P
Kitzman et al,[8] 2013	**MLwHF**					
Supervised facility based. Endurance only. 16 wk – 3 times weekly. Older, mean age 70 ± 7 y. n = 46 women (76%). Exercise (n = 32). Attention control (n = 31)	Emotional	6 ± 5	5 ± 4	4 ± 5	3 ± 4	P = .19
	Physical	17 ± 8	12 ± 8	13 ± 11	11 ± 10	P = .50
	Total	36 ± 19	26 ± 19	28 ± 23	25 ± 22	P = .50
	SF-36					
	Physical component	48 ± 18	63 ± 20	50 ± 25	53 ± 27	P = .03
	Emotional component	63 ± 30	83 ± 31	66 ± 37	62 ± 35	P = .04

Data from Refs.[5,8,23,24,53,55,56]

None of the studies resulted in lower HRQoL scores for exercise compared with control.

Examination of the trials that were negative for HRQoL[43–49] shed light on potential reasons for the lack of effect (see **Table 5**). Two of the nonsignificant trials[45,47] used a generic HRQoL measure, which may not be as sensitive or responsive as the disease-specific measures (ie, MLwHF and KCCQ). The training programs and dose of exercise may have been an influencing factor in the remaining negative trials. Two were home-based walking programs[43,44] and one was supervised, facility based for 3 months, but the frequency was only twice weekly.[49] The final negative trial was a 3-month program in a supervised facility with 30-minute, 3 times per week sessions, at 60% to 70% maximum heart rate.[48] Although this specific training program does not meet the volume of exercise (150 minutes) recommended in the Heart Failure Society of America 2010 Comprehensive Heart Failure Practice Guideline,[50] it has produced positive responses in HRQoL in other trials.

Several exercise trials have now been conducted that report HRQoL effects at 12 months or greater follow-up.[4,35–37,39,51,52] This literature allows for examination of whether the improvements in HRQoL are sustained over time as a result of exercise. Six of these 7 trials[4,35,37,39,51,52] showed sustained positive effects, which are clinically meaningful differences for the respective measures. One trial showed significant change at 3 months, which was nonsignificant at 12 months.[36] Trials that report the sustained effect were designed with specific plans and instructions for continued exercise over the follow-up period. In addition, 3 of these trials showing sustained effect were group-based exercise,[39] club-based program,[52] or facility based,[35] in which the effects of social support on HRQoL must be considered. The Davidson and colleagues[36] (2010) trial, with the lack of a sustained effect, was a cardiac rehabilitation program over the first 3 months and maintenance program over the remaining 9 months. The number of patients who continued to exercise in the maintenance program after completion of the cardiac rehabilitation program was not identified.

Most exercise training studies have been in patients with HFrEF, and few have reported findings from trials involving patients with HFpEF. The Taylor and colleagues[6] 2012 meta-analysis of training effects in patients with HFpEF on HRQoL included 4 studies[5,23,24,53] and resulted in higher HRQoL in exercise compared with control (fixed effects mean difference, −7.3 points; 95% CI, −11.4 to −3.3; P<.0001).[6] A recent randomized trial by Kitzman and colleagues[8] (2013), which was not included in this meta-analysis, is presented in **Table 6** and summarizes the findings for HFpEF. Two additional studies were found that included patients with either HFrEF or HFpEF,[36,44] but no separate analysis was performed. Smart and colleagues[54] (2007) reported a subgroup analysis to compare HRQoL between HFpEF and HFrEF exercise trained patients (no comparison with control is reported, so this study is not included in **Table 6**). This analysis showed consistently higher HRQoL in the patients with HFpEF compared with HFrEF at baseline (P<.001) and a significant difference between the groups in HRQoL at 16 weeks (P = .006).[54] The within-group analysis for the HFpEF trained patients showed a nonsignificant effect (P = .07).[54]

Studies in HFpEF comparing exercise training with control are short duration, between 12 and 16 weeks, with the longest follow-up being 24 weeks. Small sample sizes (n = 32–67) result in inadequately powered studies to detect change in HRQoL. The gender distribution in HFpEF studies shows a predominance of women, which contrasts with HFrEF studies, with most men in the sample. The MLwHF questionnaire and the SF-36 are the 2 measures that have been used to assess HRQoL in HFpEF studies. The total MLwHF scores from the Gary 2006[55] study show significant and clinically meaningful improvement of greater than 17 points in the exercise trained group compared with control, and this effect is sustained at 24 weeks. The remaining 4 studies are nonsignificant for between-group change in MLwHF total score.[5,8,23,24] However, when the subscale scores are reported, there is a significant effect for the physical subscale but not the emotional subscale.[8,23,56] The same findings occur for the SF-36, with the physical component score significant but not the emotional component.[8,56]

SUMMARY

Exercise training studies in HFrEF show some inconsistency but overall indicate a positive effect on HRQoL. The HFrEF trials include larger sample sizes, with reportedly less bias and longer follow-up.[17] Findings in HFpEF are limited but do suggest positive effect, although samples sizes are small, and there have been no adequately powered trials to detect effects on HRQoL as a primary or even secondary end point. Findings from Smart and colleagues[54] in 2007 suggest that baseline HRQoL scores may be higher in HFpEF compared with HFrEF. Trials in HFpEF include more women and older patients, so effects by gender and age may be important to consider. The HF-ACTION trial (including only patients with HFrEF)[4] is the only exercise trial with reported subgroup interaction tests for HRQoL, and there were no significant subgroup interactions for age ($P = .44$) or gender ($P = .26$).[4] Across all studies of exercise in HF, there is wide variation in training programs (ie, type of training, setting, frequency, duration, and intensity), which could have a direct effect or serve as a mediator on perceived HRQoL.

This review does not include results from newer training strategies, such as high-intensity interval training, which may also uniquely affect HRQoL, resulting in a differing dose of exercise (ie, type of training, setting, frequency, duration, and intensity) and potential differences in perceived HRQoL. The effects related to dose of exercise on HRQoL are unclear. Keteyian and colleagues[20] (2012) have reported that dose or volume of exercise is associated with change in peak Vo_2 and risk for clinical events, but they do not report effects on HRQoL. The meta-regression from the 2014 Cochrane review showed that average exercise dose per study was not associated with HRQoL.[17] The planned individual participant data (IPD) meta-analysis by the ExTraMATCH II collaborators[57] may help to elucidate some of the questions that remain concerning the impact of exercise training on HRQoL and the potential effects of age, gender, and exercise capacity on this impact. Results from an IPD meta-analysis have greater statistical power and therefore are more likely to provide definitive estimation of overall and subgroup effects from exercise training in HF than have been obtained from aggregate data meta-analyses such as the 2014 Cochrane review and from analyses of single trials.[57]

REFERENCES

1. Sullivan MJ, Higginbotham MB, Cobb FR. Exercise training in patients with severe left ventricular dysfunction. Hemodynamic and metabolic effects. Circulation 1988;78:506–15.
2. Smart N, Marwick TH. Exercise training for patients with heart failure: a systematic review of factors that improve mortality and morbidity. Am J Med 2004; 116:693–706.
3. O'Connor CM, Whellan DJ, Lee KL, et al. Efficacy and safety of exercise training in patients with chronic heart failure. JAMA 2009;301:1439–50.
4. Flynn KE, Pina IL, Whellan DJ, et al. Effects of exercise training on health status in patients with chronic heart failure: HF-ACTION randomized controlled trial. JAMA 2009;301:1451–9.
5. Edelmann F, Gelbrich G, Dungen HD, et al. Exercise training improves exercise capacity and diastolic function in patients with heart failure with preserved ejection fraction: results of the Ex-DHF (Exercise training in Diastolic Heart Failure) pilot study. J Am Coll Cardiol 2011;58:1780–91.
6. Taylor RS, Davies EJ, Dalal HM, et al. Effects of exercise training for heart failure with preserved ejection fraction: a systematic review and meta-analysis of comparative studies. Int J Cardiol 2012;162:6–13.
7. Haykowsky MJ, Timmons MP, Kruger C, et al. Meta-analysis of aerobic interval training on exercise capacity and systolic function in patients with heart failure and reduced ejection fractions. Am J Cardiol 2013;111:1466–9.
8. Kitzman DW, Brubaker PH, Herrington DM, et al. Effect of endurance exercise training on endothelial function and arterial stiffness in older patients with heart failure and preserved ejection fraction: a randomized, controlled single-blind trial. J Am Coll Cardiol 2013;62:584–92.
9. Lee AP, Ice R, Blessey R, et al. Long-term effects of physical training on coronary patients with impaired ventricular function. Circulation 1979;60:1519–26.
10. Cohn EH, Williams RS, Wallace AG. Exercise responses before and after physical conditioning in patients with severely depressed left ventricular function. Am J Cardiol 1982;49:296–300.
11. Klocek M, Kubinyi A, Bacior B, et al. Effect of physical training on quality of life and oxygen consumption in patients with congestive heart failure. Int J Cardiol 2005;103:323–9.
12. Passino C, Serverino S, Poletti R, et al. Aerobic training decreases B-type natriuretic peptide expression and adrenergic activitation in patients with heart failure. J Am Coll Cardiol 2006;47: 1835–9.
13. Mueller L, Myers J, Kottman W, et al. Exercise capacity, physical patterns and outcomes six years after cardiac rehabilitation in patients with heart failure. Clin Rehabil 2007;21:923–31.
14. Pina IL, Bittner V, Clare RM, et al. Effects of exercise training on outcomes in women with heart failure. Analysis of HF-ACTION by sex. JACC Heart Fail 2014;2:180–6.
15. Beckie TM, Mendoca MA, Flethcher GF, et al. Examining the challenges of recruiting women into a cardiac rehabilitation program. J Cardiopulm Rehab Prev 2009;29:13–21.
16. Grace SL, Gravely-Witte S, Kayaniyil S, et al. A multisite examination of sex differences in cardiac rehabilitation barriers by participation status. J Womens Health 2009;18:209–16.
17. Taylor RS, Sagar VA, Davies EJ. Exercise-based rehabilitation for heart failure. Cochrane Database Syst Rev 2014;(4):CD003331.
18. Wisloff U, Stoylen A, Loennechen JP, et al. Superior cardiovascular effect of aerobic interval training

versus moderate continuous training in heart failure patients: a randomized study. Circulation 2007; 115:3086–94.

19. Ismail H, McFarlane JR, Nojoumian AH, et al. Clinical outcomes and cardiovascular responses to different exercise training intensities in patients with heart failure. A systematic review and meta-analysis. JACC Heart Fail 2013;1:514–22.

20. Keteyian SJ, Leifer ES, Houston-Miller N, et al. Relation of volume of exercise and clinical outcomes in patients with heart failure. J Am Coll Cardiol 2012;60:1899–905.

21. Haykowsky MJ, Liang Y, Pechter D, et al. A meta-analysis of the effect of exercise training on left ventricular remodeling in heart failure patients: the benefit depends on the type of training performed. J Am Coll Cardiol 2007;49:2329–36.

22. Haykowski MJ, Kitzman DW. Exercise physiology in heart failure and preserved ejection fraction. Heart Failure Clin 2014;10:445–52.

23. Kitzman DW, Brubaker PH, Morgan TM, et al. Exercise in older patients with heart failure and preserved ejection fraction. Circ Heart Fail 2010;3: 659–67.

24. Smart NA, Haluska B, Jeffriess L, et al. Exercise training in heart failure with preserved systolic function: a randomized controlled trial of the effects on cardiac function and functional capacity. Congest Heart Fail 2012;18:295–301.

25. Alves AJ, Ribeiro F, Goldhammer E, et al. Exercise training improves diastolic function in heart failure patients. Med Sci Sports Exerc 2012;44:776–85.

26. Butler J, Fonarow GC, Zile MR, et al. Developing therapies for heart failure with preserved ejection fraction: current state and future directions. JACC Heart Fail 2014;2:97–112.

27. Selig SE, Carey MF, Menzies DG, et al. Moderate-intensity resistance training in patients with chronic heart failure improves strength, endurance, heart rate variability, and forearm blood flow. J Card Fail 2004;10:21–30.

28. Levinger I, Bronks R, Cody DV, et al. Resistance training for chronic heart failure patients on beta blocker medications. Int J Cardiol 2005;102:493–9.

29. Levinger I, Bronks R, Cody DV, et al. The effect of resistance training on left ventricular function and structure with chronic heart failure. Int J Cardiol 2005;105:159–63.

30. Savage PA, Shaw AO, Miller MS, et al. Effect of resistance training on physical disability in chronic heart failure. Med Sci Sports Exerc 2011;43:1379–86.

31. American College of Sports Medicine. ACSM's guidelines for exercise testing and training. 9th edition. Philadelphia: Wolters Kluwer Williams & Wilkins; 2014.

32. Williams MA, Haskell WL, Ades PA, et al. Resistance exercise in individuals with and without cardiovascular disease: 2007 update: a scientific statement from the American Heart Association. Circulation 2007;116:572–84.

33. Davies EJ, Moxham T, Rees K, et al. Exercise based rehabilitation for heart failure. Cochrane Database Syst Rev 2010;(4):CD003331. http://dx.doi.org/10.1002/14651858.CD003331.pub3.

34. Austin J, Williams R, Ross L, et al. Randomised controlled trial of cardiac rehabilitation in elderly patients with heart failure. Eur J Heart Fail 2005;7: 411–7. pii:S1388-9842(04)00282-X.

35. Belardinelli R, Georgiou D, Cianci G, et al. Randomized, controlled trial of long-term moderate exercise training in chronic heart failure: effects on functional capacity, quality of life, and clinical outcome. Circulation 1999;99:1173–82.

36. Davidson PM, Cockburn J, Newton PJ, et al. Can a heart failure-specific cardiac rehabilitation program decrease hospitalizations and improve outcomes in high-risk patients? Eur J Cardiovasc Prev Rehabil 2010;17(4):393–402. http://dx.doi.org/10.1097/HJR.0b013e328334ea56.

37. Jolly K, Taylor RS, Lip GY, et al. A randomized trial of the addition of home-based exercise to specialist heart failure nurse care: the Birmingham rehabilitation uptake maximisation study for patients with congestive heart failure (BRUM-CHF) study. Eur J Heart Fail 2009;11:205–13. http://dx.doi.org/10.1093/eurjhf/hfn029.

38. Koukouvou G, Kouidi E, Iacovides A, et al. Quality of life, psychological and physiological changes following exercise training in patients with chronic heart failure. J Rehabil Med 2004;36:36–41.

39. Nilsson BB, Westheim A, Risberg MA. Long-term effects of a group-based high-intensity aerobic interval-training program in patients with chronic heart failure. Am J Cardiol 2008;102:1220–4. http://dx.doi.org/10.1016/j.amjcard.2008.06.046.

40. Yeh GY, McCarthy EP, Wayne PM, et al. Tai chi exercise in patients with chronic heart failure: a randomized clinical trial. Arch Intern Med 2011;171: 750–7. http://dx.doi.org/10.1001/archinternmed.2011.150.

41. Bocalini DS, dos Santos L, Serra AJ. Physical exercise improves the functional capacity and quality of life in patients with heart failure. Clinics (Sao Paulo) 2008;63:437–42. pii:S1807-59322008000400005.

42. Norman JF, Pozehl BJ, Duncan KA, et al. Effects of exercise training versus attention on plasma B-type natriuretic peptide, 6-minute walk test and quality of life in individuals with heart failure. Cardiopulm Phys Ther J 2012;23:19–25.

43. Dracup K, Evangelista LS, Hamilton MA, et al. Effects of a home-based exercise program on clinical outcomes in heart failure. Am Heart J 2007; 154(5):877–83. http://dx.doi.org/10.1016/j.ahj.2007.07.019.

44. Gary RA, Dunbar SB, Higgins MK, et al. Combined exercise and cognitive behavioral therapy improves outcomes in patients with heart failure. J Psychosom Res 2010;69:119–31. http://dx.doi.org/10.1016/j.jpsychores.2010.01.013.

45. Zwisler AD, Soja AM, Rasmussen S, et al. Hospital-based comprehensive cardiac rehabilitation versus usual care among patients with congestive heart failure, ischemic heart disease, or high risk of ischemic heart disease: 12-month results of a randomized clinical trial. Am Heart J 2008;155:1106–13. http://dx.doi.org/10.1016/j.ahj.2007.12.033.

46. Zwisler AD, Schou L, Soja AM, et al. A randomized clinical trial of hospital-based, comprehensive cardiac rehabilitation versus usual care for patients with congestive heart failure, ischemic heart disease, or high risk of ischemic heart disease (the DANREHAB trial)–design, intervention, and population. Am Heart J 2005;150:899.e7–16. http://dx.doi.org/10.1016/j.ahj.2005.06.010.

47. Jonsdottir S, Andersen KK, Sigurosson AF, et al. The effect of physical training in chronic heart failure. Eur J Heart Fail 2006;8:97–101. pii:S1388-9842(05)00129-7.

48. McKelvie RS, Teo KK, Roberts R, et al. Effects of exercise training in patients with heart failure: the exercise rehabilitation trial (EXERT). Am Heart J 2002;144:23–30. pii:S000287030200039X.

49. Witham MD, Gray JM, Argo IS, et al. Effect of a seated exercise program to improve physical function and health status in frail patients > or = 70 years of age with heart failure. Am J Cardiol 2005;95:1120–4. pii:S0002-9149(05)00201-8.

50. Heart Failure Society of America, Lindenfeld J, Albert NM, Boehmer JP, et al. HFSA 2010 comprehensive heart failure practice guideline. J Card Fail 2010;16:e1–194. http://dx.doi.org/10.1016/j.cardfail.2010.04.004.

51. Austin J, Williams WR, Ross L, et al. Five-year follow-up findings from a randomized controlled trial of cardiac rehabilitation for heart failure. Eur J Cardiovasc Prev Rehabil 2008;15(2):162–7. http://dx.doi.org/10.1097/HJR.0b013e3282f10e87.

52. Belardinelli R, Georgiou D, Cianci G, et al. 10-year exercise training in chronic heart failure: a randomized controlled trial. J Am Coll Cardiol 2012;60:1521–8. http://dx.doi.org/10.1016/j.jacc.2012.06.036.

53. Gary R. Exercise self-efficacy in older women with diastolic heart failure: results of a walking program and education intervention. J Gerontol Nurs 2006;32:31–9.

54. Smart N, Haluska B, Jeffriess L, et al. Exercise training in systolic and diastolic dysfunction: effects on cardiac function, functional capacity, and quality of life. Am Heart J 2007;153:530–6. pii:S0002-8703(07)00056-7.

55. Gary RA, Sueta CA, Dougherty M, et al. Home-based exercise improves functional performance and quality of life in women with diastolic heart failure. Heart Lung 2004;33:210–8. pii:S0147956304000433.

56. Nolte K, Herrmann-Lingen C, Wachter R, et al. Effects of exercise training on different quality of life dimensions in heart failure with preserved ejection fraction: the ex-DHF-P trial. Eur J Prev Cardiol 2014. http://dx.doi.org/10.1177/2047487314526071.

57. Taylor RS, Piepoli MF, Smart N, et al. Exercise training for chronic heart failure (ExTraMATCH II): protocol for an individual participant data meta-analysis. Int J Cardiol 2014;174:683–7. http://dx.doi.org/10.1016/j.ijcard.2014.04.203.

58. Willenheimer R, Rydberg E, Cline C. Effects on quality of life, symptoms and daily activity 6 months after termination of an exercise training programme in heart failure patients. Int J Cardiol 2001;77(1):25–31.

Prognosis
Does Exercise Training Reduce Adverse Events in Heart Failure?

Jonathan Myers, PhD[a],*, Clinton A. Brawner, PhD[b],
Mark J.F. Haykowsky, PhD[c], Rod S. Taylor, PhD[d,e]

KEYWORDS

- Prognosis • Oxygen uptake • Aerobic capacity • Cardiac rehabilitation • Cardiac output

KEY POINTS

- Exercise training in patients with heart failure (HF) is associated with numerous physiologic benefits.
- The HF-ACTION (Heart Failure: A Controlled Trial Investigating Outcomes of Exercise Training) trial along with systematic reviews and meta-analyses using the Cochrane database have greatly enhanced our understanding of the outcome benefits associated with endurance exercise training in patients with HF.
- Recent studies demonstrate that the benefits of training are similar between men and women with HF.

INTRODUCTION

Exercise intolerance, frequently exhibited by fatigue or shortness of breath with a minimal degree of exertion, is a hallmark of chronic heart failure (HF). Quantifying exercise intolerance has profound implications for the determination of disability, quality of life (QOL), prognosis, and the capacity to perform daily activities in patients with HF. One of the principal goals of treatment in HF is therefore to improve exercise capacity; therapies designed to improve exercise capacity in patients with HF are thus critical to improving outcomes. The pathophysiologic features of HF that underlie reduced exercise tolerance have been the focus of numerous investigations for several decades.[1,2] These features involve both central (cardiac) and peripheral (skeletal muscle and vascular) abnormalities, including impaired

cardiac output responses to exercise, abnormal redistribution of blood flow, reduced mitochondrial volume and density, abnormal oxidative enzyme activity, impaired vasodilatory capacity, heightened systemic vascular resistance, and autonomic nervous system changes.[1–4] Until the late 1980s, patients with HF were commonly excluded from exercise programs because of concerns over safety, whether training caused further harm to an already damaged myocardium, and questions as to whether these patients could benefit from exercise. These concerns have been allayed by numerous studies performed over the last 25 years documenting that exercise training in stable patients with HF is safe; that training causes no further damage to the myocardium; and that training is associated with numerous physiologic, musculoskeletal, and psychosocial benefits.[1,4,5] Many studies preformed over the last 2 decades

[a] Cardiology Division, Palo Alto VA Health Care System, Stanford University, Cardiology 111C, 3801 Miranda Avenue, Palo Alto, CA 94304, USA; [b] Division of Cardiovascular Medicine, Henry Ford Hospital, 6525 Second Avenue, Detroit, MI 48202, USA; [c] Alberta Cardiovascular and Stroke Research Centre (ABACUS), Mazankowski Alberta Heart Institute, University of Alberta, 3-16 Corbett Hall, Edmonton, AB T6G 2G4, Canada; [d] Graduate School of Education, University of Exeter Medical School, Veysey Building, Salmon Pool Lane, Exeter EX2 4SG, UK; [e] National Institute of Public Health, University of Southern Denmark, Campusvej 55, DK-5230, Odense M, Denmark
* Corresponding author.
E-mail address: drj993@aol.com

Heart Failure Clin 11 (2015) 59–72
http://dx.doi.org/10.1016/j.hfc.2014.08.012
1551-7136/15/$ – see front matter Published by Elsevier Inc

have also demonstrated improved clinical outcomes following exercise training in HF, including reductions in morbidity, mortality, and hospitalization, along with enhanced QOL.[1,4,6,7] This article provides an overview of the benefits of exercise training in HF and the implications of these benefits for improving outcomes. The application of recent meta-analyses, novel observations on exercise training and outcomes among women, and recent findings from the landmark HF-ACTION (Heart Failure: A Controlled Trial Investigating Outcomes of Exercise Training) trial are discussed.

MECHANISMS OF BENEFIT WITH EXERCISE TRAINING AND IMPLICATIONS FOR IMPROVING OUTCOMES

Potential mechanisms by which exercise training may improve exercise capacity and reduce cardiac events in HF are outlined in **Table 1**; importantly, the extent to which one or a combination of these mechanisms may affect an individual patient's exercise tolerance varies considerably. Peak oxygen consumption (Vo_2) is strongly related to prognosis in patients with HF, and exercise training generally improves peak Vo_2 in the range of 10% to 25%[1,4]; however, even small changes in peak Vo_2 are associated with significantly improved outcomes.[8] Numerous central and peripheral factors influence peak Vo_2, but increases in peak Vo_2 and related benefits from training are fundamentally related to the combination of an improvement in peak cardiac output, improved vascular reactivity, better utilization of oxygen through metabolic changes in the skeletal muscle, and more efficient ventilation. These mechanisms are outlined in the following section.

Central Adaptations

A general consensus exists that the benefits of exercise training in patients with HF are caused largely by adaptations in the peripheral vasculature and skeletal muscle rather than the heart itself.[4,9] Although the focus of these studies has been on patients with HF and reduced ejection fraction (HFrEF), this also seems to be the case among patients with HF and preserved EF (HFpEF).[10] This consensus evolved in part because of the recognition that EF is poorly correlated with exercise capacity.[1,3,4] However, although the preponderance of studies have reported that EF and other measures of contractility show minimal change following training, several studies have reported significant improvements in these indices.[11–14] Most of these studies have focused on resting EF, and less is known regarding indices of contractility during exercise. Because of the difficulty measuring cardiac output directly, it has not been widely reported; but studies using thermodilution techniques have reported increases in maximal cardiac output following training in the range of 5% to 20%.[15] A meta-analysis of 104 patients reported a mean increase in maximal cardiac output of 2.5 L/min, corresponding to a 21% increase.[9] Whether this increase in cardiac output is a result of increases in maximal heart rate or stroke volume is unclear;

Table 1
Potential mechanisms by which exercise training improves outcomes

System	Response to Training	Effect on Outcomes
Cardiac function	• Increased cardiac output • Increase or no change in contractility • Increased peak Vo_2 • Improved ventilatory efficiency	• Increased exercise capacity • Improved QOL • Reduced mortality • Reduced hospitalizations
Regional blood flow	• Increased vasodilatory capacity • Improved endothelial function • Improved redistribution of flow	• Increased exercise capacity
Skeletal muscle	• Increased aerobic enzymes • Increased mitochondrial volume and density • Increased capillary density • Decreased muscle receptor sensitivity	• Increased exercise capacity • Improved physical function • Reduced ventilatory response • Reduced mortality
Autonomic nervous system	• Decrease in plasma norepinephrine • Increased heart rate variability • Reduced chemoreceptor and ergoreceptor sensitivity • Reduced ventilatory response	• Reduced cardiac rhythm disturbances • Reduced or no change in mortality

Abbreviation: Vo_2, peak oxygen consumption.

studies have reported small improvements in both indices as well as no change.[15] When changes in maximal cardiac output do occur, they have been attributed to some combination of small changes in peak heart rate, stroke volume, and afterload reduction (caused by enhanced endothelial-dependent vasodilation).[1,13,15,16]

Vascular Adaptations

Numerous recent studies have characterized abnormal endothelial function in HF, and favorable adaptations in endothelial function have been consistently reported after rehabilitation programs.[1,2,13,17,18] Exercise training decreases circulating catecholamine levels in patients with HF, has antiinflammatory and antioxidative effects, reduces natriuretic peptide concentrations, and increases shear stress and nitric oxide bioavailability,[18–22] all leading to reduced peripheral vasoconstriction, improved endothelial function, and enhanced endothelial repair.[16,17,23,24] These adaptations result in better skeletal muscle perfusion during exercise. There have been dozens of such studies over the last 2 decades, and the volume of work by Hambrecht and colleagues[24] is particularly notable. They reported that a regimen using handgrip exercise training 6 times per day significantly improved endothelial-dependent vasodilation after 4 weeks in patients with HF; the effects of training were similar to those of the potent vasodilator L-arginine. Circulating progenitor cells, which have the ability to differentiate and exhibit endothelial properties and enhance endothelial function, increase following training in HF.[16,19,24,25] Numerous studies have reported that changes in endothelium-dependent peripheral blood flow after training are paralleled by improvements in peak V_{O_2}.[25–27]

Skeletal Muscle Adaptations

Metabolic changes in the skeletal muscle with aerobic training include increases in aerobic enzymes, increases in mitochondrial size and density, and increases in capillary density.[1,2,4,17–21] Muscle biopsy studies have demonstrated shifts from type II to type I muscle fibers after training.[28] Cytochrome c oxidase–positive mitochondria, an important rate-limiting enzyme in oxidative phosphorylation, was demonstrated to increase 41% after 6 months of training.[29] ^{31}P MRI spectroscopy has been used to document abnormalities in skeletal muscle metabolism in HF, including early intracellular acidification, accumulation of inorganic phosphate (Pi), accelerated utilization of phosphocreatine (PCr), and delayed PCr during recovery from exercise.[30–34] Exercise training has been demonstrated to partially reverse these abnormalities in oxidative metabolism measured by MRI and near-infrared spectroscopy techniques, including a slower increase in Pi, a decline in phosphocreatine, a decrease in Pi/creatine phosphate (CP) versus power output, and faster recovery of O_2 stores after exercise.[35,36] Regular exercise also reduces muscle wasting and helps restore the anabolic/catabolic imbalance that is common in HF.[37,38]

Ventilatory Adaptations

Ventilatory inefficiency has been demonstrated to be strongly associated with morbidity and mortality in HF; in fact, studies performed over the last 15 years have shown that markers of ventilatory inefficiency, such as the minute ventilation/carbon dioxide production (VE/V_{CO_2}) slope and oxygen uptake efficiency slope (OUES), are more powerful predictors of risk for adverse outcomes than many clinical and cardiopulmonary exercise test responses in HF.[39] Application of these indices for the identification of high-risk patients has been recommended in recent guidelines on the evaluation and management of HF[40]; the influence of training on these indices is, therefore, important to document. Excessive ventilation in patients with HF has been associated with ventilation/perfusion mismatching caused by impaired cardiac output responses to exercise, early lactate accumulation (which stimulates ventilation through the buffering of lactate), and chemoreceptor and muscle receptor hyperactivity.[39–41] Improvements in abnormal ventilation after training involves some combination of hemodynamic changes (reduced pulmonary pressures or improved ventilation-perfusion mismatching), metabolic changes reflected by a delay in lactate accumulation, a change in ventilatory control, and a change in the ventilatory pattern that makes breathing more efficient. Recent studies have reported that these indices respond favorably to training.[42,43] In addition, a growing number of studies have demonstrated that specific training of the respiratory muscles results in improved ventilatory dynamics and exercise performance.[44,45] Improvement in the ventilatory response to exercise is a critically important mechanism underlying the enhanced functional capabilities and outcomes following training in patients with HF.

Studies have also identified a pathophysiologic mechanism unique to HF that underlies abnormal ventilation and that responds favorably to training. This mechanism involves specific ventilatory signals arising from the exercising muscle, which are abnormally enhanced in HF (termed an *ergoreflex* contribution to ventilation).[46,47] These signals have been demonstrated to contribute to the abnormal hemodynamic, autonomic, and ventilatory responses to exercise that characterize HF. Afferent fibers present in skeletal muscle (ergoreceptors) are sensitive to metabolic changes that occur during muscular work. These receptors seem to mediate circulatory adaptations occurring in the early stages of exercise, are stimulated by metabolic acidosis, and are partially responsible for sympathetic vasoconstriction.[46-48] It has also been demonstrated that hypoxic chemosensitivity is increased in HF and that this heightened chemosensitivity is correlated with the VE/VCO$_2$ slope. The results of these enhanced ergoreflex and chemoreceptor responses are hyperventilation and heightened sympathetic outflow, which cause an increase in peripheral resistance and, thus, a decrease in muscle perfusion. These muscle receptors are less sensitive to stimulation after training; it has been demonstrated that after a 6-week forearm training protocol, the ergoreflex contribution to exercise ventilation was reduced by 58%.[48] These salutary effects on ventilatory control are an additional mechanism by which outcomes are improved with regular exercise in HF.

EXERCISE TRAINING AND OUTCOMES IN HEART FAILURE

By 2004, there had been more than 80 published trials (30 randomized controlled trials [RCTs]) of exercise training in patients with HFrEF.[49] Based on a meta-analysis of these studies, exercise training in patients with HFrEF seemed to be safe and effective.[49] In spite of this, adoption of exercise training for these patients in clinical practice was slow because of the limited sample size of these trials, the lack of data from a large multicenter trial, and limited data on safety. As a result, in the United States, although cardiac rehabilitation (CR) was a covered benefit for beneficiaries of Medicare and many private health insurances for several heart disease–related diagnoses (eg, acute myocardial infarction, valve disease, cardiac transplant), HFrEF was not a CR-eligible diagnosis.

Implications from Heart Failure: A Controlled Trial Investigating Outcomes of Exercise Training (HF-ACTION)

To address this gap, HF-ACTION was designed and funded by the US National Heart, Lung, and Blood Institute (NHLBI). Investigators randomized patients with HFrEF (EF <35%, New York Heart Association [NYHA] class II–IV) to endurance exercise training or usual care.[50] Patients randomized to exercise participated in 3 months of supervised exercise training (3 days per week), with exercise intensity prescribed at 60% to 70% of the measured heart rate reserve. Patients were transitioned from supervised exercise to 5 days per week of home-based exercise training. These patients were provided a heart rate monitor to guide exercise intensity and a leg ergometer or treadmill for their home. Patients in the usual-care group were provided secondary prevention education, including information on the importance of regular physical activity. Both groups were contacted every 2 to 4 weeks. The primary outcome was a composite end point of incident all-cause mortality or all-cause hospitalization. The study was designed to detect an 11% reduction in this end point at 2 years based on enrollment of 3000 subjects.[50]

Although the study was designed to enroll 3000 subjects, a planned interim analysis revealed that, because of a higher-than-expected event rate, 2300 subjects would be sufficient to evaluate the primary outcome.[50] In the end, between 2003 and 2007, HF-ACTION investigators randomized 2331 patients (median age = 59 years, 27%–30% women) with HFrEF from 82 sites in the United States, Canada, and France. In an intent-to-treat analysis, exercise training was associated with an 11% lower adjusted risk (hazard ratio [HR] 0.89; 95% confidence interval [CI] 0.81, 0.99) for incident all-cause mortality/hospitalization and a 15% lower adjusted risk (HR 0.85; 95% CI 0.74, 0.99) for incident cardiovascular-related mortality or HF hospitalization. This effect was seen in spite of significant crossover between groups. Only 30% of the patients in the exercise group achieved the goal of 120 minutes per week of exercise, and 22% to 28% of the patients in the usual-care group self-reported regular exercise participation.[50]

In a planned secondary analysis, Keteyian and colleagues[51] examined the dose-response relationship between the volume of exercise performed and clinical outcomes among patients randomized to the exercise group in HF-ACTION. They reported a reverse J-shaped relationship between the volume of exercise performed (ie, product of exercise time and workload expressed in metabolic equivalents [METs]) and adjusted risk for all-cause mortality/hospitalization as well as cardiovascular-related mortality or HF hospitalization. The lowest risk for both outcomes was observed among patients who performed 3 to 5 MET-hours per week and 5 to 7 MET-hours per week of exercise compared with patients who did not exercise (ie, 0 to 1 MET-hours per week of exercise).[51]

In spite of the lower risk for clinical events observed among patients in the exercise group compared with the control group of HF-ACTION, patients in the exercise group showed only a mild improvement in exercise capacity. On average, peak V_{O_2} increased just 0.6 mL/kg/min at 3 months after randomization ($P<.001$, compared with change in control group).[50] Swank and colleagues[8] evaluated whether the change in peak V_{O_2} at 3 months was associated with a lower risk for mortality/hospitalization, regardless of group assignment. Among patients who were event free through 3 months after randomization, every 6% (eg, ~1 mL/kg/min) increase in peak V_{O_2} at 3 months was associated with a 5% lower adjusted risk (HR = 0.95; 95% CI 0.93, 0.98) for all-cause mortality/hospitalization, a 4% lower adjusted risk (HR = 0.96; 95% CI 0.94, 0.99) for cardiovascular-related mortality/hospitalization, and a 7% lower adjusted risk (HR = 0.93; 95% CI 0.90, 0.97) for all-cause mortality.[8]

In another analysis of data from the HF-ACTION trial, Reed and colleagues[52] evaluated the cost-effectiveness of the exercise training intervention as it was applied in the trial. Consistent with other economic evaluations of health care interventions, the investigators considered all patient-level direct costs, including the patients' time to travel to and from the exercise facility and to perform the exercise (center or home based), and staff time to perform follow-up phone calls intended to promote adherence. Importantly, this was a cost analysis of the intervention delivered in the HF-ACTION trial, which was more comprehensive than a typical CR program. Reed and colleagues[52] used a patient-to-staff ratio of 1.7 in the analysis. This ratio contrasts with the recommended ratio of up to 5 patients per staff member in CR programs.[53] According to the investigators,[52] with the exception of the patients' time, the cost of the exercise intervention was considered relatively low for the health care system. The total health care cost during follow-up was not significantly different between the exercise and control groups, and there was no consistent difference in medical resource utilization. The investigators concluded that cost may be improved if these patients are incorporated into a standard CR program whereby patient-to-staff ratios are more efficient. The investigators concluded that intervention costs may be reduced if patients were incorporated into a more standard CR program whereby patient-to-staff ratios are more efficient than in the trial.

With a final enrollment of 2331 patients[54] and a total cost exceeding $37.5 million,[55] HF-ACTION was the largest and most expensive trial of exercise training to be funded by the US National Institutes of Health. Results from the HF-ACTION trial confirmed the safety and clinical benefit of moderate-intensity cardiorespiratory exercise training for patients with HFrEF. These data were helpful in persuading the US Centers for Medicare and Medicaid to approve coverage of phase 2 CR for Medicare beneficiaries with HFrEF beginning in 2014. In addition, as stated by Michael Lauer, MD (director of the Division of Cardiovascular Sciences at the NHLBI), HF-ACTION investigators demonstrated that large, multisite, end-point driven behavioral trials (such as exercise training) can be successfully conducted (comments following the initial presentation of the primary results during the HF-ACTION investigators meeting in conjunction with the 2008 American Heart Association Scientific Sessions).

EXERCISE TRAINING AND OUTCOMES IN WOMEN WITH HEART FAILURE
Impaired Exercise Tolerance in Women with Heart Failure

Women with HF have reduced exercise tolerance, measured objectively as decreased peak V_{O_2} and distance walked in 6 minutes (6MWD).[56] Data from the HF-ACTION trial revealed that the baseline peak V_{O_2} and 6MWD were 10% and 7% lower, respectively, in clinically stable women (n = 661) compared with men (n = 1670) with HFrEF.[56,57] Scott and associates[58] extended these findings to patients with HFpEF and reported that peak V_{O_2} was 16% lower in women compared with men.[58] Given that peak V_{O_2} is inversely associated with all-cause death in men and women,[59,60] a consequence of the impaired exercise tolerance is that women with HF may have reduced survival compared with men with similar health status and ventricular function. Moreover, peak V_{O_2} in women with HF is less than the minimal threshold level required for full and independent living.[61] Accordingly, therapies that improve exercise tolerance may be especially relevant to maintaining functional independence and improving survival in women with HF.

Exercise Training and Improvement in Exercise Tolerance and Quality of Life in Women with Heart Failure

Women with HF have been underrepresented in exercise intervention trials.[57,61] Indeed, to date, only 4 RCTs have examined the efficacy of exercise training on health-related outcomes in women with HF (total sample size, n = 84).[62–65]

Tyni-Lenne and colleagues[64] performed the first randomized cross-over trial comparing 8 weeks of knee extensor exercise training (3 days per week at 65%–75% peak power output × 15 minutes) versus an 8-week control (no training) period on peak Vo_2, 6MWD, skeletal muscle metabolic capacity, and QOL in 16 women with clinically stable HFrEF (mean age = 62 years). Compared with control subjects, 8 weeks of exercise training significantly increased peak Vo_2, 6MWD, quadriceps muscle citrate synthase, lactate dehydrogenase, along with physical and psychosocial QOL.

Pu and colleagues[63] compared 10 weeks of high-intensity upper and lower extremity strength training (3 sets × 8 repetitions at 82% maximal strength) versus low-intensity stretching on peak 6MWD, peak Vo_2, muscle strength and endurance, skeletal muscle mass and morphology, and cardiac function in 16 older women (mean age = 77 years) with HFrEF. No adverse events were found with the strength-training program; this mode of training was associated with a significant increase in 6MWD, lower extremity maximal strength, and endurance compared with controls. No significant difference was found for peak Vo_2, skeletal muscle fiber distribution or oxidative capacity, or global systolic or diastolic function. In addition, it seemed that the improved aerobic endurance was mediated by favorable skeletal muscle adaptations because the increase in vastus lateralis type I (oxidative) fiber area and citrate synthase activity were positively related to the increase in 6WMD.

Haykowsky and colleagues[62] examined the effects of 6 months (3 months supervised followed by 3 months unsupervised) aerobic and strength training (n = 10) versus aerobic training alone (n = 10) on peak Vo_2, muscle strength, and QOL in older women with HFrEF (mean age = 72 years). Supervised (cycle) training was performed 2 days per week at 60% to 70% of the heart rate reserve, whereas unsupervised (walking) training was performed 2 days per week at a rate of perceived exertion between 12 and 14. The combined group also performed 1 to 2 sets of supervised upper and lower extremity strength training at 50% to 70% of maximal strength and unsupervised upper and lower extremity strength training using handheld and leg weights.[62] The main finding of this study was that 3 months of supervised aerobic or combined aerobic and strength training increased peak Vo_2 and leg press maximal strength that was not maintained with unsupervised training.[62] No significant change was found in QOL after exercise training.

Gary and colleagues[65] performed the first exercise RCT in women with HFpEF (mean age = 68 years; mean EF = 55%). Subjects were randomly assigned to 12 weeks of unsupervised exercise (walking 3 days per week at 40%–60% peak heart rate) plus an education program (HF disease management and women's health) versus an education program alone. The primary outcomes were 6MWD and QOL. The investigators reported that the intervention group had a significantly greater improvement in 6MWD and QOL compared with the control group after 12 weeks.

Although there has been a relative paucity of studies in women, taken together, these findings suggest that supervised aerobic training is an effective therapy to improve peak Vo_2, 6MWD, and QOL, whereas supervised strength training performed alone or in combination with aerobic training improves muscle strength in women with HF.

Exercise Training, All-Cause Mortality, and Hospitalization in Women with Heart Failure

Pina and colleagues[57] recently reported findings from an exploratory analysis on the effects of exercise training on peak Vo_2 and a combined end point of all-cause mortality and hospital stay in women (exercise group, n = 290; usual care group, n = 229) and men (exercise group, n = 682; usual care group, n = 668) from the HF-ACTION trial. Despite adherence to endurance training being higher among men (45% of men maintained a goal of 90 minutes of exercise per week vs 37% of women), the mean difference between exercise and usual-care participants was similar in men (0.5 mL/kg/min, 95% CI 0.22–0.79) and women (0.73 mL/kg/min, 95% CI 0.27–1.19) after 3 months of training. Endurance training was also associated with a 26% reduction in the combined end point in women, whereas there was no decrease in men (estimated effect in women: 0.74 95% CI 0.59–0.92; estimated effect in men: 0.99 95% CI 0.86–1.13; P value for interaction = .027). Accordingly, the findings from this subanalysis provide proof of concept that the endurance training–mediated increase in peak Vo_2 may be associated with favorable improvements in all-cause mortality and hospitalization in women with HF. Despite this potential benefit, a limitation of the HF-ACTION trial is that the median age of participants was lower than the age at first diagnosis of HF in population-based studies (59 years vs ≥70 years, respectively).[66–68]

Summary and Future Directions

Women with either HFpEF or HFrEF have severely reduced peak Vo_2. The mechanisms responsible for the reduced peak Vo_2 in women with HF have not been studied extensively; however, it is likely caused by impaired cardiac, vascular, and skeletal muscle function that result in reduced convective or diffusive O_2 transport and/or by abnormalities in oxygen utilization by the active muscles. Regular aerobic training improves peak Vo_2 and 6MWD in women with HF. Moreover, strength training alone or in combination with aerobic training improves maximal muscular strength in women with HFrEF. The mechanisms responsible for the improvement in exercise tolerance have not been well studied, but the limited data to date suggest that they may be related to favorable changes in skeletal muscle oxidative capacity.[63,64] Finally, the increased peak Vo_2 in women with HFrEF with short-term training may be associated with a greater reduction in all-cause mortality and hospital stay than men with similar health status and ventricular function. Future prospective trials are required to determine whether the increase in peak Vo_2 is associated with favorable improvements in survival and hospitalization in older women with HF.

META-ANALYSES OF EXERCISE TRAINING AND OUTCOMES IN HEART FAILURE: THE 2014 COCHRANE REVIEW

The latest update of the Cochrane systematic review and meta-analysis of RCTs of exercise-based CR for HF was published in April 2014.[69,70] In brief, the methods of this review were as follows: MEDLINE, EMBASE, and the Cochrane Library were searched up to January 2013 for RCTs that included adults (≥18 years) with HFpEF or HFrEF and reported follow-up for 6 months or more after randomization; further trials were retrieved through a manual search of references including studies and recent reviews; there was no language restriction; trials were pooled when possible using either fixed or random effects meta-analysis.

This review included 33 RCTs in a total of 4740 patients predominantly with HFrEF and NYHA class II to III (**Table 2**). Most trials were small (<100 participants) and single center (30 trials), with the HF-ACTION trial[2,3] contributing approximately 50% (2331 participants) of all included patients. The mean age of patients across the trials ranged from 51 to 81 years. Although there was evidence of more women recruited in recent trials, most patients were predominantly men (median 87%). Eleven trials reported follow-up in excess of 12 months. All trials evaluated a cardiorespiratory exercise training intervention, and 11 also included resistance training. Exercise training was most commonly delivered in either an exclusively center-based setting or a center-based setting in combination with some home exercise sessions. A small number of studies (N = 5) were conducted in an exclusively home-based setting. The dose of exercise training ranged widely across studies, with session durations of 15 to

Table 2
Selected characteristics of the 33 trials in the Cochrane meta-analysis

Characteristic	Number (%) or Median (Range)
Exercise-only CR	10 (30)
Setting	
Center based	14 (43)
Home based	5 (15)
Both	13 (39)
Unspecified	1 (3)
Sample size	52 (19–2331)
Publication date	
1990–99	5 (15)
2000–09	22 (66)
2010 or later	6 (18)
Single center	30 (91)
Study location	
Europe	20 (60)
North America[a]	11 (33)
Other	2 (6)
Sex	
Men only	12 (36)
Women only	0 (0)
Both	20 (61)
Unspecified	1 (3)
Age (years)	60.5 (51–81)
Diagnosis	
HFrEF only	29 (88)
HFpEF only	0 (0)
Both	4 (12)
Left ventricular EF (%)	29 (21–41)
Included NYHA IV	6 (18)
NYHA class unspecified	4 (12)

[a] HF-ACTION trial also included 6 French centers (out of 82 centers).

Data from Taylor RS, Sagar VA, Davies EJ, et al. Exercise-based rehabilitation for heart failure. Cochrane Database Syst Rev 2014;4:CD003331. http://dx.doi.org/10.1002/14651858.CD003331.pub4.

120 minutes, 1 to 7 sessions per week, intensity of 40% to 80% of maximal heart rate (or equivalent of 50%–85% of peak Vo_2 or Borg rating of 12–18), delivered over 15 to 120 weeks. The main outcomes of the Cochrane review are summarized in the following section.

Mortality

There was no significant difference in pooled mortality up to 12 months follow-up between exercise training and control groups (25 trials; fixed-effect relative risk [RR] 0.92, 95% CI 0.67–1.26; *P* = .67; heterogeneity (I²) = 0%; **Fig. 1A**). There was a trend toward a reduction in all-cause mortality when pooled across the longest follow-up point of the 6 trials with more than 12 months follow-up (fixed-effect RR 0.80, 95% CI 0.75 to 1.02; *P* = .09; I² = 34%, **Fig. 1B**).

Hospital Admissions

There were reductions in the number of patients experiencing all hospital admissions with exercise compared with control up to 12 months of follow-up (15 trials; fixed-effect RR 0.75, 95% CI 0.62 to 0.92; *P* = .005; I² = 0%; **Fig. 2A**) and

HF-specific admissions (12 trials; fixed-effect RR 0.61, 95% CI 0.46 to 0.8; *P* = .0004; I² = 34%; **Fig. 2C**). There was no difference in all hospital admissions in trials with more than 12 months of follow-up (5 trials, random-effect RR 0.92, 95% CI 0.66 to 1.29; *P* = .63; I² = 63%; **Fig. 2B**).

Health-Related Quality of Life

A total of 18 trials reported a validated health-related QOL measure. Although most of the studies (13 studies) used the disease-specific Minnesota Living with Heart Failure questionnaire, the HF-ACTION trial used the Kansas City Cardiomyopathy Questionnaire.[2] Generic health-related QOL was assessed using the EuroQoL, Short-Form 36,

A

Study or Subgroup	Treatment Events	Total	Control Events	Total	Weight	Risk Ratio M-H, Fixed, 95% CI
Austin 2005	5	100	4	100	5.3%	1.25 [0.35, 4.52]
DANREHAB 2008	4	45	3	46	3.9%	1.36 [0.32, 5.75]
Davidson 2010	4	53	11	52	14.8%	0.36 [0.12, 1.05]
Dracup 2007	9	87	8	86	10.7%	1.11 [0.45, 2.75]
Gary 2010 (comp)	0	18	1	19	1.9%	0.35 [0.02, 8.09]
Gary 2010 (exalone)	1	20	0	17	0.7%	2.57 [0.11, 59.30]
Giannuzzi 2003	0	45	1	45	2.0%	0.33 [0.01, 7.97]
Gielen 2003	0	10	0	10		Not estimable
Gottlieb 1999	1	17	1	16	1.4%	0.94 [0.06, 13.82]
Hambrecht 1995	1	12	0	10	0.7%	2.54 [0.11, 56.25]
Hambrecht 1998	1	10	1	10	1.3%	1.00 [0.07, 13.87]
Hambrecht 2000	3	36	2	37	2.6%	1.54 [0.27, 8.69]
Jolly 2009	7	84	5	85	6.6%	1.42 [0.47, 4.29]
Keteyian 1996	0	21	1	19	2.1%	0.30 [0.01, 7.02]
Klecha 2007	0	25	0	25		Not estimable
McKelvie 2002	19	90	20	91	26.5%	0.96 [0.55, 1.68]
Myers 2000	1	12	0	13	0.6%	3.23 [0.14, 72.46]
Nilsson 2008	2	40	1	40	1.3%	2.00 [0.19, 21.18]
Norman 2012	1	22	0	20	0.7%	2.74 [0.12, 63.63]
Pozehl 2007	0	15	1	6	2.8%	0.15 [0.01, 3.16]
Wall 2010	1	9	1	10	1.3%	1.11 [0.08, 15.28]
Willenheimer 2001	3	27	2	27	2.7%	1.50 [0.27, 8.28]
Witham 2005	1	41	3	41	4.0%	0.33 [0.04, 3.07]
Witham 2012	2	53	1	54	1.3%	2.04 [0.19, 21.81]
Yeh 2011	0	50	3	50	4.7%	0.14 [0.01, 2.70]
Total (95% CI)		**942**		**929**	**100.0%**	**0.93 [0.69, 1.27]**
Total events	66		70			

Heterogeneity: Chi² = 12.60, df = 22 (*P* = .94); I² = 0%
Test for overall effect: Z = 0.43 (*P* = .67)

0.005 0.1 1 10 200
Favours exercise Favours control

B

Study or Subgroup	Experimental Events	Total	Control Events	Total	Weight	Risk Ratio M-H, Fixed, 95% CI
Austin 2005	31	100	38	100	13.6%	0.82 [0.56, 1.20]
Belardinelli 1999	9	50	20	49	7.2%	0.44 [0.22, 0.87]
Belardinelli 2012	4	63	10	60	3.7%	0.38 [0.13, 1.15]
HF ACTION 2009	189	1159	198	1171	70.5%	0.96 [0.80, 1.16]
Jónsdóttir 2006	2	21	2	22	0.7%	1.05 [0.16, 6.77]
Mueller 2007	9	25	12	25	4.3%	0.75 [0.39, 1.46]
Total (95% CI)		**1418**		**1427**	**100.0%**	**0.88 [0.75, 1.02]**
Total events	244		280			

Heterogeneity: Chi² = 7.54, df = 5 (*P* = .18); I² = 34%
Test for overall effect: Z = 1.69 (*P* = .09)

0.02 0.1 1 10 50
Favours experimental Favours control

Fig. 1. (*A*) All-cause mortality up to 12 months' follow-up. (*B*) All-cause mortality more than 12 months' follow-up. DANREHAB, danish rehabilitation trial; M-H, mantel-haenszel. (*From* Taylor RS, Sagar VA, Davies EJ, et al. Exercise-based rehabilitation for heart failure. Cochrane Database Syst Rev 2014;4:CD003331. http://dx.doi.org/10.1002/14651858.CD003331.pub4; with permission.)

A

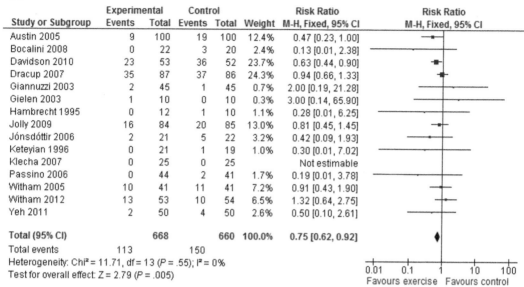

Study or Subgroup	Experimental Events	Total	Control Events	Total	Weight	Risk Ratio M-H, Fixed, 95% CI
Austin 2005	9	100	19	100	12.4%	0.47 [0.23, 1.00]
Bocalini 2008	0	22	3	20	2.4%	0.13 [0.01, 2.38]
Davidson 2010	23	53	36	52	23.7%	0.63 [0.44, 0.90]
Dracup 2007	35	87	37	86	24.3%	0.94 [0.66, 1.33]
Giannuzzi 2003	2	45	1	45	0.7%	2.00 [0.19, 21.28]
Gielen 2003	1	10	0	10	0.3%	3.00 [0.14, 65.90]
Hambrecht 1995	0	12	1	10	1.1%	0.28 [0.01, 6.25]
Jolly 2009	16	84	20	85	13.0%	0.81 [0.45, 1.45]
Jónsdóttir 2006	2	21	5	22	3.2%	0.42 [0.09, 1.93]
Keteyian 1996	0	21	1	19	1.0%	0.30 [0.01, 7.02]
Klecha 2007	0	25	0	25		Not estimable
Passino 2006	0	44	2	41	1.7%	0.19 [0.01, 3.78]
Witham 2005	10	41	11	41	7.2%	0.91 [0.43, 1.90]
Witham 2012	13	53	10	54	6.5%	1.32 [0.64, 2.75]
Yeh 2011	2	50	4	50	2.6%	0.50 [0.10, 2.61]
Total (95% CI)		**668**		**660**	**100.0%**	**0.75 [0.62, 0.92]**
Total events	113		150			

Heterogeneity: Chi² = 11.71, df = 13 (P = .55); I² = 0%
Test for overall effect: Z = 2.79 (P = .005)

0.01 0.1 1 10 100
Favours exercise Favours control

B

Study or Subgroup	Treatment Events	Total	Control Events	Total	Weight	Risk Ratio M-H, Random, 95% CI
Austin 2005	53	100	38	100	31.0%	1.39 [1.02, 1.90]
Belardinelli 1999	5	50	14	49	9.7%	0.35 [0.14, 0.90]
HF ACTION 2009	729	1159	760	1171	41.9%	0.97 [0.91, 1.03]
Jónsdóttir 2006	7	21	11	22	13.9%	0.67 [0.32, 1.39]
Mueller 2007	2	25	3	25	3.5%	0.67 [0.12, 3.65]
Total (95% CI)		**1355**		**1367**	**100.0%**	**0.92 [0.66, 1.29]**
Total events	796		826			

Heterogeneity: Tau² = 0.07; Chi² = 10.90, df = 4 (P = .03); I² = 63%
Test for overall effect: Z = 0.48 (P = .63)

0.1 0.2 0.5 1 2 5 10
Favours exercise Favours control

C

Study or Subgroup	Treatment Events	Total	Control Events	Total	Weight	Risk Ratio M-H, Fixed, 95% CI
Belardinelli 1999	5	50	14	49	14.5%	0.35 [0.14, 0.90]
Belardinelli 2012	8	63	25	60	26.3%	0.30 [0.15, 0.62]
Dracup 2007	35	87	37	86	38.3%	0.94 [0.66, 1.33]
Giannuzzi 2003	2	45	1	45	1.0%	2.00 [0.19, 21.28]
Hambrecht 1995	0	12	1	10	1.7%	0.28 [0.01, 6.25]
Jolly 2009	4	84	2	85	2.0%	2.02 [0.38, 10.75]
Jónsdóttir 2006	0	21	3	22	3.5%	0.15 [0.01, 2.73]
Mueller 2007	2	25	3	25	3.1%	0.67 [0.12, 3.65]
Myers 2000	0	12	2	13	2.5%	0.22 [0.01, 4.08]
Passino 2006	0	44	2	41	2.7%	0.19 [0.01, 3.78]
Willenheimer 2001	0	23	3	27	3.3%	0.17 [0.01, 3.07]
Witham 2012	1	53	1	54	1.0%	1.02 [0.07, 15.87]
Total (95% CI)		**519**		**517**	**100.0%**	**0.61 [0.46, 0.80]**
Total events	57		94			

Heterogeneity: Chi² = 16.70, df = 11 (P = .12); I² = 34%
Test for overall effect: Z = 3.52 (P = .0004)

0.005 0.1 1 10 200
Favours exercise Favours control

Fig. 2. (*A*) All hospital admissions up to 12 months' follow-up. (*B*) All hospital admissions more than 12 months' follow-up. (*C*) HF-related hospital admissions up to 12 months' follow-up. Two trials reported no deaths in either exercise CR or control arms. M-H, mantel-haenszel. (*From* Taylor RS, Sagar VA, Davies EJ, et al. Exercise-based rehabilitation for heart failure. Cochrane Database Syst Rev 2014;4:CD003331. http://dx.doi.org/10.1002/14651858.CD003331.pub4; with permission.)

A

Study or Subgroup	Treatment Mean	SD	Total	Control Mean	SD	Total	Weight	Mean Difference IV, Random, 95% CI
Austin 2005	22.9	14.7	95	36.9	21.3	94	10.0%	-14.00 [-19.22, -8.78]
Belardinelli 1999	40	19	48	51	22	46	7.3%	-11.00 [-19.33, -2.67]
Davidson 2010	52.9	15.7	50	56.4	18.3	42	8.3%	-3.50 [-10.54, 3.54]
Dracup 2007	35.7	23.7	86	43.2	27.3	87	7.9%	-7.50 [-15.12, 0.12]
Gary 2010 (comp)	24.2	16.3	15	34.3	23.6	16	4.0%	-10.10 [-24.30, 4.10]
Gary 2010 (exalone)	25.6	19.7	17	28.9	29.9	14	2.7%	-3.30 [-21.55, 14.95]
Jolly 2009	37.6	21	80	34.9	24.8	77	8.2%	2.70 [-4.50, 9.90]
Koukouvou 2004	34.1	13	16	45.2	9	19	7.9%	-11.10 [-18.65, -3.55]
McKelvie 2002	-3.4	18.1	57	-3.3	13.9	67	9.5%	-0.10 [-5.86, 5.66]
Nilsson 2008	23	14	35	28	20	37	7.6%	-5.00 [-12.94, 2.94]
Passino 2006	32	26.5	44	53	32	41	4.7%	-21.00 [-33.54, -8.46]
Witham 2012	15.4	14.8	43	11.3	12.1	44	9.5%	4.10 [-1.59, 9.79]
Yeh 2011	13	4	50	18	6	50	12.5%	-5.00 [-7.00, -3.00]
Total (95% CI)			**636**			**634**	**100.0%**	**-5.83 [-9.21, -2.44]**

Heterogeneity: Tau² = 22.85; Chi² = 40.24, df = 12 (P<.0001); I² = 70%
Test for overall effect: Z = 3.37 (P = .0007)

-20 -10 0 10 20
Favours exercise　Favours control

B

Study or Subgroup	Exercise Mean	SD	Total	Control Mean	SD	Total	Weight	Mean Difference IV, Random, 95% CI
Austin 2005	35.5	21.7	57	37.1	24.9	55	30.0%	-1.60 [-10.26, 7.06]
Belardinelli 1999	44	21	48	54	22	46	29.9%	-10.00 [-18.70, -1.30]
Belardinelli 2012	43	12	63	58	14	60	40.1%	-15.00 [-19.62, -10.38]
Total (95% CI)			**168**			**161**	**100.0%**	**-9.49 [-17.48, -1.50]**

Heterogeneity: Tau² = 35.87; Chi² = 7.33, df = 2 (P = .03); I² = 73%
Test for overall effect: Z = 2.33 (P = .02)

-20 -10 0 10 20
Favours exercise　Favours control

C

Study or Subgroup	Treatment Mean	SD	Total	Control Mean	SD	Total	Weight	Std. Mean Difference IV, Random, 95% CI
Austin 2005	22.9	14.7	95	36.9	21.3	94	6.2%	-0.76 [-1.06, -0.47]
Belardinelli 1999	40	19	48	51	22	46	5.5%	-0.53 [-0.94, -0.12]
Bocalini 2008	-87	4	22	-81	6	20	4.0%	-1.17 [-1.83, -0.51]
DANREHAB 2008	-42.7	9.1	19	-37.4	11.4	15	3.8%	-0.51 [-1.20, 0.18]
Davidson 2010	52.9	15.7	50	56.4	18.3	42	5.5%	-0.20 [-0.62, 0.21]
Dracup 2007	35.7	23.7	86	43.2	27.3	87	6.2%	-0.29 [-0.59, 0.01]
Gary 2010 (comp)	24.2	16.3	15	34.3	23.6	16	3.7%	-0.48 [-1.20, 0.23]
Gary 2010 (exalone)	25.6	19.7	17	28.9	29.9	14	3.7%	-0.13 [-0.84, 0.58]
HF ACTION 2009	72.39	20.46	906	71.24	21.48	850	7.1%	0.05 [-0.04, 0.15]
Jolly 2009	37.6	21	80	34.9	24.8	77	6.1%	0.12 [-0.20, 0.43]
Jónsdóttir 2006	-47.55	8.7	21	-44.1	14.04	20	4.2%	-0.29 [-0.91, 0.32]
Klocek 2005 (const)	-109	23.5	14	-71.7	23.5	7	2.4%	-1.52 [-2.57, -0.48]
Klocek 2005 (Prog)	-99	23.5	14	-71.7	23.5	7	2.6%	-1.12 [-2.10, -0.13]
Koukouvou 2004	34.1	13	16	45.2	9	19	3.7%	-0.99 [-1.69, -0.28]
McKelvie 2002	-3.4	18.1	57	-3.3	13.9	67	5.9%	-0.01 [-0.36, 0.35]
Nilsson 2008	23	14	35	28	20	37	5.2%	-0.29 [-0.75, 0.18]
Norman 2012	-81	18.2	19	-77.9	11.6	18	4.1%	-0.20 [-0.84, 0.45]
Passino 2006	32	26.5	44	53	32	41	5.3%	-0.71 [-1.15, -0.27]
Willenheimer 2001	-0.7	0.8	20	0	1	17	3.9%	-0.76 [-1.44, -0.09]
Witham 2005	-69	13	36	-65	10	32	5.1%	-0.34 [-0.82, 0.14]
Yeh 2011	13	4	50	18	6	50	5.5%	-0.97 [-1.39, -0.56]
Total (95% CI)			**1664**			**1576**	**100.0%**	**-0.46 [-0.66, -0.26]**

Heterogeneity: Tau² = 0.14; Chi² = 94.85, df = 20 (P<.00001); I² = 79%
Test for overall effect: Z = 4.58 (P<.00001)

-4 -2 0 2 4
Favours exercise　Favours control

Fig. 3. (*A*) Minnesota Living with Heart Failure score up to 12 months' follow-up. (*B*) Minnesota Living with Heart Failure score more than 12 months' follow-up. (*C*) All health-related quality outcomes. IV, instrumental variable; DANREHAB, danish rehabilitation trial; SD, standard deviation. (*From* Taylor RS, Sagar VA, Davies EJ, et al. Exercise-based rehabilitation for heart failure. Cochrane Database Syst Rev 2014;4:CD003331. http://dx.doi.org/10.1002/14651858.CD003331.pub4; with permission.)

Psychological General Wellbeing index, Patient's Global Assessment of QOL, and Spritzer's QOL Index. Across the studies reporting the total Minnesota Living with Heart Failure questionnaire score up to 12 months of follow-up, there was evidence of a clinically important improvement with exercise (random-effects weighted mean difference (WMD) −5.8, 95% CI −9.2 to −2.4; P = .0007; I^2 = 70%; **Fig. 3**A). This benefit was also seen in the 3 trials that reported follow-up of more than 12 months (random-effect WMD −9.5, 95% CI −17.5 to −1.5; P = .022; I^2 = 73%; **Fig. 3**B). Pooling across all studies, regardless of the outcome measure used, showed a significant improvement in QOL with exercise (random-effects standardized mean difference [SMD] −0.46, 95% CI −0.66 to −0.26; P<.0001; I^2 = 79%; **Fig. 3**C).

SUMMARY

Regular exercise training reduces adverse events in patients with either HFrEF or HFpEF. Studies performed over the last 3 decades have provided extensive insights into both the health outcome benefits of exercise training and the physiologic mechanisms underlying these benefits. Physiologic adaptations that occur following exercise training involve both central and peripheral mechanisms that include increases in peak cardiac output, improved vascular reactivity, better utilization of oxygen through metabolic changes in the skeletal muscle, changes in autonomic function, and more efficient ventilation.

Although women have been underrepresented in previous studies, the available data indicate that women generally achieve physiologic benefits from exercise training to an extent that is similar to men. Using the combined end point of mortality and hospitalization, some evidence exists that women may even derive outcome benefits from CR that are greater than those of men.[57] The landmark HF-ACTION trial has had a major impact on our understanding of the effects of endurance exercise training on health outcomes in patients with HF. This knowledge has provided insight not only into the benefits of CR in HF but has also provided a clearer understanding of the dose-response relationship between the volume of exercise performed and clinical outcomes, the cost-effectiveness of training in HF, and the difficulties associated with conducting such a large and ambitious multicenter trial. The results of HF-ACTION have had an important impact on the recent approval of coverage for CR for patients with HFrEF by US Centers for Medicare and Medicaid.

Systematic reviews and meta-analyses using the Cochrane database have provided level 1 evidence (evidence obtained from properly designed RCTs) that exercise-based rehabilitation is associated with important reductions in hospitalization and improvements in health-related QOL of participants with HF. Moreover, these benefits seem to be consistent across patients regardless of age, sex, disease severity, and CR program characteristics (exercise only vs comprehensive CR). Exercise interventions seem to be safe for patients with HF with no increased mortality in the short-term, and there is some evidence supporting reductions in mortality in the longer-term (>12 months of follow-up). Although more recent trials have recruited patients with HFpEF and NHYA class IV and include a greater proportion of women and older patients, these groups remain underrepresented and need to be the focus of future clinical trials. Future trials also need to evaluate interventions to enhance the long-term maintenance of exercise-based CR for HF and the outcomes, costs, and cost-effectiveness of programs delivered exclusively in a home-based setting.

REFERENCES

1. Downing J, Balady GJ. The role of exercise training in heart failure. J Am Coll Cardiol 2011; 58:561–9.
2. Piepoli MF, Guazzi M, Boriani G, et al. Exercise intolerance in chronic heart failure: mechanisms and therapies. Part 1. Eur J Cardiovasc Prev Rehabil 2010;17:637–42.
3. Myers J, Froelicher VF. Hemodynamic determinants of exercise capacity in chronic heart failure. Ann Intern Med 1991;115:377–86.
4. Pina IL, Apstein CS, Balady GJ, et al. Exercise and heart failure: a statement from the American Heart Association Committee on exercise, rehabilitation, and prevention. Circulation 2003;107:1210–25.
5. Haykowsky M, Scott J, Esch B, et al. A meta-analysis of the efforts of exercise training on left ventricular remodeling following myocardial infarction: start early and go longer for greatest exercise benefits on remodeling. Trials 2011;12:92.
6. Davies EJ, Moxham T, Rees K, et al. Exercise training for systolic heart failure: Cochrane systematic review and meta-analysis. Eur J Heart Fail 2010;12:706–15.
7. Davies EJ, Moxham T, Rees K, et al. Exercise based rehabilitation for heart failure. Cochrane Database Syst Rev 2010;(4):CD003331.
8. Swank AM, Horton J, Fleg JL, et al. Modest increase in peak VO_2 is related to better clinical outcomes in chronic heart failure patients: results from heart failure and a controlled trial to investigate outcomes of exercise training (HF-ACTION). Circulation 2012;5:579–85.

9. Van Tol BA, Huijsmans RJ, Droon DW, et al. Effects of exercise training on cardiac performance, exercise capacity and quality of life in patients with heart failure: a meta-analysis. Eur J Heart Fail 2006;8:841–50.

10. Haykowsky MJ, Brubaker PH, Stewart KP, et al. Effect of endurance training on the determinants of peak exercise oxygen consumption in elderly patients with stable compensated heart failure and preserved ejection fraction. J Am Coll Cardiol 2012;60:120–8.

11. Wisloff U, Stoylen A, Leonnenchen JP, et al. Superior cardiovascular effect of aerobic interval training versus moderate continuous training in heart failure patients: a randomized study. Circulation 2007; 115:3086–94.

12. Giannuzzi P, Temporelli PL, Corra U, et al, ELVD-CHF Study Group. Antiremodeling effect of long-term exercise training in patients with stable chronic heart failure: results of the Exercise in Left Ventricular Dysfunction and Chronic Heart Failure (ELVD-CHF) trial. Circulation 2003;108:557–9.

13. Hambrecht R, Gielen S, Linke A, et al. Effects of exercise training on left ventricular function and peripheral resistance in patients with chronic heart failure: a randomized trial. JAMA 2000; 283:3095–101.

14. Erbs S, Linke A, Gielen S, et al. Exercise training in patients with severe chronic heart failure: impact on left ventricular performance and cardiac size. A retrospective analysis of the Leipzig Heart Failure Training Trial. Eur J Cardiovasc Prev Rehabil 2003; 10:336–44.

15. Mezzani A, Corra U, Gianuzzi P. Central adaptations to exercise training in patients with chronic heart failure. Heart Fail Rev 2008;13:13–20.

16. Erbs S, Hollriegel R, Linke A, et al. Exercise training in patients with advanced chronic heart failure (NYHA IIIb) promotes restoration of peripheral vasomotor function, induction of endogenous regeneration, and improvement of left ventricular function. Circ Heart Fail 2010;3:486–94.

17. Duscha BD, Schulze PC, Robbins JL, et al. Implications of chronic heart failure on peripheral vasculature and skeletal muscle before and after exercise training. Heart Fail Rev 2008;13:21–37.

18. Peipoli MF. Exercise training in chronic heart failure: mechanisms and therapies. Neth Heart J 2013;21:85–90.

19. Gielen S, Schuler G, Adams V. Cardiovascular effects of exercise training: molecular mechanisms. Circulation 2010;122:1221–38.

20. Gielen S, Adams V, Mobius-Winkler S, et al. Anti-inflammatory effects of exercise training in the skeletal muscle of patients with chronic heart failure. J Am Coll Cardiol 2003;42:861–8.

21. Tabet J, Meurin P, Driss AB, et al. Benefits of exercise training in chronic heart failure. Arch Cardiovasc Dis 2009;102:721–30.

22. Mendes-Ribeiro AC, Mann GE, Meirelles LR, et al. The role of exercise on L-arginine nitric oxide pathway in chronic heart failure. Open Biochem J 2009;3:55–65.

23. Van Craenebroeck EM, Hoymans VY, Beckers PJ, et al. Exercise training improves function of circulating angiogenic cells in patients with chronic heart failure. Basic Res Cardiol 2010;105:665–76.

24. Hambrecht MD, Hillbrich L, Erbs S, et al. Correction of endothelial dysfunction in chronic heart failure: additional effects of exercise training and oral L-arginine supplementation. J Am Coll Cardiol 2000;35:706–13.

25. Hambrecht R, Fiehn E, Weigl C, et al. Regular physical exercise corrects endothelial dysfunction and improves exercise capacity in patients with chronic heart failure. Circulation 1998;98:2709–15.

26. Linke A, Schoene N, Gielen S, et al. Endothelial dysfunction in patients with chronic heart failure: systemic effects of lower-limb exercise training. J Am Coll Cardiol 2001;37:392–7.

27. Hornig B, Maier V, Drexler H. Physical training improves endothelial function in patients with chronic heart failure. Circulation 1996;93:210–4.

28. Hambrecht R, Fiehn E, Yu J, et al. Effects of endurance training on mitochondrial ultrastructure and fiber type distribution in skeletal muscle of patients with stable chronic heart failure. J Am Coll Cardiol 1997;29:1067–73.

29. Hambrecht R, Niebauer J, Fiehn E, et al. Physical training in patients with stable chronic heart failure: effects on cardiorespiratory fitness and ultrastructural abnormalities of leg muscles. J Am Coll Cardiol 1995;25:1239–49.

30. Kao W, Helpern JA, Goldstein S, et al. Abnormalities of skeletal muscle metabolism during nerve stimulation determined by 31P nuclear magnetic resonance spectroscopy in severe congestive heart failure. Am J Cardiol 1995;76:606–9.

31. Van Der Ent M, Jeneson JA, Remme WJ, et al. A non-invasive selective assessment of type I fibre mitochondrial function using 31P NMR spectroscopy. Evidence for impaired oxidative phosphorylation rate in skeletal muscle in patients with chronic heart failure. Eur Heart J 1998;19:124–31.

32. Stassijns G, Lysens R, Decramer M. Peripheral and respiratory muscles in chronic heart failure. Eur Respir J 1996;9:2161–7.

33. Cohen-Solal A, Laperche T, Morvan D, et al. Prolonged kinetics of recovery of oxygen consumption after maximal graded exercise in patients with chronic heart failure. Analysis with gas exchange measurements and NMR spectroscopy. Circulation 1995;91:2924–32.

34. Belardinelli R, Barstow TJ, Nguyen P, et al. Skeletal muscle oxygenation and oxygen uptake kinetics following constant work rate exercise in chronic congestive heart failure. Am J Cardiol 1997;80: 1319–24.

35. Vasileiadis I, Kravari M, Terrovitis J, et al. Interval exercise training improves tissue oxygenation in patients with chronic heart failure. World J Cardiovasc Dis 2013;3:301–7.

36. Adamopoulos S, Coats AJ, Brunotte F, et al. Physical training improves skeletal muscle metabolism in patients with chronic heart failure. J Am Coll Cardiol 1993;21:1101–6.

37. Gielen S, Sandri M, Kozarez I, et al. Exercise training attenuates MuRF-1 expression in the skeletal muscle of patients with chronic heart failure independent of age: the randomized Leipzig Exercise Intervention in Chronic Heart Failure and Aging catabolism study. Circulation 2012;125: 2716–27.

38. Adams V, Doring C, Schuler G. Impact of physical exercise on alterations in the skeletal muscle in patients with chronic heart failure. Front Biosci 2008;13:302–11.

39. Arena R, Myers J, Guazzi M. The clinical and research applications of aerobic capacity and ventilator efficiency in heart failure: an evidence-based review. Heart Fail Rev 2008;13:245–69.

40. Balady GJ, Arena R, Sietsema K, et al, American Heart Association Exercise, Cardiac Rehabilitation, and Prevention Committee of the Council on Clinical Cardiology, Council on Epidemiology and Prevention, Council on Peripheral Vascular Disease, Interdisciplinary Council on Quality of Care and Outcomes Research. Clinicians guide to cardiopulmonary exercise testing in adults: a scientific statement from the American Heart Association. Circulation 2010;122:191–225.

41. Ingle L. Theoretical rationale and practical recommendations for cardiopulmonary exercise testing in patients with chronic heart failure. Heart Fail Rev 2007;12:12–22.

42. Myers J, Gademan M, Brunner K, et al. Effects of high-intensity training on indices of ventilatory efficiency in chronic heart failure. J Cardiopulm Rehabil Prev 2012;32:9–16.

43. Gademan MG, Swenne CA, Verwey HF, et al. Exercise training increases oxygen uptake efficiency slope in chronic heart failure. Eur J Cardiovasc Prev Rehabil 2008;15:140–4.

44. Cahalin LP, Semigran MJ, Dec GW. Inspiratory muscle training in patients with chronic heart failure awaiting cardiac transplantation: results of a pilot clinical trial. Phys Ther 1997;77:830–8.

45. Lin S, McElfresh J, Hall B, et al. Inspiratory muscle training in patients with heart failure: a systematic review. Cardiopulm Phys Ther J 2012;23:29–36.

46. Clark AL, Piepoli M, Coats AJ. Skeletal muscle and the control of ventilation on exercise: evidence for metabolic receptors. Eur J Clin Invest 1995;25: 299–305.

47. Ponikowski PP, Chua TP, Francis DP, et al. Muscle ergoreceptor overactivity reflects deterioration in clinical status and cardiorespiratory reflex control in chronic heart failure. Circulation 2001;104:2324–30.

48. Piepoli M, Clark AL, Volterrani M, et al. Contribution of muscle afferents to the hemodynamic, autonomic, and ventilator responses to exercise in patients with chronic heart failure: effects of physical training. Circulation 1996;93:940–52.

49. Smart N, Marwick TH. Exercise training for patients with heart failure: a systematic review of factors that improve mortality and morbidity. Am J Med 2004;116(10):693–706. http://dx.doi.org/10.1016/j. amjmed.2003.11.033.

50. O'Connor CM, Whellan DJ, Lee KL, et al. Efficacy and safety of exercise training in patients with chronic heart failure: HF-ACTION randomized controlled trial. JAMA 2009;301(14):1439–50. http://dx.doi.org/10.1001/jama.2009.454.

51. Keteyian SJ, Leifer ES, Houston-Miller N, et al. Relation between volume of exercise and clinical outcomes in patients with heart failure. J Am Coll Cardiol 2012;60(19):1899–905. http://dx.doi.org/ 10.1016/j.jacc.2012.08.958.

52. Reed SD, Whellan DJ, Li Y, et al. Economic evaluation of the HF-ACTION (Heart Failure: A Controlled Trial Investigating Outcomes of Exercise Training) randomized controlled trial: an exercise training study of patients with chronic heart failure. Circ Cardiovasc Qual Outcomes 2010;3(4):374–81. http:// dx.doi.org/10.1161/CIRCOUTCOMES.109.907287.

53. Lawson GJ. Cardiac rehabilitation staffing. In: Kraus WE, Keteyian SJ, editors. Contemporary cardiology: cardiac rehabilitation. Totowa (NJ): Humana Press; 2007. p. 277–87.

54. Whellan DJ, O'Connor CM, Lee KL, et al. Heart failure and a controlled trial investigating outcomes of exercise training (HF-ACTION): design and rationale. Am Heart J 2007;153(2):201–11. http://dx. doi.org/10.1016/j.ahj.2006.11.007.

55. National Heart Lung and Blood Institute. NHLBI fact book, fiscal year 2008. [108]. Bethesda, MD: National Institutes of Health. Available at: http:// www.nhlbi.nih.gov/files/docs/factbook/FactBook 2008.pdf.

56. Pina IL, Kokkinos P, Kao A, et al. Baseline differences in the HF-ACTION by sex. Am Heart J 2009;158:S16–23.

57. Pina IL, Bittner V, Clare RM, et al. Effects of exercise training on outcomes in women with heart failure: analysis of HF-ACTION (Heart Failure-A Controlled Trial Investigating Outcomes of Exercise Training) by sex. JACC Heart Fail 2014;2:180–6.

58. Scott JM, Haykowsky MJ, Eggebeen J, et al. Reliability of peak exercise testing in patients with heart failure with preserved ejection fraction. Am J Cardiol 2012;110:1809–13.

59. Gulati M, Pandey DK, Arnsdorf MF, et al. Exercise capacity and the risk of death in women: the St James women take heart project. Circulation 2003;108:1554–9.

60. Myers J, Prakash M, Froelicher V, et al. Exercise capacity and mortality among men referred for exercise testing. N Engl J Med 2002;346:793–801.

61. Haykowsky MJ, Ezekowitz JA, Armstrong PW. Therapeutic exercise for individuals with heart failure: special attention to older women with heart failure. J Card Fail 2004;10:165–73.

62. Haykowsky M, Vonder Muhll I, Ezekowitz J, et al. Supervised exercise training improves aerobic capacity and muscle strength in older women with heart failure. Can J Cardiol 2005;21:1277–80.

63. Pu CT, Johnson MT, Forman DE, et al. Randomized trial of progressive resistance training to counteract the myopathy of chronic heart failure. J Appl Physiol (1985) 2001;90:2341–50.

64. Tyni-Lenne R, Gordon A, Jansson E, et al. Skeletal muscle endurance training improves peripheral oxidative capacity, exercise tolerance, and health-related quality of life in women with chronic congestive heart failure secondary to either ischemic cardiomyopathy or idiopathic dilated cardiomyopathy. Am J Cardiol 1997;80:1025–9.

65. Gary RA, Sueta CA, Dougherty M, et al. Home-based exercise improves functional performance and quality of life in women with diastolic heart failure. Heart Lung 2004;33:210–8.

66. Niederseer D, Thaler CW, Niederseer M, et al. Mismatch between heart failure patients in clinical trials and the real world. Int J Cardiol 2013;168:1859–65.

67. Cleland JG, Swedberg K, Follath F, et al. The Euro-heart failure survey programme– a survey on the quality of care among patients with heart failure in Europe. Part 1: patient characteristics and diagnosis. Eur Heart J 2003;24:442–63.

68. Lee DS, Gona P, Vasan RS, et al. Relation of disease pathogenesis and risk factors to heart failure with preserved or reduced ejection fraction: insights from the Framingham Heart Study of the National Heart, Lung, and Blood Institute. Circulation 2009;119:3070–7.

69. Taylor RS, Sagar VA, Davies EJ, et al. Exercise-based rehabilitation for heart failure. Cochrane Database Syst Rev 2014;(4):CD003331. http://dx.doi.org/10.1002/14651858.CD003331.pub4.

70. Flynn KE, Piña IL, Whellan DJ, et al. Effects of exercise training on health status in patients with chronic heart failure: HF-ACTION randomized controlled trial. JAMA 2009;153:1451–9.

Rehabilitation Practice Patterns for Patients with Heart Failure
The South American Perspective

Audrey Borghi-Silva, PhD, PT[a],*, Renata Trimer, PhD, PT[a],
Renata G. Mendes, PhD, PT[a], Ross A. Arena, PhD, PT[b],
Pedro V. Schwartzmann, PhD, MD[c]

KEYWORDS

- Chronic heart failure • Rehabilitation • Chagas cardiomyopathy • Referral • Cardiovascular disease

KEY POINTS

- The incidence and prevalence of heart failure (HF) in South America (SA) is currently a significant concern and will continue to be so for the foreseeable future.
- Chagas heart disease represents a main cause of HF in Latin America, despite progress in transmission control.
- Cardiac rehabilitation (CR) is recognized as an integral component of comprehensive HF care; however, SA suffers from an insufficient infrastructure to support current needs.
- It is essential to expand CR delivery and develop new strategies that could allow more HF patients to have access to services.
- New studies, conducted in SA, should be undertaken to assess the safety and efficacy of novel CR models, particularly in patients with Chagas HF.

HEART FAILURE INCIDENCE AND PREVALENCE IN SOUTH AMERICA

In most South American (SA) countries, the primary health concern has shifted from infectious diseases to noncommunicable chronic diseases.[1,2] Noncommunicable diseases are projected to continue to increase, especially in low- and middle-income countries. In addition, cardiovascular disease (CVD) is responsible for the largest proportion of current noncommunicable chronic disease incidence and prevalence, a trend that will continue into the future.[3–5]

Heart failure (HF) is an important public health issue in SA countries owing to its high incidence and prevalence, cost of care, and morbidity and mortality. The social, labor, and broader economic impacts are also substantial.[6] Demographic risk factors for the development of HF include older age, male sex, ethnicity, and low socioeconomic status.[7]

HF prevalence is related to, among other things, comorbidities and CVD risk factors, underlying disease state (eg, cardiomyopathy, hypertension, valve disease), and therapeutic advances for ischemic heart disease and other conditions that

[a] Cardiopulmonary Physiotherapy Laboratory, Federal University of Sao Carlos, Rod Washington Luis Km 235 - SP - 310, Sao Carlos, Sao Paulo 13565-90, Brazil; [b] Integrative Physiology Laboratory, Department of Physical Therapy, College of Applied Health Sciences, University of Illinois Chicago, 1918 West Taylor Street, Chicago, IL 60612, USA; [c] Clinical Hospital, Rehabilitation Institute Lucy Montoro, Ribeirao Preto School of Medicine, University of Sao Paulo, Monte Alegre, Ribeirão Preto, Sao Paulo 14048-900, Brazil
* Corresponding author. Cardiopulmonary Physiotherapy Laboratory, Department of Physical Therapy, Federal University of Sao Carlos, Rodovia Washington Luis Km 235, Sao Carlos, Sao Paulo, Brazil.
E-mail address: audrey@ufscar.br

Heart Failure Clin 11 (2015) 73–82
http://dx.doi.org/10.1016/j.hfc.2014.08.004
1551-7136/15/$ – see front matter © 2015 Elsevier Inc. All rights reserved.

may lead to HF.[2,6] Rheumatic heart disease and Chagas' heart disease are still often attributed to HF in SA countries.[2]

Although HF is currently acknowledged as an important public health problem,[2,6,8] some studies indicate that the true impact this chronic condition has in SA countries remains unknown. Epidemiologic data are scarce and related to clinical trials, hospital-based studies, and reference centers.[9] Also, the prevalence of HF-reduced ejection fraction and HF-preserved ejection fraction is not well documented. The most relevant knowledge about HF is provided by North American and European studies; therefore, more studies are needed to guide the most appropriate and effective interventions in other countries as those in SA.

The Brazilian Public Health System Database (DATASUS) indicates there are currently 2 million patients with HF and 240,000 new cases being diagnosed each year. Moreover, HF is considered a major cause of hospitalization among patients diagnosed with CVD disease in the Brazilian Public Health System.[8,10,11]

In 1 Brazilian analysis of patients admitted to the hospital for decompensated HF, an ischemic etiology (30%) was the most common, followed by hypertensive (21%), valvular (15%), and Chagas (15%) etiologies.[12] Another Brazilian study, however, demonstrated that Chagas disease (41%) was the more frequent etiology for patients admitted with decompensated HF. The authors attributed this latter result to location, with the Midwest region of Brazil being one of the most prevalent areas for Chagas disease in Brazil.[8]

According to the National Register of HF in Chile, the main etiologies for HF were ischemic heart disease and hypertension, with elderly patients comprising the majority of those hospitalized for this condition. Noncompliance with diet or medical prescriptions and infections were important risk factors associated with HF decompensation.[13] Mean hospital stay was 10 ± 9 days and mortality was 5.6%,[14] with a significant proportion of cases having HF-preserved ejection fraction.[15] In Argentina, an ischemic etiology also seems to be more prevalent, with a lower prevalence of Chagas HF (10.5%).[16] This also seems to be the case in Colombia.[17]

Regarding hospital admissions, in 2007 the Brazilian Ministry of Health attributed 39.4% to HF (70% in the age group >60 years).[18] In-hospital mortality ranged from 6.58% to 6.95% and the average hospital stay was 5.8 days.[19] In Argentina, severe presentation on admission (eg, cardiogenic shock, acute pulmonary edema, anasarca) occurred in 30% of the cases. The median hospital stay was 7 days and in-hospital mortality 8%. After 90 days, readmittance was 24.5%, and post discharge mortality was 12.8%.[20] In general, the total number of HF hospital admissions has been decreasing. However, when hospitalized, patients are presenting with greater disease severity and poorer myocardial function, and are at greater risk of death.[21–23]

Mortality data from São Paulo State (Brazil) in 2006 demonstrated that HF or etiologies associated with HF were responsible for 15,336 deaths, 6.3% of the total.[24] Actually, mortality data associated with HF in Brazil as a whole has been declining,[25] although some regions have not demonstrated this trend.[26] This overall mortality reduction trend is likely associated with improvement in HF prevention and treatment.

THE CURRENT CARDIAC REHABILITATION DELIVERY MODEL IN SOUTH AMERICA

Despite major advances in HF therapies, most patients continue to experience exercise intolerance owing to intrinsic abnormalities in cardiac function coupled with varying degrees of maladaptive changes in the skeletal and respiratory musculature, vasculature, and pulmonary circulation. In this context, numerous studies demonstrate that regular exercise is safe and associated with substantial benefits in appropriately selected HF patients.[27] Cardiac rehabilitation (CR) programs are considered as an integral component to the comprehensive care of the patients with HF.[27] Exercise training (ET) and HF disease-related self-care counseling are both recommended by the American Heart Association and the American College of Cardiology,[27] as well as the Brazilian Society of Cardiology.[28]

The majority of CR centers in SA countries include resting and exercise assessments, physical activity counseling, ET, and education on nutrition and risk factor management. CR is traditionally divided into 4 phases that extend from a hospital-based stage to a maintenance phase, commonly numbered from I to IV.[29–31] CR programs for HF can be located within a hospital as part of a cardiology department, medical center, or in an off-site location. Staffing for CR typically comprises a multidisciplinary team that includes at least 2 health care professionals; a majority of the centers have a cardiologist, a physical therapist, and a nutritionist.[32]

An important study was carried out to assess the characteristics and current level of CR program implementation in SA countries by Cortes-Bergoderi and colleagues.[32] The investigators conducted a survey assessing the density of CR programs and demonstrated an extremely low number in SA countries. Specifically, they identified only 160 programs in 9 of the 10 countries represented in the SA Society of Cardiology. These CR programs provided services to a median of 180 patients per year and were commonly led by cardiologists and physical therapists.[32]

A physical exercise program is highly recommended and safe for HF patients.[33–35] The principal studies with HF patients conducted in SA countries are listed in **Table 1**. A typical training session used in these studies consisted of a warmup (10–15 min), training phase (15–30 min), and cool down (3–6 min).[33–39,42–45] Endurance training was usually carried out on a stationary bike, treadmill, or over ground walking. Resistance exercises were commonly prescribed in centers with phase II programs using free weights or other resistance systems.[34,35,37,41,42,45]

The Borg scale is a simple, practical, and inexpensive method of exercise monitoring in HF and

Table 1
South American studies that evaluated cardiac rehabilitation programs in patients with heart failure

Study	Subjects	Intensity and Components of Exercise Intervention	Program Duration	Main Results
Carvalho et al,[36] 2009	HF patients	AE on a treadmill monitored by HR at 80%–90% of the AT	8 wk	Significant improvement in peak Vo₂ and no significant changes in values of 24-h blood pressure
Ueno et al,[37] 2009	HF patients with CSA and OSA	AE monitored by HR corresponding with AT on an EB and local strengthening	16 wk	Reduced MSNA and increased forearm blood flow, peak Vo₂, and HRQOL in all groups.
Lima et al,[38] 2010	HF patients with chronic Chagas disease	Walking for up to 30 min at 55%–65% of peak HR	12 wk	Improvement in functional capacity and HRQOL
Santos et al,[39] 2010	HF patients with left ventricular dysfunction	AE monitored by HR levels corresponding with AT on an EB and local strengthening	16 wk	Improvement in myocardial blood flow
Mendes et al,[40] 2011	HF patients post CABG	Progressive exercises at 2–4 METs	5 d	Significant cardiac autonomic improvement
Fialho et al,[41] 2012	HF patients with chronic Chagas disease	AE and resistance exercises according to the Borg scale	24 wk	Significant improvement in peak Vo₂
de Araújo et al,[42] 2012	HF patients with left ventricular dysfunction admitted to the ward	Respiratory, lower and upper limbs exercises + neuromuscular electrostimulation	16 d	improvement in 6 min walk test distance
Ricca-Mallada et al,[43] 2012	HF patients	AE on an EB at 80% of HR achieved at peak incremental exercise	24 wk	Significant increase of RR interval, high- and low-frequency power of HRV, and the magnitudes of deceleration capacity and acceleration capacity
da Silva Souza et al,[44] 2013	HF patients with chronic Chagas disease	AE monitored by HR on a treadmill and resistance training	24 wk	No changes in HRV

Abbreviations: AE, aerobic exercise; AT, anaerobic threshold; CABG, cardiac artery bypass grafting; CSA, central sleep apnea; EB, ergometric bike; HF, heart failure; HR, heart rate; HRQOL, healthy related quality of life; HRV, heart rate variability; METs, metabolic equivalents; MSNA, muscle sympathetic neural activity; OSA, obstructive sleep apnea; Vo₂, oxygen consumption.
Data from Refs.[36–44]

is the most frequently used method to define the intensity of ET in SA countries.[32–34] Another inexpensive and relatively easy way to monitor and prescribe ET is heart rate (HR) monitoring.[36–46] The advantage of using HR as a variable for exercise prescription and monitoring is its close relation to oxygen consumption in healthy individuals[47,48] and in patients with HF.[49]

Initial improvements in physical capacity, perceived symptoms, and muscle strength are normally seen after 4 weeks of ET, assuming an appropriate upward titration of exercise volume (ie, duration, frequency, intensity).[33,34] Most CR programs in HF entails at least 12 weeks of training, during which time patients receive close exercise monitoring and counseling.

The number of CR programs in SA countries seems to be insufficient for the population, particularly given the currently high and growing burden of CVD. In addition, there seems to be a significant need for standardization of CR program components and services in the region.

HEART FAILURE SECONDARY TO CHAGAS DISEASE IN SOUTH AMERICA

Chagas disease represents a main cause of HF in SA countries, despite progress in transmission control,[50] and is responsible for many deaths, hospital admissions and poor functional status. Chagas disease is caused by the protozoan *Trypanosoma cruzi* and the World Health Organization estimates that 8 to 10 million people are infected worldwide.[51,52] The cardiac form is the most serious and frequent manifestation of chronic Chagas disease and it develops in 20% to 30% of individuals afflicted with this condition.[50]

The detrimental effects of Chagas disease include parasite persistence, a chronic inflammatory response, an autoimmune response, damage to the parasympathetic system causing sympathetic hyperactivity, and microvascular abnormalities.

Although the benefits of ET in HF are well established, patients with Chagas disease are often excluded from randomized trials analyzing therapy for HF, especially nonpharmacologic treatment. In general, all recommendations for the management of chronic Chagas disease are supported by C-level evidence, which is derived from case series and expert opinions.

Currently, there is only a small, randomized, controlled ET trial in 40 patients with HF owing to Chagas disease, showing a significant improvement in functional capacity and health-related quality of life in the ET group.[38,53] Specifically, although the authors included only a limited number of patients over a short-term follow-up, there was a clear demonstration of an increase in exercise time, 6-minute walk test distance, estimated peak oxygen consumption, and quality of life in the Chagas HF ET group. Lima and colleagues[38] demonstrated that ET is feasible, effective, and did not result in significant adverse, events in patients with Chagas HF.

In Brazil, despite the clear benefits of outpatient CR, there are large regional inequalities with respect to CR program availability[54] and most of the programs are focused on primary and secondary prevention of ischemic heart disease. There are incipient initiatives to improve CR, but they lack availability for HF, especially for Chagas patients.

CARDIAC REHABILITATION FOR PATIENTS WITH HEART FAILURE SECONDARY TO CHAGAS DISEASE

Chagas cardiomyopathy is a heterogeneous entity with a wide variation in clinical course and prognosis. Chagas HF is associated with a cluster of unique traits, such as high frequency of arrhythmias, early cardiac denervation, atrioventricular and intraventricular blocks, and sudden cardiac death. These deleterious traits may unfavorably alter the clinical course of the disease in comparison to patients with HF other than that caused by Chagas disease.[55] Accordingly, previous studies have demonstrated that patients with Chagas HF have poor long-term outcomes.[56,57]

Indeed, some characteristics present in patients with Chagas HF are relevant to CR (**Table 2**). First, Chagas disease is considered an arrhythmogenic cardiomyopathy with a wide variety of abnormalities of the conduction system, associated with both bradyarrhythmias and tachyarrhythmias. Polymorphic or monomorphic ventricular premature beats, and runs of nonsustained ventricular tachycardia are a common finding on Holter monitoring and exercise testing,[58] the latter being an independent predictor of mortality.[59,60] Sustained ventricular tachycardia can also occur, and is the main trigger of sudden death in Chagas HF.[61] Moreover, the severity of ventricular arrhythmias tends to correlate with the degree of left ventricular dysfunction, but can also occur in patients with preserved ventricular function.[62] In addition, Chagas HF is usually a primary cause of atrioventricular block and sinus node dysfunction; these patients are frequently candidates for the implantation of pacemakers.[28] Taken together, all these rhythm disturbances are a concern during CR and should be carefully monitored and treated according to current guidelines. Particularly, despite a scarcity of evidence from randomized controlled

Table 2
Characteristics of Chagas disease that may be present and should be evaluated before initiation of cardiac rehabilitation

Parameter	Particularities of Chagas Disease
Electrocardiogram	Right bundles-branch block often associated with left anterior hemiblock, ST-T changes, abnormal Q waves, low voltage of QRS
Echocardiogram	Apical left ventricular aneurysm, mural thrombus, segmental left ventricular wall motion abnormalities and associated involvement of the right ventricle
Myocardial scintillography	Perfusion defects without obstructive coronary disease
Involvement of the digestive system	Mega-esophagus and/or megacolon
Thromboembolism	Relatively frequent; brain embolism is most common
Arrhythmias	Wide variety of abnormalities of the conduction system; bradyarrhythmias (sinus node dysfunction, atrioventricular blocks), ventricular premature beats and tachycardia and ventricular tachycardia
Dysautonomia	Vagal dysfunction and cardiac sympathetic denervation

Adapted from Refs.[50,52,53]

trials, some observational data suggest that amiodarone could improve survival in patients with ischemic heart disease who are at high risk of death because of malignant arrhythmias.[50]

Second, dysautonomia manifested as a vagal dysfunction may occur early in the course of the disease and before the development of left ventricular dysfunction.[63,64] Because these patients have a reduced vagal modulation over the sinus node, reduction of the HR response to physiologic stimuli may be present. However, in the Lima and colleagues[38] study, response of HR, systemic blood pressure, calculated peak oxygen consumption, and 6-minute walking test distance in patients with Chagas HF was comparable with results of ET in other etiologies with low use of β-blockers.[65,66]

Third, thromboembolic events are relatively frequent in Chagas HF and represent another cause of death in these patients.[61] Brain embolism is the most common clinically recognized event, followed by limb and pulmonary embolisms.[52] Therefore, proper anticoagulation therapy should be evaluated in selected patients before starting CR.[53] Finally, treatment of patients with Chagas HF has traditionally been extrapolated from guidelines developed for the management of HF from other causes, including guidance on CR programming.

A very important issue for CR in patients with Chagas HF is the appropriate selection of patients. Beyond traditional criteria for the evaluation of patients with HF at high risk and worse prognosis, there is a validated score for predicting mortality specifically in those with Chagas HF. Variables included in this scoring system are (1) abnormal electrocardiogram, (2) low QRS voltage, (3) cardiomegaly presented on chest x-ray, (4) segmental or global wall motion abnormalities on the echocardiogram, (5) the presence of nonsustained ventricular tachycardia on 24-hour electrocardiogram monitoring, (6) male sex, and (7) poor functional capacity.[67,68] The scoring system is listed in **Table 3**. This score may additionally help to stratify prognosis and should be considered, together

Table 3
Rassi score for prediction of total mortality

Risk Factor	Points
NYHA class III or IV	5
Cardiomegaly (chest radiograph)	5
Segmental or global wall motion abnormality (2D echocardiogram)	3
Nonsustained ventricular tachycardia (24-h Holter)	3
Low QRS voltage (ECG)	2
Male sex	2

Total Points	Total Mortality 5 y (%)	Total Mortality 10 y (%)	Risk
0–6	2	10	Low
7–11	18	44	Intermediate
12–20	63	84	High

Abbreviations: ECG, Electrocardiogram; NYHA, New York Heart Association.
From Rassi A Jr, Rassi A, Marin-Neto JA. Chagas disease. Lancet 2010;375(9723):1397; with permission.

with clinical evaluation, to objectively quantify the risk of future events and individualize the CR supervision strategy for each patient.

According to the classification of the I Latin American Guidelines for the Diagnosis and Treatment of Chagas Cardiomyopathy,[67] which classifies Chagas cardiomyopathy into acute and chronic phases, exercise should be avoided in the acute phase owing to a high level of parasitemia and inflammation. The early stage of the chronic phase is where it is most appropriate to implement CR and ET. In stage D, which includes patients with symptoms of HF at rest and refractory to maximized medical therapy, CR should not be implemented. **Table 4** summarizes the stages in the development of HF owing to Chagas disease.

ADHERENCE FOR AND BARRIERS TO CARDIAC REHABILITATION IN PATIENTS WITH CHAGAS HEART FAILURE IN SOUTH AMERICA

Cortes-Bergoderi and colleagues[32] identified 160 centers that offered CR in 9 of 10 countries represented by the South American Society of Cardiology; 116 responded to a survey. Based on these data, it was estimated that there is 1 CR program for every 2,319,312 inhabitants in SA countries. Fewer than half of the centers offered a phase I CR; 91% had phase II, 89% phase III, and 57% phase IV programs. The most commonly perceived barriers to participation in a CR program were lack of referral from the cardiologist or primary care physician, as reported by 70% of the CR program directors, lack of economic resources (12.8%), space availability (6.2%), and transportation issues (2.5%).

Concerning adherence and compliance, only a few Brazilian studies have addressed this issue. Lima and colleagues,[38] studying the effects of ET in HF patients owing Chagas disease, obtained 95% adherence in those participating in ET, which has been recognized as fundamental to achieve treatment goals.[69] In another ET study in patients with Chagas HF, participation was much lower (ie, 23%); however, for those who participated, there were no dropouts during the study.[44]

Despite the well-recognized beneficial effects of CR,[70,71] it is necessary for future studies to assess factors surrounding adherence and compliance with CR in patients with Chagas HF. In addition, strategies to promote referral, attendance, and adherence to CR in these patients in SA countries,[65] as well as in others parts of the world, is necessary, because CR adherence is well below optimal levels.[72]

Indeed, the eligibility for CR in patients with Chagas HF is perceived as being considerably low.[38,41] Reasons for ineligibility include high severity of the disease, clinical instability,[70,73] low adherence to pharmacotherapy, and other comorbidities.

Low sociocultural and educational level, lack of understanding of the potential positive effects of physical activity, older age, and being a woman have all been identified as barriers for attendance and adherence to CR.[74] Other reasons include lack of time, program availability, or difficulties regarding transportation. In this context, recent studies focusing on home-based education and care as well as self-monitoring have demonstrated promise in patients with Chagas HF.[75,76] Implementation of these approaches may also prove useful CR strategies to improve participation and compliance.

Table 4 Stages in the development of heart failure owing to Chagas disease	
Stages	**Findings**
A	Patients present with no symptoms of HF and no structural heart disease (normal ECG and chest X-ray)
B1	Asymptomatic patients with ECG changes (arrhythmias or conduction disorders); mild echocardiographic contractile abnormalities, possibly with normal global ventricular function
B2	Patients with decreased left ventricular ejection fraction who have never had any signs or symptoms of HF
C	Patients with left ventricular dysfunction and prior or current symptoms of HF
D	Patients with symptoms of HF at rest, refractory to maximized medical therapy (NYHA functional class IV) that require specialized and intensive interventions

Abbreviations: ECG, electrocardiogram; HF, heart failure; NYHA, New York Heart Association.

From Andrade JP, Marin-Neto JA, Paola AA, et al. I Latin American guidelines for the diagnosis and treatment of Chagas cardiomyopathy. Arq Bras Cardiol 2011; 97(2 Suppl 3):1–48; with permission.

CHALLENGES FOR THE FUTURE OF CARDIAC REHABILITATION IN SOUTH AMERICA

The incidence and prevalence of HF owing to Chagas disease is still highly prevalent in SA counties,[77] despite government efforts to control the disease. Therefore, strategies to reduce the risk of HF are imperative and constitute the first step.[2] In relation to barriers to CR referral, participation, and adherence, a primary challenge for the future in SA countries is to effectively engage HF outpatients in formal CR programs, and, in parallel, consistently encouraging patients to maintain optimized medication and proper nutrition.[78]

The expansion and access to formal CR programs is a major challenge, given the large territory comprising SA countries and that most regions consist of rural areas.[79,80] The current availability of formal CR programs is insufficient and they are primarily only available in larger cities of a given SA country,[54] too far for many patients living in rural areas to attend. In this context, home-based CR program strategies have been tested[81]; however, the effectiveness and safety of this approach needs to be assessed by additional research before it can be supported clinically. More recently, however, emphasis has been given to home-based telemonitoring programs using Internet and mobile phone technology.[82] In SA countries, these strategies may be a viable approach and should be explored further.

Programs focused on education not only in HF patients to manage self-care but also to conduct caregiver training is an important goal, mainly for palliative care in patients with end-stage HF.[83] In this context, strategies can be conducted by an appropriately trained, local, multiprofessional team, in close proximity to where a patient lives, creating an opportunity to implement local, home- or community-based CR programming. Additionally, training local health professionals may allow for the expanded delivery of formal outpatient CR programs in small hospitals with a basic CR team (ie, physician, exercise scientist or physical therapist, psychologist, and nutritionist)[54] could be safe and feasible, especially for high-risk patients.

Finally, in HF patients hospitalized for an acute decompensation, low-intensity ET and respiratory exercises[84,85] have shown to be safe[86] and improve exercise capacity,[87] even in patients undergoing intravenous inotropic support.[88] The goal of this approach is to preserve muscle mass, minimize the risk of complications, and accelerate time to discharge, reducing costs and preparing the patient for outpatient CR.[86]

SUMMARY

The incidence and prevalence of HF in SA countries is currently a significant concern and will continue to be so for the foreseeable future. CR programming, although clearly beneficial for patients with HF, suffers from an insufficient infrastructure to support current needs. In addition, referral, attendance, and adherence issues are all concerns in SA counties for eligible patients who can actually attend a CR program. It is therefore essential to expand CR delivery and develop new strategies that could allow more HF patients to have access to CR services. Finally, new studies, conducted in SA countries, should be undertaken to assess the safety and efficacy of CR, particularly in patients with Chagas HF.

REFERENCES

1. Yusuf S, Reddy S, Ounpuu S, et al. Global burden of cardiovascular diseases: part I: general considerations, the epidemiologic transition, risk factors, and impact of urbanization. Circulation 2001; 104(22):2746–53.
2. Bocchi EA. Heart failure in South America. Curr Cardiol Rev 2013;9(2):147–56.
3. Gersh BJ, Sliwa K, Mayosi BM, et al. Novel therapeutic concepts: the epidemic of cardiovascular disease in the developing world: global implications. Eur Heart J 2010;31(6):642–8.
4. World Health Organization. WHO global status report on no communicable diseases. Geneva (Switzerland): World Health Organization; 2011.
5. Mansur Ade P, Favarato D. Mortality due to cardiovascular diseases in Brazil and in the metropolitan region of São Paulo: a 2011 update. Arq Bras Cardiol 2012;99(2):755–61.
6. Braunwald E. Heart failure. JACC Heart Fail 2013; 1(1):1–20.
7. Schocken DD, Benjamin EJ, Fonarow GC, et al. Prevention of heart failure: a scientific statement from the American Heart Association Councils on Epidemiology and Prevention, Clinical Cardiology, Cardiovascular Nursing, and High Blood Pressure Research; Quality of Care and Outcomes Research Interdisciplinary Working Group; and Functional Genomics and Translational Biology Interdisciplinary Working Group. Circulation 2008;117: 2544–65.
8. Nogueira PR, Rassi S, Corrêa Kde S. Epidemiological, clinical e therapeutic profile of heart failure in a tertiary hospital. Arq Bras Cardiol 2010;95(3): 392–8.
9. Mendez GF, Cowie MR. The epidemiological features of heart failure in developing countries; a review of the literature. Int J Cardiol 2001;80:213–9.
10. Ministério da Saúde. Datasus. Informações de Saúde. Estatísticas vitais. Disponível em: http://www.datasus.gov.br. Accessed February 10, 2014.
11. Sociedade Brasileira de Cardiologia. Revisão das II Diretrizes da Sociedade Brasileira de Cardiologia

para o diagnóstico e tratamento da insuficiência cardíaca. Arq Bras Cardiol 2002;79(suppl 4):1–30.

12. Mangini S, Silveira FS, Silva CP, et al. Descompensated heart failure in the emergency department. Arq Bras Cardiol 2008;90(6):400–6.

13. Castro P, Vukasovic JL, Garcés E, et al. Insuficiencia Cardíaca: Registro y Organización. Cardiac failure in Chilean hospitals: results of the National Registry of Heart Failure, ICARO. Rev Med Chil 2004;132(6):655–62.

14. Castro GP, Verdejo PH, Vukasovic RJ, et al. Predictors of hospital death and prolonged hospitalization in patients with cardiac failure in Chilean hospitals. Rev Med Chil 2006;134(9):1083–91.

15. Vukasovic RJ, Castro GP, Sepúlveda ML, et al. Characteristics of heart failure with preserved ejection fraction: results of the Chilean national registry of heart failure, ICARO. Rev Med Chil 2006;134(5):539–48.

16. Doval HC, Nul DR, Grancelli HO, et al. Grupo de Estudio de la Sobrevida en la Insuficiencia Cardiaca en Argentina (GESICA). Randomised trial of low-dose amiodarone in severe congestive heart failure. Lancet 1994;344(8921):493–8.

17. Cubillos-Garzón LA, Casas JP, Morillo CA, et al. Congestive HF in Latin America: the next epidemic. Am Heart J 2004;147:412–7.

18. Bocchi EA, Guimarães G, Tarasoutshi F, et al. Cardiomyopathy, adult valve disease and Heart failure in South America. Heart 2008;95:181–9.

19. Bocchi EA, Vilas-Boas F, Perrone S, Grupo de Estudos de Insuficiência Cardíaca, Brazilian Society of Cardiology, Argentine Federation of Cardiology, Argentine Society of Cardiology, Chilean Society of Cardiology, Costa Rican Association of Cardiology, Colombian Society of Cardiology, Equatorian Society of Cardiology, Guatemalan Association of Cardiology, Peruvian Society of Cardiology, Uruguayan Society of Cardiology, Venezuelan Society of Cardiology, Mexican Society of Cardiology, Mexican Society of Heart Failure, Interamerican Society of Heart Failure. I Latin America guidelines for the assessment and management of decompensated heart failure. Arq Bras Cardiol 2005;85(Suppl 3):1–48 [in English, Portuguese].

20. Fairman E, Thierer J, Rodríguez L, et al. Registro Nacional de Internación por Insuficiencia Cardíaca 2007 National registry of hospitalization for heart failure 2007. Rev Argent Cardiol 2009;77:33–9.

21. BREATHE Investigators. Rationale and design: BREATHE registry—I Brazilian Registry of Heart Failure. Arq Bras Cardiol 2013;100(5):390–4.

22. Albanesi Filho FM. What is the current scenario for heart failure in Brazil? Arq Bras Cardiol 2005;85(3):155–6.

23. Godoy HL, Silveira JA, Segalla E, et al. Hospitalization and mortality rates for heart failure in public hospitals in São Paulo. Arq Bras Cardiol 2011;97(5):402–7.

24. Fundação Sistemo Edstadual. Portal de estatísticas do Estado de São Paulo. Available at: http://www.seade.gov.br. Accessed February 10, 2014.

25. Gaui EN, Klein CH, Oliveira GM. Mortality due to heart failure: extended analysis and temporal trend in three states of Brazil. Arq Bras Cardiol 2010;94(1):55–61.

26. Gaui EN, Oliveira GM, Klein CH. Mortality by heart failure and ischemic heart disease in Brazil from 1996 to 2011. Arq Bras Cardiol 2014;102(6):557–65.

27. Ades PA, Keteyian SJ, Balady GJ, et al. Cardiac rehabilitation exercise and self-care for chronic heart failure. JACC Heart Fail 2013;1(6):540–7.

28. Bocchi EA, Braga FG, Ferreira SM, et al. III Brazilian guidelines on chronic heart failure. Arq Bras Cardiol 2009;93(1 Suppl 1):3–70 [in Portuguese].

29. Taylor RS, Brown A, Ebrahim S, et al. Exercise-based rehabilitation for patients with coronary heart disease: systematic review and meta-analysis of randomized controlled trials. Am J Med 2004;116:682–92.

30. Witt BJ, Jacobsen SJ, Weston SA, et al. Cardiac rehabilitation after myocardial infarction in the community. J Am Coll Cardiol 2004;44:988–96.

31. Squires RW, Gau GT, Miller TD, et al. Cardiovascular rehabilitation: status. Mayo Clin Proc 1990;65:731–55.

32. Cortes-Bergoderi M, Lopez-Jimenez F, Herdy AH, et al. Availability and characteristics of cardiovascular rehabilitation programs in South America. J Cardiopulm Rehabil Prev 2013;33:33–41.

33. Working Group on Cardiac Rehabilitation and Exercise Physiology and Working Group on Heart Failure of the European Society of Cardiology. Recommendations for exercise testing in chronic heart failure patients. Eur Heart J 2001;22:37–45.

34. Pina IL, Apstein CS, Balady GJ, et al. Exercise and heart failure. A statement from the American Heart Association Committee on exercise, rehabilitation, and prevention. Circulation 2003;107:1210–25.

35. Dickstein K, Cohen-Solal A, Filippatos G, et al. ESC Guidelines for the diagnosis and treatment of acute and chronic heart failure 2008. The Task Force for the Diagnosis and Treatment of Acute and Chronic Heart Failure 2008 of the European Society of Cardiology. Developed in collaboration with the Heart Failure Association of the ESC (HFA) and endorsed by the European Society of Intensive Care Medicine (ESICM). Eur Heart J 2008;29:2388–442.

36. Carvalho VO, Ciolac EG, Guimarães EV, et al. Effect of exercise training on 24-Hour ambulatory blood pressure monitoring in heart failure patients. Congest Heart Fail 2009;15:176–80.

37. Ueno LM, Drager LF, Rodrigues AC, et al. Effects of exercise training in patients with chronic heart failure and sleep apnea. Sleep 2009;32(5):637–47.

38. Lima MO, Rocha MO, Nunes MC, et al. A randomized trial of the effects of exercise training in Chagas cardiomyopathy. Eur J Heart Fail 2010; 12:866–73.

39. Santos JM, Kowatsch I, Tsutsui JM, et al. Effects of exercise training on myocardial blood flow reserve in patients with heart failure and left ventricular systolic dysfunction. Am J Cardiol 2010;105:243–8.

40. Mendes RG, Simões RP, Costa FS, et al. Left-ventricular function and autonomic cardiac adaptations after short-term in patient cardiac rehabilitation: a prospective clinical trial. J Rehabil Med 2011;43:720–7.

41. Fialho PH, Tura BR, de Sousa AS, et al. Effects of an exercise program on the functional capacity of patients with chronic Chagas' heart disease, evaluated by cardiopulmonary testing. Rev Soc Bras Med Trop 2012;45(2):220–4.

42. de Araújo CJ, Gonçalves FS, Bittencourt HS, et al. Effects of neuromuscular electrostimulation inpatients with heart failure admitted to ward. J Cardiovasc Surg 2012;7:124.

43. Ricca-Mallada R, Migliaro ER, Piskorski J, et al. Exercise training slows down heart rate and improves deceleration and acceleration capacity in patients with heart failure. J Electrocardiol 2012;45:214–9.

44. da Silva Souza MV, Soares CC, de Oliveira JR, et al. Heart rate variability: analysis of time-domain indices in patients with chronic Chagas disease before and after an exercise program. Rev Port Cardiol 2013;32(3):219–27.

45. Myers J. Principles of exercise prescription for patients with chronic heart failure. Heart Fail Rev 2008;13:61–8.

46. Carvalho VO, Rodrigues Alves RX, Bocchi EA, et al. Heart rate dynamic during an exercise test in heart failure patients with different sensibilities of the carvedilol therapy: heart rate dynamic during exercise test. Int J Cardiol 2010;142:101–4.

47. Carvalho VO, Guimaraes GV. An overall view of physical exercise prescription and training monitoring for heart failure patients. Cardiol J 2010; 17(6):644–9.

48. Swain DP, Leutholtz BC, King ME, et al. Relationship between heart rate reserve and VO2 reserve in treadmill exercise. Med Sci Sports Exerc 1998; 30:318–21.

49. Carvalho VO, Guimaraes GV, Bocchi EA. The relationship between heart rate reserve and oxygen uptake reserve in heart failure patients on optimized and non-optimized beta-blocker therapy. Clinics (Sao Paulo) 2008;63:725–30.

50. Rassi A Jr, Rassi A, Marin-Neto JA. Chagas disease. Lancet 2010;375(9723):1388–402.

51. Schmunis GA, Yadon ZE. Chagas disease: a Latin American health problem becoming a world health problem. Acta Trop 2010;115(1–2):14–21.

52. Nunes MC, Dones W, Morillo CA, et al. Chagas disease: an overview of clinical and epidemiological aspects. J Am Coll Cardiol 2013;62(9):767–76.

53. Ribeiro AL, Nunes MP, Teixeira MM, et al. Diagnosis and management of Chagas disease and cardiomyopathy. Nat Rev Cardiol 2012;9(10):576–89.

54. Borghi-Silva A, Mendes RG, Trimer R, et al. Current trends in reducing cardiovascular disease risk factors from around the world: focus on cardiac rehabilitation in Brazil. Prog Cardiovasc Dis 2014;56(5): 536–42.

55. Bestetti RB, Muccillo G. Clinical course of Chagas' heart disease: a comparison with dilated cardiomyopathy. Int J Cardiol 1997;60(2):187–93.

56. Vilas Boas LG, Bestetti RB, Otaviano AP, et al. Outcome of Chagas cardiomyopathy in comparison to ischemic cardiomyopathy. Int J Cardiol 2013;167(2):486–90.

57. Freitas HF, Chizzola PR, Paes AT, et al. Risk stratification in a Brazilian hospital-based cohort of 1220 outpatients with heart failure: role of Chagas' heart disease. Int J Cardiol 2005;102(2):239–47.

58. Rassi Junior A, Gabriel Rassi A, Gabriel Rassi S, et al. Ventricular arrhythmia in Chagas disease. Diagnostic, prognostic, and therapeutic features. Arq Bras Cardiol 1995;65(4):377–87.

59. Ribeiro AL, Cavalvanti PS, Lombardi F, et al. Prognostic value of signal-averaged electrocardiogram in Chagas disease. J Cardiovasc Electrophysiol 2008;19(5):502–9.

60. Rassi A Jr, Rassi A, Little WC, et al. Development and validation of a risk score for predicting death in Chagas' heart disease. N Engl J Med 2006; 355(8):799–808.

61. Rassi A Jr, Rassi SG, Rassi A. Sudden death in Chagas' disease. Arq Bras Cardiol 2001;76(1): 75–96.

62. Carrasco HA, Guerrero L, Parada H, et al. Ventricular arrhythmias and left ventricular myocardial function in chronic chagasic patients. Int J Cardiol 1990;28(1):35–41.

63. Ribeiro AL, Moraes RS, Ribeiro JP, et al. Parasympathetic dysautonomia precedes left ventricular systolic dysfunction in Chagas disease. Am Heart J 2001;141(2):260–5.

64. Villar JC, Leon H, Morillo CA. Cardiovascular autonomic function testing in asymptomatic T. cruzi carriers: a sensitive method to identify subclinical Chagas' disease. Int J Cardiol 2004;93(2–3):189–95.

65. Bocchi EA. Exercise training in Chagas' cardiomyopathy: trials are welcome for this neglected heart disease. Eur J Heart Fail 2010;12(8):782–4.

66. Silva MS, Bocchi EA, Guimaraes GV, et al. Benefits of exercise training in the treatment of

heart failure: study with a control group. Arquivos brasileiros de cardiologia 2002;79(4):351–62.

67. Andrade JP, Marin-Neto JA, Paola AA, et al. I Latin American guidelines for the diagnosis and treatment of Chagas cardiomyopathy. Arquivos brasileiros de cardiologia 2011;97(2 Suppl 3):1–48.

68. Rassi A Jr, Rassi A, Rassi SG. Predictors of mortality in chronic Chagas disease: a systematic review of observational studies. Circulation 2007;115(9): 1101–8.

69. O'Connor CM, Whellan DJ, Lee KL, et al. Efficacy and safety of exercise training in patients with chronic heart failure: HF-ACTION randomized controlled trial. JAMA 2009;301:1439–50.

70. Salvetti XM, Oliveira JA, Servantes DM, et al. How much do the benefits cost? Effects of a home-based training programme on cardiovascular fitness, quality of life, programme cost and adherence for patients with coronary disease. Clin Rehabil 2008;22(10–11):987–96.

71. Kühr EM, Ribeiro RA, Rohde LE, et al. Cost-effectiveness of supervised exercise therapy in heart failure patients. Value Health 2011;14(5 Suppl 1): S100–7.

72. Barbour KA, Miller NH. Adherence to exercise training in heart failure: a review. Heart Fail Rev 2008;13:81–9.

73. Bocalini DS, dos Santos L, Serra AJ. Physical exercise improves the functional capacity and quality of life in patients with heart failure. Clinics (Sao Paulo) 2008;63(4):437–42.

74. Ghisi GL, Santos RZ, Schveitzer V, et al. Development and validation of the Brazilian Portuguese version of the cardiac rehabilitation barriers scale. Arq Bras Cardiol 2012;98(4):344–52.

75. Domingues FB, Clausell N, Aliti GB, et al. Education and telephone monitoring by nurses of patients with heart failure: randomized clinical trial. Arq Bras Cardiol 2011;96(3):233–9.

76. Mussi CM, Ruschel K, de Souza EN, et al. Home visit improves knowledge, self-care and adhesion in heart failure: randomized clinical trial HELEN-I. Rev Lat Am Enfermagem 2013;21(Spec No):20–8.

77. Bimbi BJ, Unger P, Vandenbossche JL, et al. Chagas disease: don't forget it in Latin American patients with heart block! Acta Cardiol 2014;69(2): 206–8.

78. Rabelo ER, Aliti GB, Goldraich L, et al. Non-pharmacological management of patients hospitalized with heart failure at a teaching hospital. Arq Bras Cardiol 2006;87(3):352–8.

79. de Melo Ghisi GL, Oh P, Benetti M, et al. Barriers to cardiac rehabilitation use in Canada versus Brazil. J Cardiopulm Rehabil Prev 2013;33(3):173–9.

80. Ghisi GL, dos Santos RZ, Aranha EE, et al. Perceptions of barriers to cardiac rehabilitation use in Brazil. Vasc Health Risk Manag 2013;9:485–91.

81. Servantes DM, Pelcerman A, Salvetti XM, et al. Effects of home-based exercise training for patients with chronic heart failure and sleep apnoea: a randomized comparison of two different programmes. Clin Rehabil 2012;26(1):45–57.

82. Scherr D, Kastner P, Kollmann A, et al. Effect of home-based telemonitoring using mobile phone technology on the outcome of heart failure patients after an episode of acute decompensation: randomized controlled trial. J Med Internet Res 2009; 11(3):e34.

83. Abete P, Testa G, Della-Morte D, et al. Treatment for chronic heart failure in the elderly: current practice and problems. Heart Fail Rev 2013; 18(4):529–51.

84. Reis MS, Arena R, Archiza B, et al. Deep breathing heart rate variability is associated with inspiratory muscle weakness in chronic heart failure. Physiother Res Int 2014;19(1):16–24.

85. Reis MS, Deus AP, Simões RP, et al. Autonomic control of heart rate in patients with chronic cardiorespiratory disease and in healthy participants at rest and during a respiratory sinus arrhythmia maneuver. Rev Bras Fisioter 2010;14(2):106–13.

86. Rossi Caruso FC, Arena R, Mendes RG, et al. Heart rate autonomic responses during deep breathing and walking in hospitalised patients with chronic heart failure. Disabil Rehabil 2011;33(9):751–7.

87. Houchen L, Watt A, Boyce S, et al. A pilot study to explore the effectiveness of "early" rehabilitation after a hospital admission for chronic heart failure. Physiother Theory Pract 2012;28(5):355–8.

88. Arena R, Humphrey R, Peberdy MA. Safety and efficacy of exercise training in a patient awaiting heart transplantation while on positive intravenous inotropic support. J Cardiopulm Rehabil 2000; 20(4):259–61.

Exercise Therapy for Heart Failure Patients in Canada

James A. Stone, MD, PhD, FRCPC[a,b,*],
Trina Hauer, BPAS, MSc[a], Mark Haykowsky, PhD[c],
Sandeep Aggarwal, MD, FRCPC[a,b]

KEYWORDS

• Functional capacity • Disability • Aerobic capacity • Muscular strength • Muscular endurance

KEY POINTS

- Contemporary heart failure (HF) pharmacologic therapies are intended to improve ventricular function and reduce ventricular afterload.
- HF patients have significant central and peripheral deconditioning.
- Incidence of HF in Canada is similar to other industrialized countries.
- HF patients require carefully tailored, individualized exercise programs.
- Exercise therapy for HF patients, both aerobic and resistance training, should start with ultrashort episodes of exercise activity, gradually increasing the frequency and duration of the exercise episodes.

INTRODUCTION

Time was when a diagnosis of congestive heart failure (HF) gave rise to the treatment of patients with digoxin and diuretics. Although these therapies almost invariably acutely improved patient's symptoms, mostly through a reduction in volume overload, decades later they were shown to probably hasten mortality, possibly through increased sympathetic activation.[1] In contemporary cardiology practice, beta blockers for severe left ventricular (LV) systolic dysfunction, once contraindicated; ace inhibitors or angiotensin receptor blockers; aldosterone inhibitors; and judicious use of diuretics, often on an as-needed basis based on weight and symptoms, have become the mainstays of pharmacologic therapy.[2] Despite these significant and substantial advances in medical therapy, with subsequent significant and substantial reductions in mortality, many patients remain significantly debilitated from a functional capacity perspective.

What has not been generally appreciated in the medical community, even the cardiology community or the wider associated health care professions, is the massive deconditioning influence of systolic HF on skeletal muscle aerobic function, along with reductions in capillary density, and thus aerobic capacity.[3] Many individuals, despite optimal pharmacologic therapy, continue to have significant functional impairment with concomitant shortness of breath during exertion. The general assumption is that these individuals are short of breath secondary to reduced cardiac output from their LV systolic dysfunction, even in the absence of volume overload or elevations in b-type natriuretic peptide (BNP) levels. Decades of medical dogma dictated that if patients can improve their LV function, they could reduce their symptoms of exertional breathlessness. Like most dogma, it

[a] Cardiac Wellness Institute of Calgary, Calgary, Alberta, Canada; [b] Libin Cardiovascular Institute of Alberta, University of Calgary, Calgary, Alberta, Canada; [c] Department of Physical Therapy, University of Alberta, Edmonton, Alberta, Canada
* Corresponding author. Suite 306, 803 1st Avenue Northeast, Calgary, Alberta T2E 7C5, Canada.
E-mail address: JStone@totalcardiology.ca

Heart Failure Clin 11 (2015) 83–88
http://dx.doi.org/10.1016/j.hfc.2014.08.011
1551-7136/15/$ – see front matter © 2015 Elsevier Inc. All rights reserved.

was based on personal and professional beliefs rather than hard science.

In reality, patients with significant LV systolic dysfunction are often deconditioned from an aerobic capacity perspective, because of a significant reduction in oxidative enzymes within skeletal muscle. With reductions in forward blood flow, as a consequence of reduced cardiac output from LV systolic function, there is less tissue oxygenation of skeletal muscle (**Fig. 1**).[3,4] At a very simplistic level, the reduction in tissue oxygenation eventually translates into a reduction in oxidative enzymes within skeletal muscle. Interestingly, in the same manner that deprivation of myocardial blood flow can produce a reduction in myocyte function and subsequent hibernating myocardium, the same deprivation of oxygen at the skeletal muscle level may result in the reduced

formation of oxidative enzymes in order to protect skeletal muscle from oxidative injury.[5]

From a patient perspective, it makes little difference whether their exertional shortness of breath and physical incapacitation are secondary to diminished cardiac output or secondary to diminished oxidative enzymes and energy production within the working skeletal muscles. Patients understand that within hours, even days, after a major cardiac insult that reduces cardiac output, anything other than minimal exertion causes significant shortness of breath. In hyperacute and acute situations, this is almost certainly a manifestation of poor cardiac output. Very quickly, however, the reduced cardiac output translates into reduced oxidative enzymes, reduced capillary density, and reduced energy production at the level of the skeletal muscle.

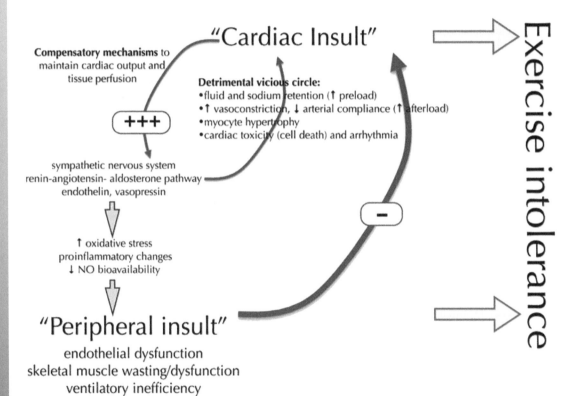

Fig. 1. Determinants of exercise intolerance in patients with chronic heart failure. Reduced cardiac performance will trigger compensatory neuro-hormonal mechanisms to preserve cardiac output, blood pressure and organ perfusion; these include the renin-angiotensinaldosterone pathway, the sympathetic nervous system, increased levels of endothelin and vasopressin. However, as these compensatory systems become chronically stimulated, they initiate a vicious circle and cause cardiotoxicity, myocyte hypertrophy/death, changes in peripheral and coronary artery compliance and excessive fluid retention. Progressively, other detrimental pathways are turned on, leading to oxidative stress, a pro-inflammatory status and reduced nitric oxide (NO) bioavailability, which initiate peripheral maladaptations, such as peripheral endothelial dysfunction, skeletal muscle wasting and ventilator inefficiency occur. Both central cardiac and hemodynamic changes, as well as these peripheral abnormalities will determine the heart failure phenotype and will culminate in symptoms of exercise intolerance. (*From* Conraads VM, Van Craenenbroeck EM, De Maeyer C, et al. Unraveling new mechanisms of exercise intolerance in chronic heart failure. Role of exercise training. Heart Fail Rev 2013;18:66; with permission.)

Contemporary pharmacotherapy of HF, particularly with beta-blockers and renin angiotensin aldosterone system antagonists, can frequently result in increases in cardiac output.[2] However, as already pointed out, this is only half of the exercise intolerance equation. The other half of the equation is what happens at the level of the skeletal muscle. Furthermore, it is overly simplistic to look at cardiac output and the oxidative generation of skeletal muscle energy as the only 2 major components contributing to an individual's functional capacity. Exercise training not only increases levels of oxidative enzymes within skeletal muscle, it also increases motor unit recruitment within skeletal muscle, thereby increasing muscle efficiency. In addition, exercise training also reduces sympathetic tone and tends to increase parasympathetic tone, both of these alterations having favorable effects on outcomes and exercise capacity. Along with these favorable changes in a patient's neurohormonal status and central nervous system tone, is the favorable influence of exercise training on ventricular–vascular coupling. Exercise training in persons with HF may promote improved afterload reduction, and improved ventricular–vascular coupling, through increased peripheral vasodilation in working skeletal muscles, as a consequence of exercise.[3] Indeed, improvements in ventricular–vascular coupling, as a result of exercise training, are likely to have a much more significant contribution to improvements in functional capacity in patients with HF than has been appreciated previously.[6]

This article will examine the current incidence of HF in Canada, recommendations for the treatment of HF in Canada, and recommendations for the use of exercise therapy in patients with HF in Canada.

INCIDENCE OF HEART FAILURE IN CANADA

The prevalence of HF in the general adult population in Canada is estimated to be in the range of 1.5%, with an annual incidence of approximately 0.5%.[7] Large, diagnostic code-based government databases do not differentiate between those with significant LV systolic dysfunction as the etiology of their HF versus those with preserved LV ejection fractions. Historically, most patients with HF were felt to have significant LV systolic dysfunction. However, with the general aging of the baby boomer population, approximately 50% of patients now seen in HF clinics in Canada have HF with preserved LV ejection fractions.[2] Once a diagnosis of HF has been established, most patients in Canada will eventually undergo an imaging study to differentiate HF

secondary to ventricular systolic dysfunction versus HF with a preserved ejection fraction.[2] As with most westernized medical models, the diagnosis of HF is based on a combination of symptoms, exertional breathlessness, orthopnea, paroxysmal nocturnal dyspnea (PND), nocturnal cough, peripheral edema, physical examination evidence of volume overload, elevated jugular venous pressure (JVP), wet lung crackles, peripheral edema, as well as ancillary imaging test such as chest radiographs and echocardiograms. Following these investigations, those patients appropriate for revascularization therapy will generally undergo invasive revascularization. In the last decade, the use of BNP levels has increased significantly and has been used to help to establish the diagnosis of HF, particularly in circumstances in which clinical or imaging evaluation is ambiguous.[2]

TREATMENT RECOMMENDATIONS FOR HEART FAILURE IN CANADA

For almost a decade, practitioners in Canada have had the benefit of using evidence-informed clinical practice guidelines for the diagnosis and management of HF.[2] These guidelines emphasize the importance of appropriate diagnosis, investigation, treatment, ongoing monitoring, and optimal patient disposition (eg, HF clinics, family practice, internal medicine, and cardiology practice). Recommended pharmacologic therapies and interventions include as-needed diuretics acutely and chronically to relieve volume overload, the use of aldosterone antagonists, the use of beta-blockers, and, where clinically indicated, supplemental inclusion of digoxin, hydralazine, and long-acting nitrates. In addition, depending on the patient's clinical circumstances, the implantation of an implantable cardioverter defibrillator (ICD) may be appropriate, as is the institution of pacemaker-mediated cardiac resynchronization therapy.[2]

In 2004, the Canadian Association of Cardiac Rehabilitation (CACR) issued the first Canadian evidence-informed guidelines on the use of exercise therapy in patients with a history of congestive HF.[8] At that point in time, the benefits of exercise therapy in patients with HF were mostly limited to clinical trials demonstrating improvements in functional capacity, improvements in skeletal muscle mitochondrial size and density, improvements in skeletal muscle oxidative enzymes, reductions in arterial endothelial dysfunction, decreases in circulating catecholamines, and improvements in exertional breathlessness, general fatigue, sleep disturbances, and muscle weakness.[8] The Heart

Failure - A Controlled Trial Investigating Outcomes of Exercise Training (HF-ACTION) trial was published in 2009.[9] In Canada, as elsewhere around the world, the lack of a clearly demonstrable improvement in hard outcomes, without adjusting for baseline patient characteristics, observed within the largest randomized controlled trial of exercise therapy in patients with documented systolic dysfunction, was to say the least disappointing. Not surprisingly, many practitioners in the field of cardiac rehabilitation and exercise therapy simply refused to believe the results and questioned the adherence of patients to the prescribed intervention. Indeed, subsequent analysis of the HF-ACTION exercise training intervention indicated that, at any point during the study, only 30% of the patients in the intervention group were reaching their targeted weekly exercise times, compared with a similar number of patients in the nonintervention group.[10]

The 2009 CACR guideline provided specific recommendations concerning the use of aerobic training and resistance training and highlighted the need for enhanced patient surveillance, principally with increased numbers of exercise therapists supervising limited numbers of patients, as well as the importance of closer hemodynamic, rhythm, and rate of perceived exertion monitoring.[11]

TREATMENT RECOMMENDATIONS FOR USE OF EXERCISE THERAPY IN HEART FAILURE PATIENTS

In addition to the evidence-informed treatment investigations from the CACR, in 2013, the Canadian Cardiovascular Society Heart Failure Guidelines Working Group issued similar recommendations.[10] These guidelines were, however, specifically targeted at a physician population, principally internal medicine specialists and cardiologists. These guidelines, like the CACR guidelines, encourage the use of exercise training in patients with documented HF. Taking into account the significant shortcomings of the HF-ACTION trial as the definitive statement on the benefits, or lack thereof, of exercise therapy in patients with HF, these guidelines emphasize the important contribution exercise therapy may have in improving patients functional capacity and quality of life. With respect to aerobic training, these guidelines acknowledge the clinical fact documented in previous exercise and HF guidelines, and observed by practitioners in the field, that patients with acute, chronic, and acute-on-chronic HF may only be capable of sustaining aerobic or resistance training exercises for a very short period of time (ie, seconds to minutes).

However, with patience and diligence, 10-second bouts of aerobic training, such as walking, can turn into 20 seconds, which can turn into 30 seconds, and so on. The key in this patient population is not to push patients too hard and not to become frustrated with an apparent lack of progression. As indicated in the opening paragraphs, most of these patients are tremendously deconditioned from a skeletal muscle aerobic activity perspective, even when their cardiac function has been maximized, and thus it will take 10 to 12 weeks or longer, to obtain clinically obvious improvements in functional capacity. The exercise mantra for this patient population is absolutely, "Start with low exercise interval durations and increase the duration slowly."

In noncardiac populations, interval training, using bouts of higher intensities interspersed with bouts at lower intensities, is regarded by many as an optimal training method for obtaining higher increases in aerobic capacity. What limits most patient populations, cardiac patients and healthy individuals alike, is the effort required during high-intensity exercise. Not surprisingly, however, it is precisely this high-intensity effort that provides greater improvements in functional capacity. For patients with coronary artery disease, high-intensity interval training looks very attractive and may potentially lead to long-term reductions in major adverse cardiac events.[12] The use of high-intensity interval training in patients with HF is not commonplace in Canadian rehabilitation practices; if practitioners are generally fearful of performing high-intensity interval training in cardiac populations with documented coronary artery disease, they are even more leery in patients with HF. Initial evidence indicates the same may be true for patients with HF.[13] Specifically, a recent major meta-analyses by Haykowsky and colleagues[14] demonstrated that high-intensity interval training was significantly more effective than typical moderate-intensity continuous exercise training in patients with HF. Specifically, of 168 HF patients randomized to usual exercise therapy or high-intensity interval training, patients in the high-intensity interval training group obtained significantly higher increases in their maximal oxygen consumption.[14]

For patients with HF who are severely debilitated at the onset of exercise training, ultrashort, 5- to 20-second bursts of low- to moderate-intensity exercise interspersed with rest periods, may be a useful approach until a functional reserve is established. In addition, although data are limited, external support or the use of antigravity treadmills may allow for debilitated HF patients to exercise longer and thus increase functional capacity faster at the onset of an exercise training program. The use of antigravity treadmills in a very small randomized clinical trial has suggested they may be beneficial in helping morbidly obese patients attain weight loss.[15] Morbidly obese individuals are often also significantly deconditioned from a skeletal muscle aerobic capacity perspective. It is interesting to speculate that antigravity treadmills or externally supported walking with harnesses could significantly improve, potentially in a much shorter period of time, aerobic capacity in HF patients with severe disability.

Patients with HF may also benefit from resistance training.[8,10,11] Resistance training in this patient population may improve the ability to perform activities of daily living and quality of life; it may also increase skeletal muscle mass and strength, and potentially as a consequence of the increase in muscle mass, may also improve insulin resistance.[8,10,11] As with aerobic training, HF patients should start with light weights that easily facilitate higher numbers of repetitions (ie, 15–20 repetitions). As an alternative to the use of dumbbells, many patients may benefit from utilizing thera-bands as an alternative. Thera-bands have the advantage of being relatively inexpensive and portable; additionally, they may allow HF patients, particularly elderly ones, to perform resistance training activities within their own daily living environment.

SUMMARY

The diagnosis and management of HF in Canada is not significantly different from most industrialized countries throughout the world. Significant advances in pharmacologic therapy, in conjunction with targeted revascularization therapies, have helped to significantly improve outcomes for patients with HF. However, improvements in functional capacity and quality of life have lagged behind. From a patient perspective, quality of life is extremely important. Individuals with HF look forward to mobilizing on a daily basis without being extremely short of breath and fatigued. Exercise therapy for patients with HF, both aerobic training and resistance training, may significantly improve patient symptoms. Those patients who participate in an exercise program may also see significant improvements in their longevity and reductions in rehospitalization for HF. The exercise modalities available for patients with HF are changing rapidly. In particular, high-intensity interval training may become the preferred mode of exercise therapy for certain HF patients. In addition, helping severely debilitated HF patients improve their aerobic capacity through partially supported

weight exercise therapies, such as aquasize or use of antigravity treadmills or harnesses, may also lead to significant exercise improvements. Fortunately, the prognosis for HF patients in Canada has never been more optimistic and has never looked brighter. In the management of patients with HF in Canada, exercise therapy is one of the cornerstones to the attainment of enhanced longevity and improved quality of life.

REFERENCES

1. Hasselblad V, Stough WG, Shah MR, et al. Relation between dose of loop diuretics and outcomes in a heart failure population: results of the ESCAPE trial. Eur J Heart Fail 2007;9:1064–9.
2. McKelvie RS, Moe GW, Ezekowitz JA, et al. The 2012 Canadian Cardiovascular Society heart failure management guidelines update: focus on acute and chronic heart failure. Can J Cardiol 2012;29:168–81.
3. Arena R, Cahalin LP, Borghi-Silva A, et al. Improving functional capacity in heart failure: the need for a multi-faceted approach. Curr Opin Cardiol 2014;29:467–74.
4. Conraads VM, Van Craenenbroek EM, De Maeyer C, et al. Unraveling new mechanisms of exercise intolerance in chronic heart failure. Role of exercise training. Heart Fail Rev 2013;18:65–77.
5. Tabet JL, Meurin P, Ben Driss A, et al. Benefits of exercise training in chronic heart failure. Arch Cardiovasc Dis 2011;102:721–30.
6. Borlang BA, Kass DA. Ventricular-vascular interaction in heart failure. Cardiol Clin 2011;29:447–59.
7. Available at: www.heartandstroke.com/site/c.iklQLc MWJtE/b.3483991/k.34A8/Statistics.htm#references. Accessed July 30, 2014.
8. Haennel RG, Tomczak C, Haykowsky M, et al. Special populations. In: Stone JA, Arthur HM, editors. Canadian Association of Cardiac Rehabilitation guidelines for cardiac rehabilitation and cardiovascular disease prevention. Winnipeg (Canada): Canadian Association of Cardiac Rehabilitation; 2014. p. 258–308.
9. O'Conner CM, Whellan DJ, Lee KL, et al. Efficacy and safety of exercise training in patients with chronic heart failure: HF-ACTION randomized controlled trial. JAMA 2009;301:1439–50.
10. Moe GW, Ezekowitz JA, O'Mera E, et al. The 2013 Canadian Cardiovascular Society heart failure management guidelines update: focus on rehabilitation exercise and surgical coronary revascularization. Can J Cardiol 2014;30:249–63.
11. Haennel RG, Brassard CP, Tomczak C, et al. Special populations. In: Stone JA, Arthur HM, Suskin N, editors. Canadian Association of Cardiac Rehabilitation guidelines for cardiac rehabilitation and cardiovascular disease prevention. Winnipeg

(Canada): Canadian Association of Cardiac Rehabilitation; 2009. p. 449–515.

12. Mezzani A, Hamm LF, Jones AM, et al. Aerobic exercise intensity assessment and prescription in cardiac rehabilitation: a joint position statement of the European Association for Cardiovascular Prevention and Rehabilitation, the American Association of Cardiovascular and Pulmonary Rehabilitation, and the Canadian Association of Cardiac Rehabilitation. Eur J Prev Cardiol 2013;20:442–67.

13. Arena R, Myers J, Forman DE, et al. Should high intensity aerobic interval training become the clinical standard heart failure? Heart Fail Rev 2013;18:95–105.

14. Haykowsky MJ, Timmons MP, Kruger C, et al. meta-analysis of aerobic interval training on exercise capacity and systolic function in patients with heart failure and reduced ejection fractions. Am J Cardiol 2013;111:1466–9.

15. Available at: http://scholarworks.boisestate.edu/td/857. Accessed August 11, 2014.

Rehabilitation Practice Patterns for Patients with Heart Failure
The United States Perspective

Daniel E. Forman, MD

KEYWORDS

- Heart failure • Heart failure with reduced ejection fraction
- Heart failure with preserved ejection fraction • Exercise training • Cardiac rehabilitation • Adherence

KEY POINTS

- The United States is a leader among worldwide research initiatives showing benefits of exercise training for heart failure.
- Enrollment in cardiac rehabilitation in the United States remains poor.
- There are many impediments to cardiac rehabilitation enrollment and adherence in the United States that seem likely to persist irrespective of the fact that heart failure has recently been approved as an eligible diagnosis for cardiac rehabilitation.
- There are predominant shifts in the health care environment in the United States, particularly an increase in Accountable Care Organizations, which are placing greater priority in value of care (ie, changes that seem likely to bolster the application of cardiac rehabilitation for heart failure).

INTRODUCTION

Although many anticipate the recent decision of the US Center for Medicare Services (CMS) to expand cardiac rehabilitation (CR) reimbursement to include patients with systolic heart failure (HF) as a likely catalyst to expand use of exercise therapy for eligible HF patients,[1] this still remains uncertain. Although the United States has played a prominent role amid worldwide research and clinical evolution of CR for over 50 years, US patterns of referral to and enrollment in CR have remained poor.[2-4] Multiple studies show a generally consistent pattern of significant under-referral, under-enrollment, and high attrition. Patients with acute coronary syndromes (ACS), chronic coronary heart disease (CHD), revascularization, valvular heart disease, and heart transplant have all been eligible for CR for years (ie, eligible for enrollment and backed by insurance/Medicare), but only a small fraction of the suitable candidates participate. Such relatively ineffectual application and clinical impact of CR for CHD suggest that there are entrenched obstacles that limit the uptake of CR in the United States that may undercut its conceptual potential to benefit HF patients.[5,6]

Many specific reasons for the historical underuse of CR for CHD in the United States have been identified: logistic barriers, high co-payments, and inadequate patient understanding of potential benefits have all been implicated and particularly affect women, minorities, elderly, and those with lower socioeconomic status.[7] Commitment to CR by many administrators may also be undermined by the high costs required for the CR infrastructure and staff. Only exceptional CR programs achieve high enrollment and patient retention; more typically, programs are

Geriatric Cardiology Section, 3471 Fifth Avenue, Suite 500, Pittsburgh, PA 15213, USA
E-mail address: formand@pitt.edu

Heart Failure Clin 11 (2015) 89–94
http://dx.doi.org/10.1016/j.hfc.2014.08.010
1551-7136/15/$ – see front matter © 2015 Elsevier Inc. All rights reserved.

heartfailure.theclinics.com

undersized, fail to enroll many eligible candidates, and often struggle with the threat of closure amid financial deficits.[8] Given all these complicated dynamics, CR is often regarded by providers and patients as a superfluous adjunct to care rather than as essential component of therapy.

However, the future potential of CR is also fortified by dynamic changes in contemporary US health care. Growing emphasis on "value" of care, accountable care, patient-reported outcomes, and goals to minimize rehospitalizations are all contributing to increased interest in CR among a wide spectrum of providers, administrators, and even policyleaders.[9] These shifts portend greater prioritization and application of CR for HF patients in the near future, and even the potential to overcome many entrenched logistic, financial, and behavioral barriers.

A CARDIAC REHABILITATION LEGACY IN THE UNITED STATES

As an international academic and clinical frontrunner, the US role has fostered the science and implementation of CR for CHD and HF. The seminal research of Levine and Lown[10] to mobilize ACS patients led, for example, to the fundamental shift away from what had been strict bed rest and immobility for weeks after a myocardial infarction, and toward early mobilization and progressive activity. Likewise, the conspicuous and controversial exercise treatment used by Paul Dudley White for his renowned patient, President Dwight Eisenhower, after a myocardial infarction (during his first term in office)[11] served as a prominent endorsement of exercise therapy for ACS, and bolstered the concurrent efforts of Hellerstein and Ford,[12,13] Wenger,[14] and other US CR pioneers to organize and implement the original inpatient and out-patient CR programs.

More recently, the prominent of role of the United States in relation to exercise and HF was evident when the National Institutes of Health sponsored the large and expensive HF-ACTION trial (Heart Failure: A Controlled Trial Investigating Outcomes of Exercise Training).[15] Although CR for CHD has relied primarily on meta-analyses as the basis for claims regarding CR survival benefits,[16–18] raising criticisms of selection bias and exaggerated treatment effects, HF-ACTION attempted to provide a much more definitive and reliable analysis of exercise benefits for HF.

HF-ACTION assessed safety and efficacy of exercise training for medically optimized and stable patients with systolic HF (left ventricular ejection fraction [LVEF] $\leq$35%). The structured-exercise group began with 36 supervised training sessions

for 30 minutes of exercise 3 times per week.[15] Halfway through this period, patients were given a treadmill or stationary bicycle to use at home along with a heart-rate monitor and were advised to work out 5 times per week at moderate intensity for 40 minutes. The usual-care group, by contrast, was told at the study outset to try to exercise at moderate intensity, 30 minutes per day, as recommended by the current American College of Cardiology/American Heart Association (AHA) guidelines of the time,[19] but which were not supervised or encouraged along the way.

The composite primary endpoint of the study was all-cause mortality or all-cause hospital stay. Subjects with New York Heart Association functional class II to IV symptoms (n = 2331) were randomized to either 36 sessions of supervised, moderate-intensity training (60%–70% HR reserve) followed by home-based training or usual care. All subjects were followed for a median of 30 months. Outcomes included a nonsignificant reduction in the primary combined endpoint of all-cause mortality or hospital stay (hazard ratio: 0.93; P = .13). However, after adjustment for prespecified predictors of mortality (duration of the cardiopulmonary exercise test; LVEF; Beck Depression Inventory II score; history of atrial fibrillation), the primary endpoint became significant (hazard ratio: 0.89; $P<.03$).

Although these data were regarded as disappointing to some who had anticipated a more definitive attestation of exercise training mortality benefits, the fact remains that many key critical attributes of exercise training for HF were demonstrated. Indeed, adjusted data showed that exercise therapy reduced cardiac mortality and hospitalizations.[15] Moreover, total hospitalizations were reduced by 15% in the exercise group and safety of exercise training was demonstrated in the large, diverse HF study population. Furthermore, in a related study, Flynn and colleagues[20] reported significant improvements in self-reported health status in those in the exercise arm based on relatively greater improvements in the Kansas City Cardiomyopathy Questionnaire scores (mean, 5.21; 95% confidence interval, 4.42–6.00) compared with usual care alone (3.28; 95% confidence interval, 2.48–4.09) ($P<.001$).

Perhaps even more important, in a study published years after the original HF-ACTION report, Keteyian and colleagues[21] demonstrated the unambiguous survival benefits of exercise therapy for HF when exercise was assessed quantitatively. Exercise volume was a significant (P = .001) linear and logarithmic predictor of reduced all-cause mortality or hospitalization and cardiovascular mortality or HF hospitalization. Moderate exercise volumes of 3 to less than 5 metabolic equivalent (MET)-hours and 5 to less than 7 MET-hours per week were associated with reductions in subsequent risk that exceeded 30%.

Analysis by Keteyian and colleagues[21] not only demonstrates the clear benefit of exercise therapy for HF but also implicitly highlights how poor exercise adherence confounded results of the original trial. Notably, even while HF-ACTION was a well-funded trial that included many provisions to reinforce exercise training adherence, only about 30% of those in the exercise arm exercised at or above the target number of minutes per week. In a related HF-ACTION analysis, Reeves and colleagues[22] showed that this poor adherence was not predictable by standard criteria of assessment. Adherence is inherently problematic in HF patients, and adherence to exercise therapy may be particularly challenging.[23]

Thus, HF-ACTION essentially reflects well on the United States by showcasing its commitment to exercise and HF, but HF-ACTION also provides perspective regarding the difficulty of getting US enrollees to successfully maintain exercise behaviors. As a country struggling with widespread obesity, sedentary behaviors, poor sleep quality, and a surging demographic of very old adults who are prone to HF in the context of frailty, sarcopenia, pain, and multimorbidity, the challenge of advancing exercise training regimens as a US therapeutic standard may be particularly difficult.[6]

Ongoing research also highlights the impact of environment on exercise. Here again, exercise training goals are often inadvertently confounded by building or community designs that often fail to promote these priorities as part of the fundamental living configuration[24] and contribute to a sense of obstacle for exercise and/or general physical activity.

PERTINENT CHANGES IN UNITED STATES HEALTH CARE DYNAMICS
The Affordable Act

The Affordable Care Act (ACA) was initiated in 2010 as a means to better ensure patients receive high-value health care that better responds to patients' priorities and personal sense of wellness. Accountable Care Organizations (ACO) are models of care fostered by the ACA that better facilitate prevention strategies and systems of care to improve efficiencies and value of care. As ACOs continue to grow and become a more dominant standard of care, implications regarding the growth and impact of CR are also likely to escalate.[25] First, ACOs intrinsically facilitate improved access to CR to those who had previously been

deterred by financial constraints, particularly by eliminating copayments. The expectation is that women, minorities, elderly, and cardiac patients in lower socioeconomic brackets may be more likely to enroll and participate in CR.

Even more significant, ACOs elevate the priority accorded to disease prevention as well as to the overall value of care and placing greater emphasis on the quantitative/qualitative metrics achieved by prevention health care standards. Exercise training is an important ACO therapeutic option because it mitigates disease, extends active lives, and also improves patients' quality of life, self-efficacy, and functional capacity. Furthermore, the established utility of exercise therapy to reduce HF readmissions is an ever more powerful incentive both as a qualitative measure and as a means to moderate health care expenses.[26]

Although the ACOs are not specifically oriented to the issue of exercise training and HF, they provide a context in which this type of health care strategy is given greater emphasis as a common theme of care, that coalesce priorities of nurses, physicians, and other providers. Nevertheless, to do this most successfully, many of the current standards of CR in the United States may also need to be reconsidered. In a recent AHA Presidential Advisory, Balady and colleagues[25] articulated a need to possibly modify the process of CR care to better align the goals of ACOs with population needs.

Although CR is now structured as a relatively formulaic fee-for-service model with specific criteria required to document participation and payment, the AHA advisory called for consideration of new models of care in ways that achieve exercise training and wellness objectives that are more convenient and more likely to be successful. Although the AHA Advisory called for greater flexibility and creativity to achieve this potential, it also acknowledged the responsibility of investigators to prove efficacy in terms of costs, safety, enrollment, adherence, and qualitative/quantitative outcomes as models of CR care evolve.

PARTICULAR CHALLENGES REGARDING EXERCISE THERAPY FOR THE UNITED STATES POPULATION

Exercise therapy for HF presents notable challenges in the United States. Many candidates lack easy access to hospitals or providers and most are struggling with multiple medical problems in addition to HF with overall propensity to instability and complexity, and related risks of falls, incontinence, and other intrinsic risks from exercise therapy. Likewise, the subgroup of older adults with HF is rising particularly rapidly,[27] and these patients are particularly prone to cognitive changes that may confound exercise training process and efficacy. Cognitive changes are common among older HF patients, particularly impairments of executive cognition that may significantly diminish capacity to adapt to new health behaviors.[28]

In efforts to overcome some of these barriers, the United States has been leading multiple initiatives in which novel technologies are used to facilitate greater supervision and safety of exercise training for HF patients in localized settings (eg, home-based or community-based venues).[29] Studies using telemedicine as well as Skype, mobile devices, and other technologies are escalating with the common goals of overcoming logistic barriers and still preserving safety, adherence, and substantive long-lasting training effects.

UNITED STATES CONTRIBUTING TO EXPANDING MODELS OF EXERCISE TRAINING

As implicit in the content of this issue, the concept of exercise training for HF is also expanding in respect to the mode of training, and well beyond the once exclusive focus on aerobic exercise training. Strength training is a mode of exercise therapy that complements the relatively more traditional concept of continuous exercise training and extends logically from evolving insights regarding peripheral mechanisms of HF.[30] Compared with aerobic training, strength training has the potential to increase skeletal muscle mass and also to uniquely modify physiology and moderate disease.[31,32] It is particularly advantageous for HF patients suffering from frailty, sarcopenia, falls, or other complexities of management whereby increased strength or balance are critical for clinical improvement or even to enable initial aerobic capabilities.[6,33]

Inspiratory muscle training is a type of strength training that targets the large diaphragmatic muscle as well as the accessory musculature. Clinical improvements relate to improved capacity for air movement, and also to systemic metabolic effects achieved by muscle training.[34] Mancini and colleagues[35] and others in the United States have completed seminal work in this field.

High-intensity aerobic interval training differs from continuous exercise training by alternating intervals of high-intensity exercise with lower-intensity intervals thereafter.[36] The aggregate effect is higher training stimulation, with proven physiologic and clinical benefits that are well-tolerated in HF patients. The United States has played a prominent role in this literature as well as related work that better aligns the theoretic benefits of high-intensity interval training with clinical formats of CR.[37]

Finally, the prominent role of the United States of emphasizing the importance of education with respect to exercise training for HF merits emphasis.[38] Although exercise training was once actually contraindicated for HF, the United States has played a lead role in patient and provider education, such that updated insights regarding the therapeutic benefits of exercise training have been successfully promulgated.

HEART FAILURE WITH REDUCED EJECTION FRACTION VERSUS HEART FAILURE WITH PRESERVED EJECTION FRACTION

Despite the prominent impact of HF-ACTION in advancing CMS support for exercise and HF, these benefits have only been extended to patients with HF with reduced ejection fraction (HFrEF) consistent with the HF-ACTION study population. Similar remuneration is not being extended to the large and growing population of patients with HF with preserved ejection fraction (HFpEF). The logic for this discrepancy remains wanting because multiple studies from the United States and internationally provide substantive support for the rationale and efficacy of exercise therapy for HFpEF,[39] including improved vascular perfusion, skeletal muscle strength and efficiency, autonomic benefits, and metabolic benefits. Similarly, HFpEF is even more likely to be associated with comorbidity than HFrEF,[40] and many of these comorbid conditions (eg, diabetes, peripheral arterial disease, hypertension, CHD) are also likely to benefit from exercise therapy.

SUMMARY

Current use of exercise therapy for HF in the United States is in a state of evolution. Although there is strong rationale for exercise therapy for cardiovascular disease, it contrasts with a pattern of lackluster utilization of CR for CHD (ie, a pattern that bodes inauspiciously for the use of CR for HF). Still, major changes in US health care are evolving that will undoubtedly shift priorities and standards pertaining to exercise therapy for HF patients. There is strong precedent for US innovation and leadership in exercise therapy, which seems likely to merge with contemporary health care priorities to better facilitate applications of novel technologies and formats such that exercise therapy is more likely to become a key tool in the medical armamentarium for today's growing HF population. The recent decision of CMS to include

HF as an eligible diagnosis of CR payment is seen by many as an important step toward increased exercise therapy utilization for the HF population, but it also remains inconsistent and disappointing that this advance is limited only to HFrEF patients and not to those with HFpEF, a patient population that would also benefit.

ACKNOWLEDGMENTS

The author would like to thank David Whellan, MD, of Thomas Jefferson University, for his careful review of the document and for the beneficial comments he provided.

REFERENCES

1. Keteyian SJ, Squires RW, Ades PA, et al. Incorporating patient with chronic heart failure into outpatient cardiac rehabilitation. J Cardiopulm Rehabil Prev 2014;34:223–32.
2. Suaya JA, Shepard DS, Normand SL, et al. Use of cardiac rehabilitation by Medicare beneficiaries after myocardial infarction or coronary bypass surgery. Circulation 2007;116:1653–62.
3. Cortés O, Arthur HM. Determinants of referral to cardiac rehabilitation programs in patients with coronary artery disease: a systematic review. Am Heart J 2006;151:249–56.
4. Hammill BG, Curtis LH, Schulman KA, et al. Relationship between cardiac rehabilitation and long-term risks of death and myocardial infarction among elderly medicare beneficiaries. Circulation 2010; 121(1):63–70.
5. Gaalema DE, Higgins ST, Shepard DS, et al. State-by-state variations in cardiac rehabilitation participation are associated with educational attainment, income, and program availability. J Cardiopulm Rehabil Prev 2014;34:248–54.
6. Suaya J, Forman DE. Cardac rehabilitation for elderly cardiac patients. In: Cohen RA, Gunstad J, editors. Neuropsychology and cardiovascular disease. New York: Oxford University Press; 2010. p. 81–99.
7. Gurewich D, Prottas J, Bhalotra S, et al. System-level factors and use of cardiac rehabilitation. J Cardiopulm Rehabil Prev 2008;28:380–5.
8. Forman DE, Ades PA. Available at: http://commonhealth. wbur.org/2009/10/cardiovascular-disease-mismanagement-billions-for-acute-care-crumbs-for-prevention. Accessed October 28, 2009.
9. Available at: http://www.medicare.gov/hospitalcompare/linking-quality-to payment.html?AspxAutoDetectCookieSupport=1. Accessed September 24, 2014.
10. Levine SA, Lown B. "Armchair" treatment of acute coronary thrombosis. J Am Med Assoc 1952; 148(16):1365–9.
11. Lasby CG. Eisenhower's heart attack: how Ike beat heart disease and held on to the presidency. Lawrence (KS): University Press of Kansas; 1997.
12. Hellerstein HK, Ford AB. Rehabilitation of the cardiac patient. J Am Med Assoc 1957;164:225–31.
13. Katz LN, Bruce RA, Plummer N, et al. Rehabilitation of the cardiac patient. Circulation 1958;17: 114–26.
14. Wenger NK. The future of rehabilitation: a component of routine cardiac care. Adv Cardiol 1978;24: 197–201.
15. O'Connor CM, Whellan DJ, Lee KL, et al. Efficacy and safety of exercise training in patients with chronic heart failure: HF-ACTION randomized controlled trial. JAMA 2009;301:1439–50.
16. Oldridge NB, Guyatt GH, Fischer ME, et al. Cardiac rehabilitation after myocardial infarction. Combined experience of randomized clinical trials. JAMA 1988;260:945–50.
17. Taylor RS, Brown A, Ebrahim S, et al. Exercise-based rehabilitation for patients with coronary heart disease: systematic review and meta-analysis of randomized controlled trials. Am J Med 2004;116: 682–92.
18. Jolliffe JA, Rees K, Taylor RS, et al. Exercise-based rehabilitation for coronary heart disease. Cochrane Database Syst Rev 2000;(4):CD001800.
19. Hunt SA, Abraham WT, Chin MH, et al. ACC/AHA 2005 guideline update for the diagnosis and management of chronic heart failure in the adult: a report of the American College of Cardiology/American Heart Association Task Force on Practice Guidelines (Writing Committee to Update the 2001 guidelines for the evaluation and management of heart failure). J Am Coll Cardiol 2005;46:e1–82.
20. Flynn KE, Piña IL, Whellan DJ, et al. Effects of exercise training on health status in patients with chronic heart failure: HF-ACTION randomized controlled trial. JAMA 2009;301:1451–9.
21. Keteyian SJ, Leifer ES, Houston-Miller N, et al. Relation between volume of exercise and clinical outcomes in patients with heart failure. J Am Coll Cardiol 2012;60:1899–905.
22. Reeves GR, Houston-Miller N, Ellis SJ, et al. Predictors of adherence to exercise training in the Heart Failure: a controlled trial investing outcomes in exercise training study. Presented at the American Heart Association Scientific Session. Chicago (IL): November 17-20, 2002.
23. Knafl GJ, Riegel B. What puts heart failure patients at risk for poor medication adherence? Patient Prefer Adherence 2014;8:1007–18.
24. Van Dyck D, Cerin E, Conway TL, et al. Perceived neighborhood environmental attributes associated with adults' transport-related walking and cycling: findings from the USA, Australia and Belgium. Int J Behav Nutr Phys Act 2012;9:70.

25. Balady GJ, Ades PA, Bittner VA, et al. Referral, enrollment, and delivery of cardiac rehabilitation/secondary prevention programs at clinical centers and beyond: a presidential advisory from the American Heart Association. Circulation 2011;124:2951–60.

26. Available at: http://blog.cms.gov/2013/12/06/new-data-shows-affordable-care-act-reforms-are-leading-to-lower-hospital-readmission-rates-for-medicare-beneficiaries/. Accessed September 24, 2014.

27. Curtis LH, Whellan DJ, Hammill BG, et al. Incidence and prevalence of heart failure in elderly persons, 1994–2003. Arch Intern Med 2008;168:418–24.

28. Pressler SJ, Subramanian U, Kareken D. Cognitive deficits in chronic heart failure. Nurs Res 2010;59: 127–39.

29. Forman DE, LaFond K, Panch T, et al. Utility and Efficacy of a Smartphone Application to Enhance the Learning and Behavior Goals of Traditional Cardiac Rehabilitation: a FEASIBILITY STUDY. J Cardiopulm Rehabil Prev 2014;34(5):327–34.

30. Artero EG, Lee DC, Lavie CJ, et al. Effects of muscular strength on cardiovascular risk factors and prognosis. J Cardiopulm Rehabil Prev 2012; 32:351–8.

31. Forman DE, Larose SI, Wilson LB. Resistance-training strategies for older adults. In: Swank A, Hagerman P, editors. Resistance training for special populations. New York: Delmar Cenage Learning Publisher; 2009. p. 95–113.

32. Beniaminovitz A, Lang CC, LaManca J, et al. Selective low-level leg muscle training alleviates dyspnea in patients with heart failure. J Am Coll Cardiol 2002; 40:1602–8.

33. Sattelmair J, Pertman JH, Forman DE. Effects of physical activity on cardiovascular and non-cardiovascular outcomes in older adults. Clin Geriatr Med 2009;25:677–702.

34. Cahalin LP, Arena R, Guazzi M, et al. Inspiratory muscle training in heart disease and heart failure: a review of the literature with a focus on method of training and outcomes [review]. Expert Rev Cardiovasc Ther 2013;11(2):161–77. http://dx.doi.org/10.1586/erc.12.191 [Erratum in Expert Rev Cardiovasc Ther 2013;11:520].

35. Mancini DM, Henson D, La Manca J, et al. Benefit of selective respiratory muscle training on exercise capacity in patients with chronic congestive heart failure. Circulation 1995;91:320–9.

36. Wisløff U, Støylen A, Loennechen JP, et al. Superior cardiovascular effect of aerobic interval training versus moderate continuous training in heart failure patients: a randomized study. Circulation 2007; 115:3086–94.

37. Keteyian SJ, Hibner BA, Bronsteen K, et al. Greater improvement in cardiorespiratory fitness using higher-intensity interval training in the standard cardiac rehabilitation setting. J Cardiopulm Rehabil Prev 2014;34:98–105.

38. Balady GJ, Williams MA, Ades PA, et al. Core components of cardiac rehabilitation/secondary prevention programs: 2007 update: a scientific statement from the American Heart Association Exercise, Cardiac Rehabilitation, and Prevention Committee, the Council on Clinical Cardiology; the Councils on Cardiovascular Nursing, Epidemiology and Prevention, and Nutrition, Physical Activity, and Metabolism; and the American Association of Cardiovascular and Pulmonary Rehabilitation. J Cardiopulm Rehabil Prev 2007;27:121–9.

39. Haykowsky MJ, Kitzman DW. Exercise physiology in heart failure and preserved ejection fraction. Heart Fail Clin 2014;10:445–52.

40. Muzzarelli S, Leibundgut G, Maeder MT. Predictors of early readmission or death in elderly patients with heart failure. Am Heart J 2010;160:308–14.

Rehabilitation Practice Patterns for Patients with Heart Failure: The Asian Perspective

Xing-Guo Sun, MD[a,b],*

KEYWORDS

- Chronic heart failure • Cardiac rehabilitation • Exercise • Taiji • Qigong • Yoga • China • Japan

KEY POINTS

- More and more countries around world have begun to use cardiac rehabilitation in patients diagnosed with chronic heart failure (HF).
- Asia is the largest continent in the world and, depending on its economy, culture, and beliefs, a given Asian country differs from Western countries as well as others in Asia.
- The cardiac rehabilitation practice patterns for patients with HF are somewhat different in Asia. In addition to the formal pattern of Western practice, it also includes the special techniques and skills, such as Taiji, Qigong, and Yoga.
- However, these novel approaches are without regular design and strict monitoring for patients of HF and thus further research in the field.

INTRODUCTION

Chronic heart failure (HF) is a common and disabling syndrome that is a common final pathway for several cardiac conditions. Symptoms of HF include reductions in physical function and increased dyspnea and fatigue.[1] This chronic cardiac condition oftentimes accelerates deconditioning and the consequent vicious cycle of numerous associated disorders.[2] Extracardiac abnormalities and comorbidities, such as hypertension, atrial fibrillation, diabetes, renal or pulmonary disease, anemia, obesity, and physical inactivity, may increase the risk of HF. HF is a global epidemic, but clinical characteristics and treatment may vary for this chronic disease population across geographic regions.[3] From a global perspective, the increasing prevalence of HF is, however, universal as is the diminished quality of life (QOL)[4–6] and significant increase in morbidity and mortality associated with this condition. Currently, the lifetime risk of developing HF is 1 in 5 beginning at the age of 40.[7]

Asia is the largest continent in the world, occupying an area of 4400 square kilometers, accounting for 29.4% of global land area, with a total population exceeding 4 billion, accounting for about two-thirds of the world's total population. Asia has 48 countries and areas, and most of them are developing countries. Their national medical standards are generally associated with their economic level and cultural background. According to differences in economics and cultures,

Disclosures: None.
[a] State Key Laboratory of Cardiovascular Disease, Fuwai Hospital, National Center for Cardiovascular Diseases, Chinese Academy of Medical Sciences, Peking Union Medical College, 167 Beilishi Road, Xicheng District, Beijing 100037, People's Republic of China; [b] Respiratory and Critical Care Physiology and Medicine, Department of Medicine, St. John's Cardiovascular Research Center, Harbor-UCLA Medical Center, 1124 West Carson Street, RB2, Box 405, Torrance, CA 90502, USA
* State Key Laboratory of Cardiovascular Disease, Fuwai Hospital, National Center for Cardiovascular Diseases, Chinese Academy of Medical Sciences, Peking Union Medical College, 167 Beilishi Road, Xicheng District, Beijing 100037, People's Republic of China.
E-mail address: xgsun@labiomed.org

Heart Failure Clin 11 (2015) 95–104
http://dx.doi.org/10.1016/j.hfc.2014.09.001

Asia can be roughly divided into 4 different regions: the first one is developed countries represented by Japan. The second is the advanced developing countries or regions, such as Singapore, South Korea, Hong Kong, Macao, and Taiwan. The third is the larger population developing countries represented by China and India. The fourth is the others, which include South, Southeast, Mid, North, and West Asian areas and countries, predominantly in less developed or developing countries.

With economic development, a gradually westernized lifestyle, and urbanization, risk factors for cardiovascular disease (CVD) are also on the rise in all areas of Asia. As announced at the Chinese Heart Congress on August 7 to 10, 2014 in China, 4.5 million individuals had a HF diagnosis in 2013.[8] Coronary heart disease was the most common HF cause, followed by other conditions, such as hypertension and rheumatic heart disease. Between the ages of 35 and 74 years, the prevalence of HF in China was 0.9%, 0.7% in men, 1.0% in women.[8] The age of HF onset has become younger in recent years: 66.4 ± 14.1 years between 2000 and 2003, 64.9 ± 14.4 years between 2004 and 2006, and 64.2 ± 14.8 years between 2007 and 2010 ($P<.01$).[9] In Japan, 1.0 million individuals were estimated to have HF in 2005, and this number is expected to increase to 1.3 million by 2035.[10] According to a study carried out by the Turkish Society of Cardiology, the incidence of adult patients with heart disease in Turkey is 63 per 1000.[11]

As in Western countries, cardiac rehabilitation (CR) practice patterns include a healthy diet, smoking cessation, limited alcohol intake, weight control, stress and sleep management, and exercise training. In addition to these universal components of CR, Asian countries also commonly include other types of physical activity, including Taiji (or Tai Chi), Qigong, and Yoga.

CARDIAC REHABILITATION IN JAPAN

Japan began learning from the West since the Meiji restoration and gradually transformed into a capitalist country. In conjunction with Japan's rapid economic rise, it became the first Asian country embarking on the road of industrialization, and its health care system and health levels now are comparable to Western countries.

The inception of rehabilitation for patients suffering a myocardial infarction dates back to the 1950s in Japan.[12] Since the 1970s, Japan began to formalize the concept of CR. The CR Research Council was established in 1977 and the Japanese government implemented the National Health Promotion Strategies. Convened in 1978, the Japanese Association of CR (JACR), which was preceded by the CR Research Conference in 1955, ushered in a new era of CR in Japan, a framework similar to programs seen in Western countries.

CR became an intervention covered by health insurance in 1988, but just for those suffering an acute myocardial infarction (AMI). Since 1996, CR is covered by Japan's public health insurance system for AMI, angina pectoris, and HF. Patients undergoing a percutaneous coronary intervention or coronary artery bypass graft surgery became covered for CR in 2004.[13]

According to data from the Japanese Ministry of Health, Labor, and Welfare, the number of registered medical institutions with a CR program has been steadily increasing: from 186 institutions in 2005 to 608 in 2011.[14] However, according to JACR, the number of the medical institutions providing outpatient CR was only 325 in 2013. CR in Japan has been traditionally performed in the inpatient setting, and opportunities to participate in outpatient CR after hospital discharge remain low.

Obviously, the limited number of outpatient CR programs is a major obstacle with respect to availability for qualified patients in Japan.[14] A recent analysis found outpatient CR participation rates were estimated to be between 3.8% and 7.6% in Japan.[15] Saito and colleagues[16] emphasized the importance of individualized exercise prescription, determined by exercise testing, for exercise-based CR. Exercise testing is used to determine the anaerobic threshold (AT) and evaluate exercise tolerance. Therefore, exercise-based CR depending on individual exercise prescription could decrease adverse cardiovascular events and optimize outcomes.

In general, CR programs are performed in 3 stages (**Table 1**): acute (phase I), subacute (phase II),[17,18] and chronic (phase III).[19,20] In Japan, most CR programs are phase I, with a lower number of phase II and III programs.[17,18] Some studies suggest that self-monitoring of patient physical activity during phase I CR might effectively increase the physical activity level in preparation for entering a phase II CR program.[21] Patients with coronary artery disease in the chronic phase still have problems with physical function and coronary risk factors, especially in the elderly population.[17,18,22–24] Phase III CR was sparsely available until 2006 because of no coverage by health insurance.

Randomized phase III CR trials in Japan improved several aspects of physical fitness, coronary risk, and QOL.[19,20] These studies used

Table 1
Phases of cardiac rehabilitation in Japan

	Phase I		Phase II	Phase III
	Phase I		Phase II	Phase III
Period	Acute stage	Early subacute stage	Late subacute stage	Chronic stage
Location	ICU/CCU	General ward	Residential or regional rehabilitation facilities	Residential or regional rehabilitation facilities
Objective	Regain functional mobility	Return to society functions	Return to society, develop good habits	Maintain good habits

Abbreviations: CCU, coronary care unit; ICU, intensive care unit.
Adapted from Refs.[21–26]

weekly supervised exercise sessions at the clinic consisting of approximately 15 minutes of warm-up exercise, including stretching, followed by 20 to 60 minutes of continuous upright aerobic exercise (various combinations of walking, bicycling, jogging, and other activities), and light isotonic exercise, such as situps and squatting, using the patient's own body weight, followed by approximately 15 minutes of cool-down stretching and calisthenics. The intensity of supervised aerobic exercise sessions was at the AT level. In addition, the intervention group participating in phase III CR also performed resistance exercise training twice weekly, education on a healthy diet at the onset of the program and every 2 months thereafter, and weekly counseling at every visit for 6 months.[19,20] Some CR programs in Japan also include some forms of traditional Chinese exercise patterns, such as Taiji and Qigong, but they are less widespread than those in China.

CARDIAC REHABILITATION IN SINGAPORE, HONG KONG, TAIWAN, AND KOREA

CR practice using exercise training in Singapore, Hong Kong, Taiwan, and Korea is also similar to the Western model. In Singapore, several systematic reviews over the past 3 decades have consistently demonstrated cardio-protective effects of exercise-based CR programs.[25–28] Exercise-based CR, compared with usual care, reduces all-cause mortality by 20% (95% confidence interval, CI: 7%, 32%) and cardiac mortality by 26% (95% CI: 4%, 39%).[27] Hong Kong, because it was a Chinese colony governed by United Kingdom for 100 years, emulates Western CR programs, which have focused on a didactic provision of information for patients but less emphasis on psychosocial components.[29] In Taiwan, CR is commonly based on cardiopulmonary exercise testing (CPET). In all 3 above areas, in which the Chinese population is dominant, CR practice patterns for HF also include Chinese traditional

sports, such as Taiji and Qigong (for more details, see later discussion of CR in China).[30,31] In Korea, CR is majorly driven by symptom-limited CPET as an objective quantitative criterion for the exercise training protocol.

CARDIAC REHABILITATION IN CHINA
The Organizations, Associations, Committees, Guidelines, and Problems of Cardiac Rehabilitation in China

Before the 1970s in China, most cardiologists and clinicians thought that exercise was contraindicated in patients diagnosed with CVD.[12,32–37] Since the early 1980s, some cardiologists began to investigate the safety and efficacy of CR, initially only in 3 Chinese hospitals.[38,39] Subsequently, the number of hospitals with CR programs started to increase in the mid-1980s and early 1990s.[33–37] Currently, the hospitals with CR programs are dispersed among 20 provinces (municipalities).[12,32–37] However, the practice patterns of CR in hospital and other medical care units are still very simple and poorly standardized.

In 1978, the Chinese Medical Association (CMA) established 2 branches: the Chinese Society of Cardiology (CSC) and the Chinese Association of Physical Medicine and Rehabilitation. Then, in 2007, the CMA established its Sports Medicine Branch to promote CR practice in China. In 1991, the Chinese Association of Rehabilitation Medicine established its branch of Cardiovascular Committee (CCCARM) to promote CR practice particularly for CVD.[35–37] Since December of 2012, Dr Hu, a cardiologist, as the leader of CCCARM, has encouraged more cardiologists to promote and use CR.[30]

In comparing 4 different CMA-CSC's guidelines related with HF from 2007 to 2014,[40–43] only the last one announced that regular aerobic exercise improves cardiac function and symptoms in this chronic disease population (class I, A-level).[43] Moreover, this document stated CR is beneficial for stable HF patients (class IIa, B-level). It also endorsed a multidisciplinary management scheme, which includes cardiologists, psychologists, nutritionists, physical and exercise therapists, primary care physicians (urban and rural medical communities), nurses, patients, and their family members as part of a singular team to improve CR outcomes and to reduce the risk of rehospitalization (class I, A-level).[43,44] Unfortunately, there are still currently very few cardiologists who commonly add CR in their daily clinical practice for HF.

Last, currently in China, 3 additional major challenges limit CR practice and require attention: (1) the lack of professionals qualified to oversee a CR program; (2) those professionals currently delivering CR, a lower levels of financial compensation; and (3) limited payment support from health insurance.[38,45]

Cardiac Rehabilitation Practice Pattern in China

There were many studies in China that showed that activities such as walking, biking, running, and swimming effectively improve cardiac function and QOL in HF patients.[46–57] Beginning in 1992, Liu and colleagues[58–61] reported 2 to 4 weeks of walking 100 to 400 meters, twice a day, for AMI patients with HF was safe and beneficial. Other controlled studies[62–65] used a walking intervention in HF cohorts. The rehabilitation group exercised 10 to 30 minutes, 4 to 5 times per week, for 20 weeks, and exercise intensity was titrated by metabolic equivalents (METs). The rehabilitation exercise group significantly increased 6-minute walk distance (6MWD) and left ventricular ejection fraction (LVEF), significantly decreased b-type natriuretic peptide (BNP), left ventricular end-diastolic dimension, and significantly improved QOL scores.[62–65] Tian[66] used symptom-limited peak exercise testing to set training intensity (40%–80% of peak oxygen consumption [$\dot{V}o_2$]), for 10 to 20 minutes per session, 3 to 7 times per week, for 3 months. After 3 months, the patients significantly increased cardiac output, LVEF, stroke volume, cardiac index, and stroke index compared with the control group. A series of similar studies[55,67,68] used progressively increasing walking time for HF patients: the first week started at 5 to −10 minutes per day and then progressed to 3 ten-minute sessions per day (30 minutes total), greater than 5 days per week, at a heart rate of 50% to 70% of maximum, for the first 2 months. During the third to sixth months of training, more exercise was added, including cycling, jogging, playing volleyball, playing badminton, and other sport

activities, 30 minutes per day, more than 5 days per week. Results showed that this training program improved QOL and cardiac function as well as decreased morbidity and mortality.[55,67,68]

Other 6-month walking studies[47,54,56,69] initiated training at 80% to 90% of baseline 6MWD and then gradually increased the distance to 3000 to 5000 steps ($\approx$2–3 km), a cumulative time of 40 to 60 minutes, 4 to 6 days per week. Six months later, the walking group demonstrated a significant reduction in rehospitalization and resting heart rate as well as a significantly higher 6MWD and LVEF compared with controls. Another study with similar methods found that after CR, plasma angiotensin II and endothelin-1 decreased significantly.

Traditional Chinese Exercise Pattern for Rehabilitation

As briefly mentioned above, rehabilitation in China has a long history, and Qigong, Taiji, and other similar approaches are important components of rehabilitation.[27,70] Qigong is a mental and physical exercise that focuses on breathing control, physical movements, and meditation as the means to maintain physical fitness, prevent and cure diseases, and live healthy. Taiji is a form of martial arts, combining purposeful movements with meditation. It combines various boxing movements in conjunction with the change in the Yin (meaning of negative) and Yang (meaning of positive) in Yijing Chinese medicine meridian. It is a physically and mentally involved form of low to medium intensity aerobic exercise and is feasible and safe for HF patients.[31,70] Currently prevalent in the elderly population, Taiji combined with exercise training may synergistically further increase the benefits of training, particularly in terms of improving the QOL and mood.[71] Although Taiji and Qigong are widely used in the Chinese population, there are a limited number of investigations on its value when integrated into a CR program in China. It may be because these approaches are commonly accepted as providing a health benefit without any question. A multicenter, single-blind randomized controlled study[72] compared 12 weeks of Taiji to a control group. Even though the Taiji exercise group had no significant improvement in 6MWD and peak $\dot{V}O_2$, significant improvements in self-effectiveness (cardiac motion self-efficacy instruments), QOL, and mood state scores were reported in the training group. Zhuo and colleagues[73] studied changes in CPET parameters in the patients practicing Taiji to indicate the physiologic impact of this exercise approach. All subjects had more than a 5-year history of Taiji skillful practice history.

Cardiopulmonary exercise testing parameters, such as $\dot{V}O_2$, related metabolic parameters, heart rate, and blood pressure, were measured during a practice of Taiji (which lasted 17–25 minutes, an average of 22 minutes). The average energy consumption of the Taiji was 4.1 METs or 14.5 mL/kg/min, and the average heart rate was 134 bpm. These values suggested that the practice of Taiji can be classified as a mild to moderate form of exercise intensity, with an intensity level of no more than 50% of peak $\dot{V}O_2$. Zhou and colleagues[74] studied the positive improved effects of Qigong on blood lipids and heart functions, indicated that Chinese traditional methods play a unique important role in modern rehabilitation.

Square dance has become popular in China, particularly in the elderly female population; this is a simple, free, and easy-to-learn style of dancing pattern that allows for sustained physical activity. Similar to Taiji, square dance is a low-to-moderate intensity aerobic exercise that many elderly Chinese citizens perform to maintain fitness in public spaces. Although there is lack of scientific analysis on square-dance patterns for patients with HF, it is reasonable to posit this approach would improve functional capacity in this chronic disease population. However, future scientific analysis in this area is encouraged to support this hypothesis.

Researchers who are not from China have also assessed traditional Chinese methods for CR.[31,71,72,75–77] A challenge to integrating these findings into the local health care model is that Chinese citizens tend to put greater belief and trust from individuals sharing their culture background; this results in less scientific investigation in China and a lack of common standard use of Chinese traditional methods for CR in HF patients.

A meta-analysis on 14 studies conducted by Taylor and colleagues[27] reported that Taiji was effective in improving aerobic capacity. In a recent meta-analysis study, Pan and colleagues[31] pooled data from 4 randomized controlled trials (n = 242). The results suggested that Taiji significantly improved QOL but was not associated with a significant reduction in BNP, systolic/diastolic blood pressure, improved 6MWD, and peak $\dot{V}O_2$.

Taiji may promote cardiovascular health and can be considered an alternative exercise program for patients with HF. However, the study design and training protocols from different Taiji studies vary significantly, and hence, the results are difficult to compare. In future research, large samples, multicenter randomized controlled trials, and using standardized training protocols should be considered in accordance with the guidelines of exercise prescription for patients with HF.[78]

Cardiopulmonary Exercise Testing and New Theoretic System of "Holistic Integrative Physiology and Medicine" for Cardiac Rehabilitation in China

At present, the evaluation of HF severity and prognosis includes one or more of the following: (1) New York Heart Association functional classification; (2) some form of objective functional assessment; (3) LVEF; and (4) BNP. These evaluations are, however, not sufficient in objectively reflecting the patient's clinical presentation in a comprehensive manner.[79] Ideally, an assessment should accurately reflect disease severity, a heterogeneous phenomenon in patients with HF, as well as the magnitude of physiologic/clinical improvement following the implementation or titration of an intervention. Cardiopulmonary exercise testing satisfies all of the aforementioned desirable assessment attributes. Cardiopulmonary exercise testing merges traditional exercise testing monitoring procedures (ie, electrocardiography, hemodynamics, and subjective symptoms) with ventilator expired gas analysis. This additional technique can accurately quantify minute ventilation ($\dot{V}E$), $\dot{V}O_2$, and carbon dioxide production ($\dot{V}CO_2$) at rest and throughout exercise.[79–84]

Cardiopulmonary exercise testing is currently the gold standard for the noninvasive integrated evaluation of all systems involved in the aerobic exercise response.[80] It can be an objective and quantitative evaluation of cardiopulmonary function and exercise tolerance, better predict holistic health status, optimal parameter of selection, and management for heart transplant, and predict outcome.[81] However, many clinicians and experts, commonly based on the systemic physiology, have poor understanding of the integrative physiology and pathophysiology of CPET and clinical importance and safety of CPET.[78,81,83,84] At least in China, the standard CPET-guided CR investigation is still very rare. Since 2012, came back China to work for establishing national center of CVD, the author has been prompted to use CPET for personalized CR, and has been hold both training courses of "theoretical basic and clinical practice of CPET" and "standardizing practice for CPET" twice a year.

Rooted in the holistic concepts of Chinese traditional culture background and with the deep understanding of the principles of oxygenation in the human body described by modern medical science, Sun[78,83] established the fundamental structure of a new theoretic system of "Holistic Integrative Physiology and Medicine," which has been developed over the last 30 years, was first announced at the 2011 American Physiology

Society conference,[85] and was fully described in 2013.

Cardiopulmonary exercise testing is a continuous dynamic record of all integrated respiratory, circulatory, metabolic, and neurohumoral activities during a physical stimulus. Thus, CPET is an ideal tool to assess holistic integrative physiology and medicine as well as a unique guide and method for delivering a highly individualized CR program. In using this new theory to guide the interpretation of standardized clinical CPET, a holistic human physiologic functional assessment, diagnosis and differential diagnosis of disease, disease severity evaluation, evaluation of therapeutic efficacy, patients management and prognosis prediction can more accurately be achieved.[84,86–97] From a CR standpoint, an important perspective gained from CPET is identifying AT to pinpoint the optimal intensity for aerobic training.[88–91] Moreover, disease/dysfunction of the heart, lungs, circulatory systems, or periphery manifest specific and relatively unique abnormalities that are amplified during exercise and CPET can elegantly characterize these patterns.[84,86–97]

CARDIAC REHABILITATION IN INDIA

In India, there are mainly 2 rehabilitation practice patterns: one is the traditional Western mode and the other is Yoga. Regardless of the approach, CR in a structured manner is in a nascent stage in India, with the first phase II telemetry monitored programs being available only in the initial years of the twenty-first century. However, most hospitals across the country that care for HF patients do offer phase I CR.[98] Currently, there is limited evidence assessing CR outcomes in India. Although data from Western countries have shown that exercise training is valuable in patients with HF, the Indian context is very different. There are only 2 published studies on exercise training in HF available from India: one is a case series and the other one is a clinical trial, both with promising findings.[99,100] There is consensus that CR is effective and necessary in CVD populations,[101] and continued efforts are therefore needed to continue CR research in India and facilitate clinical applications.

Yoga is a typical exercise pattern and commonly popular in India and other areas in Southeast Asia, South Asia, and China. Yoga practice is safe, and participants experience improved physical function and symptom stability. Yoga exercise and breathing are a nonpharmacologic intervention that may ameliorate autonomic nervous system tone and skeletal muscle function in HF. In one study,[102] patients with HF were asked to complete 8 weeks of Yoga classes. Yoga classes lasted 60 minutes and were conducted twice weekly for a total of 16 classes over an 8-week period. Key findings were (1) a modified Yoga program was safe in stable HF patients; and (2) the modified Yoga program improved physical function measures, such as strength, balance, and endurance as well as perception of symptom stability and QOL.[102] In another study,[103] researchers examined the effect of 4 weeks of Yoga-type breathing training in patients with HF and found that dyspnea, exercise tolerance, and oxygenation were improved.

CARDIAC REHABILITATION IN BROADER REGIONS OF SOUTH ASIA

Including India, south Asia is the most densely populated geographic region in the world. People of South-Asian origin (ie, from India, Pakistan, Sri Lanka, and Bangladesh) have an increased risk of developing HF and experiencing cardiovascular death.[103–106] Although CR is effective, South Asians are among the least likely people to participate in these programs. There are several factors associated with this lack of participation.[107] Indeed, the emerging themes identified in the literature point toward several salient factors associated with South-Asian patients' experiences of CR that are commensurate with low uptake and adherence. In particular, structural barriers relating to referral, timing, location, and availability of transport were common, in addition to cultural and exercise-related barriers and language and translation difficulties.[108–113] There is emerging evidence to suggest that South Asian women, in particular, appear to experience unique and compounding social and cultural barriers to attending and participating in conventional CR programs.[111,112,114]

However, a few researchers have disaggregated their data by ethnic origin to describe what might best meet the needs of South Asian patients. Further research is needed to thoughtfully address issues of uptake of and compliance with CR by South Asian patients and to support the development of culturally sensitive and safe CR programs.[107]

SUMMARY

Given differences in economy, culture, race, standards of medical practice, and development status and others, it is no surprise that the practice of CR in patients with HF and local supporting evidence varies widely. There are many rehabilitation practice patterns in Asia, including not only the classical Western model but also Asia's traditional sports (eg, Taiji, Qigong, and Yoga). These latter approaches to physical activity are popular and should be included in CR programs in Asia. However, these sports are without regular design and strict monitoring for patients with HF, creating a fertile area for future research. As the objective and quantitative evaluation of cardiopulmonary function, exercise tolerance, and holistic health status, CPET is the gold standard assessment and, when available, should be used.

REFERENCES

1. Francis G. Pathophysiology of congestive heart failure. Rev Cardiovasc Med 2003;4(Suppl 2):S14–20.
2. Larsen AI, Dickstein K. Can sedentary patients with heart failure achieve the beneficial effect of exercise training without moving? Eur Heart J 2004; 25:104–6.
3. Norton C, Georgiopoulou VV, Kalogeropoulos AP, et al. Epidemiology and cost of advanced heart failure. Prog Cardiovasc Dis 2011;54:78–85.
4. Dracup K, Walden JA, Stevenson LW, et al. Quality of life in patients with advanced heart failure. J Heart Lung Transplant 1992;11:273–9.
5. Walke LM, Gallo WT, Tinetti ME, et al. The burden of symptoms among community-dwelling older persons with advanced chronic disease. Arch Intern Med 2004;164:2321–4.
6. Grady KL. Self-care and quality of life outcomes in heart failure patients. J Cardiovasc Nurs 2008;23: 285–92.
7. Roger VL, Go AS, Lloyd-Jones DM, et al, American Heart Association Statistics Committee and Stroke Statistics Subcommittee. Heart disease and stroke statistics–2012 update: a report from the American Heart Association. Circulation 2012;125:e2–220.
8. National Center of Cardiovascular Diseases of China. Report on cardiovascular disease in China. 1st edition. Beijing (China): Encyclopedia of China Publishing House; 2013. p. 1–6.
9. Yu SB, Cui HY, Qin M, et al. Characteristics of in-hospital patients with chronic heart failure in Hubei province from 2000 to 2010. Zhonghua Xin Xue Guan Bing Za Zhi 2011;39:549–52 [in Chinese].
10. Okura Y, Ramadan MM, Ohno Y, et al. Impending epidemic: future projection of heart failure in Japan to the year 2055. Circ J 2008;72:489–91.
11. Onat A. Prevalence of coronary heart disease in Turkish adults, new coronary events and frequency of cardiac death. In: Onat A, editor. Tekharf, health of heart on Turkish adults. Istanbul (Turkey): Yelken Press; 2007. p. 22–30.
12. Yang ZF. The development of cardiac rehabilitation in China. Chinese Journal of Rehabilitation Theory and Practice 2008;14(4):301–2.
13. Goto Y. Current state of cardiac rehabilitation in Japan. Prog Cardiovasc Dis 2014;56(5):557–62.
14. Koyama T. Trends in registered hospital and clinic on medical fee for cardiovascular rehabilitation. Jpn J Card Rehabil 2012;17:238–43.
15. Arena R, Myers J, Guazzi M. Cardiopulmonary exercise testing is a core assessment for patients with heart failure. Congest Heart Fail 2011;17(3): 115–9.
16. Saito M, Ueshima K, Saito M, et al, Japanese Cardiac Rehabilitation Survey Investigators. Safety of exercise-based cardiac rehabilitation and exercise testing for cardiac patients in Japan: a nationwide survey. Circ J 2014;78:1646–53.
17. Goto Y, Itoh H, Adachi H, et al. Use of exercise cardiac rehabilitation after acute myocardial infarction. Circ J 2003;67:411–5.
18. Goto Y, Saito M, Iwasaka T, et al, Japanese Cardiac Rehabilitation Survey Investigators. Poor implementation of cardiac rehabilitation despite broad dissemination of coronary interventions for acute myocardial infarction in Japan. Circ J 2007;71: 173–9.
19. Seki E, Watanabe Y, Shimada K, et al. Effects of a phase III cardiac rehabilitation program on physical status and lipid profiles in elderly patients with coronary artery disease. Circ J 2008;72: 1230–4.
20. Seki E, Watanabe Y, Sunayama S, et al. Effects of phase III cardiac rehabilitation programs on health-related quality of life in elderly patients with coronary artery disease: Juntendo Cardiac Rehabilitation Program (J-CARP). Circ J 2003; 67:73–7.
21. Izawa KP, Watanabe S, Hiraki K. Determination of the effectiveness of accelerometer use in the promotion of physical activity in cardiac patients: a randomized controlled trial. Arch Phys Med Rehabil 2012;93(11):1896–902.
22. Hellman EA, Williams MA. Outpatient cardiac rehabilitation in elderly patients. Heart Lung 1994;23: 506–12.
23. Yoshida T, Yoshida K, Yamamoto C, et al. Effects of a two-week, hospitalized phase II cardiac rehabilitation program on physical capacity, lipid profiles and psychological variables in patients with acute myocardial infarction. Jpn Circ J 2001;65:87–93.
24. Ades PA, Waldmann ML, Meyer WL, et al. Skeletal muscle and cardiovascular adaptations to exercise conditioning in older coronary patients. Circulation 1996;94:323–30.
25. O'Connor GT, Buring JE, Yusuf S, et al. An overview of randomized trials of rehabilitation with exercise after myocardial infarction. Circulation 1989;80(2): 234–44.
26. Oldridge NB, Guyatt GH, Fischer ME, et al. Cardiac rehabilitation after myocardial infarction. Combined

experience of randomized clinical trials. JAMA 1988;260(7):945–50.

27. Taylor RS, Brown A, Ebrahim S, et al. Exercise-based rehabilitation for patients with coronary heart disease: systematic review and meta-analysis of randomized controlled trials. Am J Med 2004; 116(10):682–92.

28. Heran BS, Chen JM, Ebrahim S, et al. Exercise-based cardiac rehabilitation for coronary heart disease. Cochrane Database Syst Rev 2011;(7):CD001800.

29. Davidson P, Daly J, Hancock K, et al. Perceptions and experiences of heart disease: a literature review and identification of a research agenda in older women. Eur J Cardiovasc Nurs 2003;2(4): 255–64.

30. Taylor-Piliae RE. The effectiveness of Taiji exercise in improving aerobic capacity: an updated meta-analysis. Med Sport Sci 2008;52:40–53.

31. Pan L, Yan J, Guo Y, et al. Effects of Taiji training on exercise capacity and quality of life in patients with chronic heart failure: a meta-analysis. Eur J Heart Fail 2013;15(3):316–23.

32. Liu JS. Retrospect and prospect of the development of heart disease rehabilitation in China. Chin J Cardiovasc Rehabil Med 2013;22(1):1–5.

33. Liu JS. Development and current situation of Chinese rehabilitative cardiology. Chin J Cardiovasc Rehabil Med 2008;17(5):417–27.

34. Liu JS. Development and current situation of Chinese rehabilitative cardiology. Chin J Cardiovasc Rehabil Med 2001;10(5):387–95.

35. Liu JS. Development and current situation of Chinese rehabilitative cardiology. Chin J Cardiovasc Rehabil Med 2005;14(5):409–18.

36. Liu JS. Development and current situation of Chinese rehabilitative cardiology. Chin J Cardiovasc Rehabil Med 2006;15(Suppl):12–21.

37. Liu JS. Development and current situation of Chinese rehabilitative cardiology. Chin J Rehabil Theo Prac 2010;16(5):406–7.

38. Feng JX, Liu ZY. Development and investigation of cardiac rehabilitation program. Chin J Tissue Engineering Research 2007;2(39):8002–4.

39. Qu L, Liu KS, Ma SP, et al. 25 cases of uncomplicated acute infarction rehabilitation medical report. J Clin Cardiol 1985;1(12):38.

40. Chinese Society of Cardiology of Chinese Medical Association, Editorial Board of Chinese Journal of Cardiology. Guidelines for the diagnosis and management of chronic heart failure. Zhonghua Xin Xue Guan Bing Za Zhi 2007;35(12):1076–95 [in Chinese].

41. Chinese Society of Cardiology of Chinese Medical Association, Editorial Board of Chinese Journal of Cardiology. Guideline for diagnosis and treatment of acute heart failure. Zhonghua Xin Xue Guan Bing Za Zhi 2010;38(3):195–208 [in Chinese].

42. Chinese Society of Cardiology of Chinese Medical Association, Editorial Board of Chinese Journal of Cardiology. Right heart failure diagnosis and treatment of Chinese expert consensus rule. Zhonghua Xin Xue Guan Bing Za Zhi 2012;40(6):449–61 [in Chinese].

43. Chinese Society of Cardiology of Chinese Medical Association, Editorial Board of Chinese Journal of Cardiology. The Chinese heart failure diagnosis and treatment guidelines 2014. Zhonghua Xin Xue Guan Bing Za Zhi 2014;42(2):98–122 [in Chinese].

44. Sochalski J, Jaarsma T, Krumholz HM, et al. What works in chronic care management: the case of heart failure. Health Aff (Millwood) 2009;28:179–89.

45. Hu DY. Actively explore and promote the establishment of cardiac rehabilitation and secondary prevention system. Zhonghua Xin Xue Guan Bing Za Zhi 2013;41(4):265–6 [in Chinese].

46. Sun DE. Effect of rehabilitation exercise on the elderly patients with chronic heart failure. J Gerontol 2012;32(9):1842–3.

47. Li L, Li RJ, Song LF, et al. Rehabilitation exercise improves heart function and quality in old patients with chronic heart failure. Chin J Cardiovasc Rehabil Med 2006;15(Suppl):133–6.

48. Jiang WW. Sports rehabilitation in patients with chronic heart failure. Geriatr Health Care 2009; 15(3):187–90.

49. Huang YL, Cheng XP. Clinical value of the 6-minute walking test in patients with chronic heart failure. Inte J Cardiovascular Dise 2006;33(1):21–3.

50. Yang SJ, Ma YT. Exercise therapy of chronic heart failure. Chin J Physical Med and Rehabil 2010; 32(12):958–60.

51. Peng W, Zhang XE, Cheng B. Physical training reduces peripheral markers of inflammation in patients with chronic heart failure. Chin J Phys Med Rehabil 2005;27(2):100–2.

52. Wang P. Cardiac rehabilitation Chin. J Phys Med Rehabil 2007;29(9):647–8.

53. Jing ZC. Clinical application of 6-minute walking test. Zhonghua Xin Xue Guan Bing Za Zhi 2006; 34(4):381–4 [in Chinese].

54. Li H, Chen WX, Liang R, et al. Application of 6-minute walking exercise training in the rehabilitation nursing of chronic heart failure patients. Guangxi Med J 2006;28(7):1111–3.

55. Wu Z. Study exercise rehabilitation improve heart function, exercise tolerance and quality of life in patients with chronic heart failure analysis. Hum Mov Sci 2012;2(3):15–6.

56. Zhao XJ. Effects of exercise training on the improvement of cardiac function and exercise endurance in patients with chronic heart failure. Chin J Clin Rehabil 2005;9(16):170–1.

57. Li Y, Bao LJ, Chen J. The clinical study of 6 min walking testing for heart failure patients with

normal ejection fraction. Ningxia Med J 2014; 36(4):355–8.

58. Liu JS, An K, Wang BL, et al. Exercise training in patients after acute myocardial infarction (AMI) with heart failure (with 2 cases report). Chin J Rehabil Med 1992;7(1):28–9.

59. Liu JS. Rehabilitation treatment in patients with coronary heart disease. Chin J Cardiovasc Rehabil Med 2003;12(Suppl):503–35.

60. Liu JS. Rehabilitation treatment in patients with coronary heart disease. Chin J Cardiovasc Rehabil Med 2006;15(Suppl):22–55.

61. Liu JS, Yang JX, Liu N, et al. Heart disease rehabilitation. Beijing (China): China Science and Technology Press; 1996. p. 1–308.

62. Qiao YG, Jing RF, Li H, et al. Dynamic change of brain natriuretic peptide during the improvement of heart failure. J Prac Med 2006;22(11):1253–4.

63. Zhang CY, Li FJ. Effects of exercise rehabilitation in aged patients with chronic heart failure. Chin Community Doctors 2013;15(20):81.

64. Liu H, Li YJ. Efficacy of comprehensive rehabilitation therapy observed in chronic congestive heart failure. Chin J of Trau Disabil Medicine 2006; 14(5):31–3.

65. Shi Y. Clinical effect of rehabilitation exercise on quality of life on the aged patients with chronic heart failure. Chin J Geriatric Care 2010;8(3):5–7.

66. Tian YH. The effects of moderate aerobic exercise for patients with chronic heart failure. Contemporary Medicine 2013;19(13):71–2.

67. Cai WH, Gao CX, Xie ZJ, et al. Curative effect of rehabilitation training for chronic congestive heart failure. Hebei Medicine 2007;13(2):167–9.

68. Ji XL. Effect of exercise rehabilitation on plasma brain natriuretic peptide levels in patients with chronic heart failure. Chin J Aesthetic Med 2012; 21(7):139–40.

69. Yan H, Fu CH, Zou EF, et al. Walk exercise training produces rehabilitation effects on heart function for patients with chronic heart failure. Chin J Cardiovasc Rehabil Med 2010;19(1):2–4.

70. Guo L, Li M. Research progress in the rehabilitation for patients with chronic heart failure recover. South Chin J Cardiovascular dise 2013;19(4):381–3.

71. Caminiti G, Volterrani M, Marazzi G, et al. Taiji enhances the effects of endurance training in the rehabilitation of elderly patients with chronic heart failure. Rehabil Res Pract 2011;2011: 761958.

72. Yeh GY, Mccarthy EP, Wayne PM, et al. Taiji exercise in patients with chronic heart failure: a randomized clinical trial. Arch Intern Med 2011; 171(8):750–7.

73. Zhuo DH. Cardiovascular and metabolic changes in respiratory function when practicing Taiji. Chin J Rehabil Med 1987;2(6):241.

74. Zhou SF. The impact of static Qigong on PGI2-TXA 2 and balance between systolic period of coronary heart disease. China Rehabilitation 1989;4(4):160.

75. Taylor-Piliae RE. Taiji as an adjunct to cardiac rehabilitation exercise training. J Cardiopulm Rehabil 2003;23:90–6.

76. Chan CL, Wang CW, Ho RT, et al. A systematic review of the effectiveness of qigong exercise in cardiac rehabilitation. Am J Chin Med 2012;40(2):255–67.

77. Yeh GY, Wood MJ, Wayne PM, et al. Taiji in patients with heart failure with preserved ejection fraction. Congest Heart Fail 2013;19(2):77–84.

78. Sun XG. New theoretical system of holistic integrative physiology and medicine: integration of self-regulating body functions. Chinese Circulation Journal 2013;28(2):88–92.

79. Zhao Q, Liu ZH, Sun XG, et al. Cardiopulmonary exercise testing assessment of exercise capacity in patients with chronic left heart failure. Chinese Circulation Journal 2011;26(5):370–3.

80. Mudge GH, Goldstein S, Addonizio LJ, et al. Task force 3: recipient guidelines/prioritization. J Am Coll Cardiol 1993;22(1):21–6.

81. Wsserman K, Hansen JE, Sue D, et al. Principles of exercise testing and interpretation. 5th edition. Philadelphia: Lippincott Williams & Wilkins; 2011. p. 9–61, 71–106, 194–234.

82. Sun XG, Guo ZY. New theory of breathing control: a complex mode integrates multi-systems. Journal of Federation of American Societies for Experimental Biology 2011;25:lb634.

83. Sun XG. New theoretical system of holistic control and regulation for life and cardiopulmonary exercise testing. Medicine and Philosophy 2013;4(3):22–7.

84. Tan XY, Sun XG. From clinical application of cardiopulmonary exercise testing to view the requirement for holistic integrative physiology and medicine. Medicine and Philosophy 2013;4(3):28–31.

85. Bernardi L, Spadacini G, Bellwon J, et al. Effect of breathing on oxygen saturation and exercise performance in chronic heart failure. Lancet 1998; 351:1308–11.

86. Sun XG, Hansen JE, Beshai JF, et al. Oscillatory breathing and exercise gas exchange abnormalities prognosticate early mortality and morbidity in heart failure. J Am Coll Cardiol 2010;55:1814–23.

87. Wasserman K, Sun XG, Hansen JE. Effect of biventricular pacing on the exercise pathophysiology of heart failure. Chest 2007;132(1):250–61.

88. Sun XG, Hansen JE, Stringer WW. Oxygen uptake efficiency plateau (OUEP) best predicts early death in heart failure. Chest 2012;141:1284–94.

89. Sun XG, Hansen JE, Oudiz RJ, et al. Exercise pathophysiology in patients with primary pulmonary hypertension. Circulation 2001;104:429–35.

90. Sun XG, Hansen JE, Oudiz RJ, et al. Gas exchange detection of exercise-induced right-to-left shunt in

patients with primary pulmonary hypertension. Circulation 2002;105:54–60.

91. Sun XG, Hansen JE, Ting H, et al. Comparison of exercise cardiac output by the Fick principle using O2 and CO2. Chest 2000;118:631–40.

92. Sun XG. Clinical importance and application of cardiopulmonary exercise testing in cardiovascular medicine. Zhonghua Xin Xue Guan Bing Za Zhi 2014;42(4):347–51 [in Chinese].

93. Sun XG, Hu DY. Requirements of clinical laboratory and quality control of cardiopulmonary exercise testing. Zhonghua Xin Xue Guan Bing Za Zhi 2014;42(10):817–21 [in Chinese].

94. Sun XG. The difficult issue of cardiopulmonary exercise testing: system calibration. Zhonghua Xin Xue Guan Bing Za Zhi 2014;42(11):995–6 [in Chinese].

95. Sun XG, Wang GZ, Lu J, et al. Oxygen uptake and carbon dioxide output ventilatory efficiency during exercise are reliable indexes of circulatory function in normal subjects. Zhonghua Xin Xue Guan Bing Za Zhi 2014;42(12):1020–4 [in Chinese].

96. Lu ZN, Huang J, Sun XG, et al. Clinical application of oxygen uptake and ventilation efficiency parameters of cardiopulmonary exercise testing for optimal management in patients with severe chronic heart failure. Zhonghua Xin Xue Guan Bing Za Zhi 2015;43, in press [in Chinese].

97. Lu ZN, Sun XG, Hu SS, et al. Peak oxygen consumption, NT-proBNP and Echoardiogram Assessment of Cardiac Function in Patients with Chronic Heart Failure. Zhonghua Xin Xue Guan Bing Za Zhi 2015;43, in press [in Chinese].

98. Contractor AS. Cardiac rehabilitation after myocardial infarction. J Assoc Physicians India 2011;59(Suppl):51–5.

99. Babu AS, Maiya AG, George MM, et al. The benefits of exercise based cardiac rehabilitation in congestive heart failure — a case series. Indian Heart J 2011;63:473–4.

100. Babu AS, Maiya AG, George MM, et al. Effects of early in-patient cardiac rehabilitation along with a structured home based program among patients with congestive heart failure: a randomized controlled trial. Heart Views 2011;12:99–103.

101. Madan K, Babu AS, Contractor A, et al. Cardiac rehabilitation in India. Prog Cardiovasc Dis 2014;56(5):543–50.

102. Howie-Esquivel J, Lee J, Collier G, et al. Yoga in heart failure patients: a pilot study. J Card Fail 2010;16(9):742–9.

103. Gupta M, Ananand AV, Singh N, et al. Risk factors, hospital management and outcomes after acute myocardial infarction in South Asian Canadians and matched control subjects. CMAJ 2002;166:717–22.

104. Bhopal R. Glossary of terms relating to ethnicity and race: for reflection and debate. J Epidemiol Community Health 2004;58:441–5.

105. Gupta M, Singh N, Verma S. South Asians and cardiovascular risk: what clinicians should know. Circulation 2006;113(25):e924–9.

106. McKeigue PM, Miller GJ, Marmot MG. Coronary heart disease in South Asians overseas: a review. J Clin Epidemiol 1989;42(7):597–609.

107. Galdas PM, Ratner PA, Oliffe JL. A narrative review of South Asian patients' experiences of cardiac rehabilitation. J Clin Nurs 2012;21(1–2):149–59.

108. Tod AM, Wadsworth E, Asif S, et al. Cardiac rehabilitation: the needs of South Asian cardiac patients. Br J Nurs 2001;10:1028–33.

109. Webster RA, Thompson DR, Mayou RA. The experiences and needs of Gujrati Hindu patients and partners in the first month after myocardial infarction. Eur J Cardiovasc Nurs 2002;1:69–76.

110. Jolly K, Greenfield SM, Hare R. Attendance of ethnic minority patients in cardiac rehabilitation. J Cardiopulm Rehabil 2004;24:308–12.

111. Vishram S, Crosland A, Unsworth J, et al. Engaging women from South Asian communities in cardiac rehabilitation. International Journal of Therapy and Rehabilitation 2008;15:298–304.

112. Chauhan U, Baker D, Lester H, et al. Exploring uptake of cardiac rehabilitation in a minority ethnic population in England: a qualitative study. Eur J Cardiovasc Nurs 2010;9:68–74.

113. Galdas PM, Kang HB. Punjabi Sikh patients' cardiac rehabilitation experiences following myocardial infarction: a qualitative analysis. J Clin Nurs 2010;19:3134–42.

114. Astin F, Atkin K, Darr A. Family support and cardiac rehabilitation: a comparative study of the experiences of South Asian and White-European patients and their carer's living in the United Kingdom. Eur J Cardiovasc Nurs 2008;7:43–51.

Past, Present, and Future Rehabilitation Practice Patterns for Patients with Heart Failure
The European Perspective

Valentina Labate, MD, Marco Guazzi, MD, PhD*

KEYWORDS

- Exercise training • Exercise performance • Peak V_{O_2} • Cardiopulmonary testing • Ventilation

KEY POINTS

- A recent European Society of Cardiology position paper strongly advises participation of patients with stable heart failure (HF) in structured exercise training (ET) programs.
- Three ET modalities are proposed for HF populations with variable combinations and extent of effects: (1) endurance aerobic (continuous and interval); (2) strength/resistance; (3) respiratory.
- In low-risk and stable HF patients, home-based ET is thought to be as safe and effective as center-based rehabilitation, although long-term adherence may be uncertain.
- In HF patients with only recent clinical stabilization or in the presence of multiple comorbidities, a center-based and supervised setting is preferred.
- Irrespective of ET modalities, most studies have clearly demonstrated significant improvements in exercise physiology (ie, oxygen consumption, muscle function, and ventilation), quality of life, and left ventricular function.

INTRODUCTION

The recent European Society of Cardiology position paper strongly advises participation of patients with stable heart failure (HF) in structured exercise training (ET) programs, and in most recent years considerable efforts have been put onto standardization of exercise prescription.[1]

Considering the different HF phenotypes and the wide heterogeneity of ET protocols, an individualized training approach is recommended.[1]

Currently, 3 different ET approaches are proposed for HF populations with variable combinations and extent of effects: (1) endurance aerobics (ie, continuous and interval); (2) strength/resistance; and (3) respiratory. For the 3 approaches, several ET programs are indeed available according to: (1) intensity level (ie, light to moderate, moderate to high, high to severe, and severe to extreme); (2) type (ie, endurance, resistance, and strength); (3) method (ie, continuous and intermittent/interval); (4) application (ie, systemic, regional, and respiratory muscle); (5) mode of exercise (ie, bicycle, treadmill); (6) monitoring (ie, supervised and nonsupervised); (7) setting (ie, hospital/center and home-based); and (8) application (ie, systemic, regional, and respiratory muscle).[1] Although the optimal combination and setting still need to be identified, evidence indicates that

Heart Failure Unit, IRCCS Policlinico San Donato, University of Milano, Milano, Italy
* Corresponding author. Heart Failure Unit, Department for Health for Science, IRCCS Policlinico San Donato, University of Milano, Piazza Malan 1, San Donato Milanese, Milano 20097, Italy.
E-mail address: marco.guazzi@unimi.it

Heart Failure Clin 11 (2015) 105–115
http://dx.doi.org/10.1016/j.hfc.2014.08.007
1551-7136/15/$ – see front matter © 2015 Elsevier Inc. All rights reserved.

home-based ET may be as safe and effective as center-based rehabilitation in low-risk and clinically stable patients, although long-term adherence may be uncertain. Conversely, in patients with HF with only recent clinical stabilization or in patients with multiple comorbidities, a center-based and supervised setting is preferred.[2] The current review provides the European perspective of ET in patients with HF.

CLINICAL EVIDENCE AND APPLICATIONS OF EXERCISE TRAINING PROGRAMS IN HEART FAILURE

The main ET studies performed in Europe with different protocols and ET modalities are summarized in **Table 1**.[3–20] The description of results primarily focuses on the ET effects on the maximal exercise response and gas exchange analysis by cardiopulmonary exercise testing.

Endurance Aerobic Exercise Training

Endurance aerobic ET can be either continuous or at an interval of different intensities. Continuous aerobic ET is intended as an exercise session that can be performed for at least 20 minutes with a mild or moderate sense of fatigue and is typically performed at mild-to-moderate or high-exercise intensities in steady-state conditions of aerobic energetic yield, which allows the patient to perform prolonged training sessions, ideally between 30 and 60 minutes in duration. It represents the best described and established form of ET with well-demonstrated efficacy and safety and is thus highly recommended in the European Consensus documents.[1,2]

In more deconditioned patients, it is recommended to "start low and go slow" (ie, at low intensity for 5–10 min twice a week). If well tolerated, the training duration per session first and the numbers of sessions per day later are increased, aiming at 20 to 60 minutes on 3–5 days per week at moderate-to-high intensity with indefinite program duration.

In contrast with continuous training protocols, aerobic interval training (AIT) requires the patients to perform alternate bouts (<1 min to 4 min) of moderate-to-high-intensity (50%–100% peak exercise capacity) exercise, interspersed with a recovery (<1 min to 3 min) phase, performed at low or no workload.

Since pioneering studies, mild-to-moderate continuous aerobic or endurance training (ie, on a cycle-ergometer or a treadmill) has been shown to produce major improvements in functional capacity (ie, exercise tolerance, peak oxygen consumption [Vo_2]) in patients with HF[21] and is the most investigated form of ET in this patient population. Such an approach is also recommended as a baseline activity in these patients.[1] In Europe, indoor cycling is usually preferred because it is the most versatile mode of ET for a wide spectrum of patients with HF. Low workloads are possible; power output is reproducible, and the weight of the patient is supported, reducing the risk of injuries. Exercise modes such as running or jogging are traditionally regarded as contraindicated in HF because they may be quite strenuous and often performed without supervision.[2]

Despite the fact that higher levels of physical activity may reduce cardiovascular events, a certain risk of sudden death and incurring myocardial infarction has to be considered. Thus, most planned studies have taken as reference the first ventilatory anaerobic threshold (1st VAT), occurring at 50% to 60% of peak VO as the reference ET intensity for patients with HF.[22]

However, because patients with HF (compared with normal individuals) need a higher percentage of their peak Vo_2 to perform daily life activities and because one of the main targets of ET is to allow these patients to perform daily tasks with less effort, training intensities above the 1st VAT have progressively been tested and introduced.[23] Specifically, the 2nd VAT occurs at 65% to 90% of peak Vo_2, at the respiratory compensation point (hyperventilation with respect to carbon dioxide [CO_2] metabolically produced). This level of exercise defines the so-called critical power (theoretic concept of the maximal work rate sustainable in a condition of physiologic aerobic balance),[24] which is now accepted as the limit for prolonged aerobic exercise without any additional risk. Accordingly, exercise intensities between 70% and 80% of peak Vo_2 are currently being used in some settings.[23,25,26]

With regard to the mode of exercise testing, it should be noted that the absolute values for peak Vo_2 is significantly different on a treadmill compared with a bicycle. Several studies have systematically shown a Vo_2 10% to 15% higher with treadmill tests because of the larger muscle mass involved during walking or running.[27–29]

Several lines of evidence suggest greater efficacy of high-intensity exercise compared with moderate levels in patients with coronary artery disease, pre-HF left ventricular (LV) dysfunction function, and chronic HF as well as in healthy subjects.[30–32] Nevertheless, in patients with HF with significantly reduced pretraining peak Vo_2 and/or high exercise-related risks, aerobic ET intensities as low as 40% of peak Vo_2 have been proven to be effective in increasing aerobic capacity, possibly with a more favorable risk/benefit ratio because of the lower increases in ventricular wall stress. Remarkably, this program induced an increase in peak Vo_2 of 17%, lactic threshold of 20%, and peak workload of 21%.[3]

In addition, Mezzani and colleagues,[33] have recently shown that a light-to-moderate-intensity aerobic ET stimulus suffices to significantly improve pulmonary Vo_2 on-kinetics, reducing the perturbation of metabolic homeostasis and allowing a faster attainment of steady-state metabolic levels in transitions between different energetic states, such as normally occurring during daily habitual activities.

In a landmark paper, Wisloff and colleagues[6] compared the effects of high-intensity AIT (HI-AIT), consisting of 4-minute training intervals at high intensity (90%–95% of peak heart rate [HR]), separated by 3-minute active pauses (walking at 50%–70% of peak HR), total exercise time 38 minutes, 3 times weekly, with moderate continuous training (MCT), which consisted of walking continuously at 70% to 75% of peak HR, for 47 minutes (to compare isocaloric sessions). Findings were in favor of significant improvements in aerobic capacity with peak Vo_2 increasing by 46% with HI-AIT versus 14% with MCT ($P<.001$), a reverse activity on LV remodeling, and improved endothelial function and quality of life (QoL). Other findings from HI-AIT studies confirm the efficacy of this approach[34,35] and this form of ET is now recommended by the European Society of Cardiology Position Statement on Exercise Training in HF in selected cases according to 4-minute bouts of high-intensity exercise (corresponding to 90%–95% of their maximal exercise capacity), interspersed with 3-minute recovery periods at low intensity, plus 5–10 minutes of warm-up and cool-down.[1]

An ongoing study that is challenging what is current practice in Europe for prescribing ET programs is the SMARTEX-HF study (randomized multicenter trial), which is aimed at definitively determining whether in a population ($n = 200$) of patients with HF reduced ejection fraction, a 12-week supervised HI-AIT program will result in a significant LV reverse remodeling compared with either training at MCT or a control group that is encouraged to exercise regularly without supervised sessions.[36] Secondary endpoints include peak Vo_2, biomarkers, QoL, and level of physical activity assessed by questionnaires. In addition, long-term maintenance of effects after the supervised training period will be determined.

Aerobic interval training is also proposed at low intensity (LI-AIT) and performed on an electrically braked cycle ergometer, which maximizes control over the patient's workload. The "on" and "off" segments are 30 and 60 seconds in duration, respectively, and the "on" segments are performed at 50% of the power output achieved during a ramp test or an incremental bicycle test (ie, 10 W/1-min increments to fatigue).[1]

In a recent meta-analysis, Ismail and colleagues[30] investigated the magnitude of improvement in cardiorespiratory fitness in relation to the different intensity of aerobic ET. Seventy-four studies were included, producing 76 intervention groups: 9 (11.8%) were HI-AIT, 38 (50%) vigorous-intensity, 24 (31.6%) MCT, and 5 (6.6%) LI-AIT groups, providing a total of 3265 exercising subjects and 2612 control subjects. Peak Vo_2 increased by a mean difference of 3.33 $mLO_2 \cdot kg^{-1} \cdot min^{-1}$ with HI-AIT groups compared with control groups demonstrating a 23% improvement from baseline.

For vigorous intensity, the mean difference was 2.27 $mLO_2 \cdot kg^{-1} \cdot min^{-1}$ with an 8% weighted mean; for MIT, the mean difference was 2.17 $mLO_2 \cdot kg^{-1} \cdot min^{-1}$ with a weighted mean of 13%; and for LI-AIT, the mean difference was 1.04 $mLO_2 \cdot kg^{-1} \cdot min^{-1}$ with a weighted mean of 7%.[30] Although at present, there is no consensus on what threshold constitutes a clinically relevant response to ET, it is well-known that some patients are unable to increase their exercise capacity within the expected range.[37] In 2008, Tabet and colleagues[38] showed that the absence of improvement in exercise capacity after an ET program, as defined as median change in percent-predicted peak Vo_2 less than 6%, was a predictor of poor prognosis in patients with HF, independently of peak Vo_2, B-type natriuretic peptide (BNP) level, New York Heart Association (NYHA) class, and left ventricular ejection fraction (LVEF) at admission.[38]

Schmid and colleagues[37] defined a responder as someone who achieved at least one of the following improvements: (1) increase in peak Vo_2 by greater than 5%; (2) increase in workload by greater than 10%; and (3) decrease in VE/VCO$_2$ slope by greater than 5%. They studied a cohort of 120 consecutive patients with HF with sinus rhythm participating in a 3-month outpatient cardiac rehabilitation program (aerobic endurance training on a cycle ergometer and gym/resistance training) and found that HR reserve, HR recovery at 1 min, and peak HR were significant predictors for a positive training response.

Resistance/Strength Exercise Training

Resistance/strength training (RST) is a muscle contraction performed against a specific opposing force, thereby generating resistance. Although sustained maximal isometric (static) resistive

Table 1
Main European randomized exercise training control trials performed in Europe

Study	Country	Participants	Training Characteristics	End Point
Continuous endurance training				
Low intensity				
Belardinelli et al,[3] 1995	Italy	N = 27 Exercise, n = 18, 16 m/2 f, mean age, 56 y. Control, n = 9, 7 m/2 f, mean age 57. NYHA class II/III.	Exercise: 8 wk of continuous ET, 3 sessions per week, 30 min at 40% of peak V_{O_2}. Control: no exercise.	Increase in peak V_{O_2} (17%), lactic acidosis threshold (20%), and peak workload (21%).
Moderate intensity				
Erbs et al,[4] 2010	Germany	N = 73 Exercise, n = 36. 26 with moderate HF, mean age, 55 y. Control, n = 37. NYHA class II/III.	Exercise: 24 wk of continuous ET, 7 sessions per week, 20 min per session at 70% of peak V_{O_2}. Control: no exercise.	Increase in peak V_{O_2} by 2.7 ± 2.2 vs -0.8 ± 3.1 $mLO_2 \cdot kg^{-1} \cdot min^{-1}$ in control and LVEF by 9.4 ± 6.1 vs $-0.8 \pm 5.2\%$ in control.
Laoutaris et al,[5] 2011	Greece	N = 15 (ventricular assist devices long-term post-LVAD implantation). Exercise, n = 10, mean age 37. Control, n = 5, 4 m/1 f, mean age 42.	Exercise: 10 wk of ET, 3–5 sessions per week, 45 min per session at Borg scale 12–14 plus walking for 30–45 min/d. Control: 10 wk walking for 30–45 min/d.	Improvement in peak V_{O_2} (19.3 ± 4.5 vs 16.8 ± 3.7 $mLO_2 \cdot kg^{-1} \cdot min^{-1}$) and V_{O_2} at VAT (15.1 ± 4.2 vs 12 ± 5.6 $mLO_2 \cdot kg^{-1} \cdot min^{-1}$), decrease in VE/VCO$_2$ slope (35.9 ± 5.6 vs 40 ± 6.5).
Giannuzzi et al,[8] 2003	Italy	N = 89 Exercise, n = 45, mean age, 60. Control, n = 44, mean age, 61. NYHA class II/III.	26 wk of continuous ET, 4 sessions per week, 30 min per session at 60% of peak V_{O_2} plus home-based training.	Improvement in work capacity, peak V_{O_2}, walking distance, and QoL.
Hambrecht et al,[9] 2000	Germany	N = 73 Exercise, n = 36, mean age, 54. Control, n = 37, mean age, 55, NYHA class I/II/III.	Exercise: 26 wk of continuous ET, 7 sessions per week, 20 min per session at 70% of MHR plus 1 group exercise session per week. Control: no exercise.	Increment in peak V_{O_2} by 4.8 $mLO_2 \cdot kg^{-1} \cdot min^{-1}$ vs 0.3 $mLO_2 \cdot kg^{-1} \cdot min^{-1}$.

High intensity

Study	Country	Population	Intervention	Outcomes
Wisloff et al,[6] 2007	Norway	N = 18 Exercise AIT: n = 9, 7 m/2 f, mean age, 77. Exercise MCT: n 9, 7 m/2 f, mean age, 75. Control: n = 9, 6 m/3 f, mean age, 76.	AIT: 12 wk of interval ET, 3 sessions per week, 38 min at 90%–95% peak Vo_2. MCT: 12 wk of MCT (walking continuously at 70%–75% of peak HR for 47 min each session). Control: training once every 3 wk.	Increase in peak Vo_2 (46%) LVEF (35%) and pro-brain natriuretic peptide (40%). Decrease in LV end-diastolic (18%) and end-systolic volumes (25%).
Freyssin et al,[7] 2012	France	N = 26 Exercise: n = 12, 6 m/6 f, mean age, 54. Control: n = 14, 7 m/7 f, mean age, 55.	8 wk of interval (first group) and continuous (second group) ET. First group: 6 sessions per week, 71 min. Second group: 61 min, at 50%–80% of the maximal power reached during a steep ramp test.	Increase in Vo_2 the duration of the exercise test, the O_2 at the VAT, and the distance walked during the 6 MWT.

Resistance training

Resistance exercise vs control

Study	Country	Population	Intervention	Outcomes
Cider et al,[10] 1997	Sweden	Total patients, N = 23. Exercise, n = 11, mean age, 62. Control, n = 12, mean age, 65. NYHA class II/III.	Exercise: supervised resistance training program at 60% of 1-RM (2630 repetitions) for upper and lower body, 26/wk for 20 wk. Control = usual care.	Mean changes in anaerobic threshold (5.9 vs 219.1 W, $P<.01$) and number of heel lifts (higher in E than in C; 23.7 vs 5.4 repetitions, $P<.01$). Mean changes in peak Vo_2, HR, peak isokinetic quadriceps muscle strength, and endurance. HR variability and scores on Nottingham Health Profile and Quality of Life Questionnaire Heart Failure were not significantly different.
Tyni-Lennè et al,[11] 2001	Sweden	N = 39 HF (23 IHD, 16 DCM). Exercise, n = 19 (15 men, aged 65 y, LVEF 27%). Control, n = 20 (18 men, aged 64 y, LVEF 28%). NYHA II–III	Exercise = Resistance training at moderate intensity, 30–120 s × 1 set × 6 exercises, 3/wk × 3 mo. Control = usual care.	Increase in peak Vo_2 (8%, $P<.03$) the distance walked in a 6MWT (11%, $P<.002$), the health-related QoL ($P<.001$), and plasma norepinephrine levels at rest (32%, $P<.003$), and at submaximal intensities ($P<.03$).

(continued on next page)

Table 1
(continued)

Study	Country	Participants	Training Characteristics	End Point
Combined resistance and aerobic exercise vs aerobic exercise				
Beckers et al,[12] 2008	Belgium	N = 58 HF (43 men). Exercise, n = 28; mean age, 58 y. Control, n = 30; mean age, 59 y. NYHA II/III	Exercise: supervised progressive resistance training program at 50%–60% of 1-RM (1610–2615 repetitions) alternating between trunk and upper and lower body in combination with leg cycling and treadmill walking/jogging for 8–15 min at a HR achieved at 90% of the anaerobic threshold, 36/wk for 23 wk. Control: supervised leg cycling, treadmill walking/jogging, stair or step, arm cycling, and half recumbent or reclined cycling for 8–15 min at a HR achieved at 90% of the anaerobic threshold, 36/wk for 23 wk.	Mean changes in steady-state workload (24.8 vs 15.6 W, $P = .007$) and HR over steady-state ratio (1.43 vs 0.47, $P = .002$), upper limb isotonic muscle strength (13.2 vs 5.7 kg, $P = .003$), and maximal expiratory pressure (12.5 vs 28.6% predicted, $P = .03$). The number of patients who reported a significant decrease on Health Complaints Scale (60 vs 28%, $P = .03$) were higher in E than in C. Mean changes in peak V_{O_2}, peak power output, peak HR, (submaximal) work economy, VE/VCO$_2$ slope, circulatory power, lower limb isokinetic measurements, lower limb isotonic muscle strength, maximal inspiratory pressure, NYHA classification, NT-pro-BNP, LVEF, LVEDD, LVESD, body fat percentage, fat mass, fat-free mass, BMI, and waist-hip ratio were not significantly different.
Degache et al,[13] 2007	France	Total patients, N = 23 HF. Exercise, n = 12, mean age 50 Control, n = 11, mean age, 55. NYHA II/III	Exercise: supervised progressive resistance training program at 70% of 1-RM (10,610 repetitions) on a isotonic concentric leg extensor bench in combination with leg cycling for 30 min at 65% of peak V_{O_2}, 36/wk for 8 wk. Control: leg cycling for 45 min at 65% of peak V_{O_2}, 36/wk for 8 wk.	Mean change in isokinetic knee extensor strength at 60° (0.14 vs 20.06 Nm/kg, P, .03) and 180° (0.13 vs 20.06 Nm/kg, P, .04) were higher in E than in C. Mean change in peak V_{O_2} was not significantly different. No statistical comparisons were reported between E and C for mean changes in NYHA classification, isokinetic knee flexor strength at 60 and 180 u/s, peak power output, peak HR, peak systolic blood pressure, and V_{O_2} at VAT.

Respiratory training

Threshold

Study	Country	Total patients	Training	Results
Johnson et al,[14] 1998	UK	Total patients (stable chronic HF). N = 16 Training, n = 8. Control, n = 8.	Training: threshold at 30% of MIP for 8 wk (15 min, 2×/d, 7/wk).	Improved MIP and MEP.
Hulzebos et al,[15] 2006	Netherlands	N = 26 (before CABG). Training, n = 14. Control, n = 12.	Training: threshold at 30% of MIP for 14–90 d (mean = 30).	Improvement in MIP and IME and postoperative pulmonary complications.
Bosnak-Guclu et al,[16] 2011	Turkey	N = 30 Training, n = 16. Control, n = 14.	Training: threshold at 40% of MIP for 6 wk (30 min, 7×/wk).	Improved in MIP, MEP, distance walked in a 6-min test, balance, dyspnea, depression, QoL.

TIRE

Study	Country	Total patients	Training	Results
Laoutaris et al,[17] 2004	Greece	N = 35 Training, n = 20. Control, n = 15.	Training: TIRE at 60% of MIP/SMIP for 10 wk (3×/wk).	Improved MIP, SMIP, distance walked in a 6-min test, peak Vo_2, HR, dyspnea, and QoL.
Laoutaris et al,[18] 2007	Greece	N = 47 Training, n = 15. Control, n = 32.	Training: TIRE at 60% of MIP/SMIP for 10 wk (3×/wk).	Improved MIP, SMIP, peak Vo_2, and dyspnea.
Laoutaris et al,[19] 2008	Greece	N = 23 Training, n = 14. Control, n = 9.	Training: TIRE at 60% of MIP/SMIP for 10 wk (3×/wk).	Improvement in MIP, SMIP, peak Vo_2, distance walked in a 6-min walk test, dyspnea.
Laoutaris et al,[20] 2013	Greece	N = 27 Training, n = 13. Control, n = 14.	Training: TIRE at 60% of MIP/SMIP for 12 wk (20 min, 3×/wk).	Improved MIP, SMIP, peak Vo_2, VE/VCO_2 slope, VAT, LVEF, LVESD, LVEDD, QoL.

Abbreviations: BMI, body mass index; CABG, coronary artery bypass graft; f, female; LVAD, left ventricular assist device; LVEDD, left ventricular end-diastolic diameter; LVESD, left ventricular end-systolic diameter; m, male; MEP, maximal expiratory pressure; MIP, maximal inspiratory pressure; SMIP, sustained maximal inspiratory pressure; TIRE, test of incremental respiratory endurance.
Data from Refs.[3–20]

exercise causes an excessive increase in blood pressure and lowers stroke volume and for this reason it is considered inappropriate for patients with HF, isotonic (dynamic) resistive exercises (constant or variable resistance through the range of motion using either free weights or weight machines), on the contrary, have become an integral part of contemporary ET programs for patients with low cardiovascular risk.

RST produces improvements in strength, improves muscle tone, and increases muscle and bone mass (counteracting loss of skeletal muscle mass typically found in elderly patients with HF or those with advanced HF at any age), which corresponds to type I fibers overexpression and improved oxidative activity. Moreover, RST has demonstrated anti-inflammatory effects and improved insulin resistance.[39] Given the demonstrated effects of RST, it has been proposed as an anabolic intervention to help prevent wasting syndrome and disability.[1,40]

In this regard, it is important to remember, however, that despite the many positive effects that have been demonstrated, RST is currently considered a complement to the primary rehabilitation intervention, aerobic endurance ET, and in no way a substitute for the latter.[1] On the other hand, however, QoL in these oftentimes disabled patients depends on engagement in daily life activity, which does not demand peak aerobic performance. Simple tasks such as pulling, pushing, and lifting (submaximal sustained efforts) require skeletal muscle mass and the strength of both the upper and the lower limbs. Patients with HF are advised to train smaller muscle groups (including upper and lower body muscle groups) in a dynamic way, avoiding Valsalva maneuvers (by giving breathing directions), at low-to-moderate intensity.

In 2006, Meyer[41] pointed out that dynamic RST is well tolerated in chronic stable HF when (1) initial contraction intensity is slow; (2) small muscle groups are involved; (3) work phases are kept short; (4) a small number of repetitions per set are performed; and (5) work/rest ratio is greater than 1:2. In stable patients with HF, the German Federation for cardiovascular prevention and rehabilitation advises short stress phases (10 repetitions maximum) at less than 60% of one-repetition maximum (1-RM) or maximum voluntary contraction (MVC) interrupted by phases of muscle relaxation. Usually, exercise is implemented at 40% to 60% of the MVC.[40]

Most commonly, dynamic resistive exercise is integrated in so-called circuit weight training, which involves both endurance and resistive ET, on an alternate basis.

Combination of Endurance-Resistance Exercise Training

Beckers and colleagues[12] performed the largest randomized trial comparing aerobic ET with a program that combines both aerobic ET and RST performed by a multifunctional fitness-machine according to a prespecified program. During the first 2 months, patients assigned to the combined group trained for almost 40 minutes on the RST equipment, and only 10 minutes were devoted to aerobic ET. RST was reduced to 30 minutes (9 muscle groups, 2 times 15 repetitions each) and aerobic ET was increased to 2 bouts of 8 minutes in the following months. During the last 2 months, aerobic ET was progressively up-titrated to a point where exercise times of 10, 12, and 15 minutes on 3 aerobic modalities (ie, treadmill, bicycle, stair or step, arm-ergometer, recumbent cycle) were achieved. They found that the observed increase in submaximal exercise capacity was larger in the combined versus the aerobic ET group, which was also reflected in terms of health-related QoL.

There were no adverse events/outcomes during training in the combined group. Moreover, the minute ventilation/carbon dioxide production (VE/VCO_2) slope improved significantly in patients assigned to the combined training regimen. Finally, in the combined training group, this study demonstrated no detrimental effects on LV remodeling and N-terminal-pro-BNP levels, mildly improved systolic function and the comparable outcomes in terms of mortality and morbidity, suggesting that this training approach in appropriate patients with HF is safe.

Respiratory Exercise Training

Respiratory muscle dysfunction, characterized by respiratory muscle fiber atrophy, deoxygenation, and impaired mitochondrial oxidative capacity, is often observed in advanced HF.[42,43] These changes lead to reduced inspiratory and expiratory muscle strength (IMS and EMS) and inspiratory muscle endurance (IME) defined as the ability to sustain a specific task over time. These variables significantly correlate with exercise tolerance, level of dyspnea, and peak Vo_2. Furthermore, many studies have documented the prognostic value of IMS and IME in HF.[42,44] Hence, routine screening for respiratory muscle dysfunction is advised and specific inspiratory muscle training in addition to standard aerobic ET and RST might be beneficial.[1]

Respiratory ET involves different types of respiratory muscle specific-training devices to improve respiratory muscle function. This approach has been shown to lead to a host of favorable functional and ventilatory effects (ie, improved overall aerobic exercise capacity, ventilatory efficiency, and QoL as well as reduced dyspnea).[2,45–47] Collectively, European guidelines suggest if a pressure loading threshold device is used, respiratory training should be initiated at 30% of the maximal inspiratory pressure (PI_{max}) and to readjust the intensity every 7 to 10 days up to a maximum of 60%. Training duration should be 20 to –30 min/d with a frequency of 3 to 5 sessions per week for a minimum of 8 weeks.[1,2]

Laoutaris and coworkers[17–19] have conducted a set of nonrandomized controlled trials of inspiratory muscle training in patients with HF using a device set at 60% of the sustained PI_{max}, with 3 sessions per week for 10 weeks. This incremental respiratory endurance regimen led to a 32% to 35% improvement in PI_{max} and a 12% to 16% increase in peak Vo_2. Significant improvements in 6-minute walk test (6MWT) distance and scores of QoL were also observed. However, there were no significant changes in ventilatory efficiency during incremental exercise, evaluated by the VE/VCO_2 slope. Recently, Smart and colleagues[48] performed a systematic review and meta-analysis to determine the magnitude of change in peak Vo_2, 6MWT distance, QoL, PI_{max}, and the VE/VCO_2 slope with inspiratory muscle training in patients with HF. The authors showed that this form of training improves cardiorespiratory fitness and QoL to a similar magnitude compared with conventional ET but may provide an initial alternative to the more severely deconditioned patients with HF who may then transition to conventional ET.

Moreover, combining inspiratory muscle training with other forms of ET could add to the effect of either approach alone. Winkelmann and colleagues[49] demonstrated that 30 minutes of daily threshold inspiratory muscle training performed at 30% of PI_{max} combined with aerobic ET resulted in additional significant improvements in maximal PI_{max}, peak Vo_2, ventilatory efficiency, and recovery oxygen kinetics. Finally, Laoutaris and colleagues[20] combining aerobic ET with RST and inspiratory muscle training in a complete exercise model called ARIS (combined aerobic/resistance/inspiratory muscle training) found that ARIS training was safe and resulted in incremental benefits in both peripheral and respiratory muscle weakness, cardiopulmonary function, and QoL compared with aerobic ET alone.

SUMMARY

In conclusion, ET in patients with HF is a well-accepted intervention in Europe, with a robust body of supporting evidence and supporting clinical guidelines. The traditional approach to aerobic ET, MCT, is being challenged by HI-AIT, and the latter approach may supplant the former in appropriate patients diagnosed with this chronic condition. In addition, evidence clearly demonstrates the important role of RST and respiratory ET in patients with HF. In fact, a combined approach may be optimal.

REFERENCES

1. Piepoli MF, Conraads V, Corra U, et al. Exercise training in heart failure: from theory to practice. A consensus document of the Heart Failure Association and the European Association for Cardiovascular Prevention and Rehabilitation. Eur J Heart Fail 2011;13(4):347–57.
2. Vanhees L, Rauch B, Piepoli M, et al. Importance of characteristics and modalities of physical activity and exercise in the management of cardiovascular health in individuals with cardiovascular disease (Part III). Eur J Prev Cardiol 2012;19(6):1333–56.
3. Belardinelli R, Georgiou D, Scocco V, et al. Low intensity exercise training in patients with chronic heart failure. J Am Coll Cardiol 1995;26(4):975–82.
4. Erbs S, Hollriegel R, Linke A, et al. Exercise training in patients with advanced chronic heart failure (NYHA IIIb) promotes restoration of peripheral vasomotor function, induction of endogenous regeneration, and improvement of left ventricular function. Circ Heart Fail 2010;3(4):486–94.
5. Laoutaris ID, Dritsas A, Adamopoulos S, et al. Benefits of physical training on exercise capacity, inspiratory muscle function, and quality of life in patients with ventricular assist devices long-term postimplantation. Eur J Cardiovasc Prev Rehabil 2011;18(1): 33–40.
6. Wisloff U, Stoylen A, Loennechen JP, et al. Superior cardiovascular effect of aerobic interval training versus moderate continuous training in heart failure patients: a randomized study. Circulation 2007; 115(24):3086–94.
7. Freyssin C, Verkindt C, Prieur F, et al. Cardiac rehabilitation in chronic heart failure: effect of an 8-week, high-intensity interval training versus continuous training. Arch Phys Med Rehabil 2012;93(8):1359–64.
8. Giannuzzi P, Temporelli PL, Corra U, et al. Antiremodeling effect of long-term exercise training in patients with stable chronic heart failure: results of the Exercise in Left Ventricular Dysfunction and Chronic Heart Failure (ELVD-CHF) Trial. Circulation 2003; 108(5):554–9.
9. Hambrecht R, Gielen S, Linke A, et al. Effects of exercise training on left ventricular function and peripheral resistance in patients with chronic heart failure: a randomized trial. JAMA 2000;283(23): 3095–101.

10. Cider A, Tygesson H, Hedberg M, et al. Peripheral muscle training in patients with clinical signs of heart failure. Scand J Rehabil Med 1997;29(2):121–7.

11. Tyni-Lennè R, Dencker K, Gordon A, et al. Comprehensive local muscle training increases aerobic working capacity and quality of life and decreases neurohormonal activation in patients with chronic heart failure. Eur J Heart Fail 2001;3(1):47–52.

12. Beckers PJ, Denollet J, Possemiers NM, et al. Combined endurance-resistance training vs. endurance training in patients with chronic heart failure: a prospective randomized study. Eur Heart J 2008; 29(15):1858–66.

13. Degache F, Garet M, Calmels P, et al. Enhancement of isokinetic muscle strength with a combined training programme in chronic heart failure. Clin Physiol Funct Imaging 2007;27(4):225–30.

14. Johnson PH, Cowley AJ, Kinnear WJ. A randomized controlled trial of inspiratory muscle training in stable chronic heart failure. Eur Heart J 1998;19(8):1249–53.

15. Hulzebos EH, Helders PJ, Favie NJ, et al. Preoperative intensive inspiratory muscle training to prevent postoperative pulmonary complications in high-risk patients undergoing CABG surgery: a randomized clinical trial. JAMA 2006;296(15):1851–7.

16. Bosnak-Guclu M, Arikan H, Savci S, et al. Effects of inspiratory muscle training in patients with heart failure. Respir Med 2011;105(11):1671–81.

17. Laoutaris I, Dritsas A, Brown MD, et al. Inspiratory muscle training using an incremental endurance test alleviates dyspnea and improves functional status in patients with chronic heart failure. Eur J Cardiovasc Prev Rehabil 2004;11(6):489–96.

18. Laoutaris ID, Dritsas A, Brown MD, et al. Immune response to inspiratory muscle training in patients with chronic heart failure. Eur J Cardiovasc Prev Rehabil 2007;14(5):679–85.

19. Laoutaris ID, Dritsas A, Brown MD, et al. Effects of inspiratory muscle training on autonomic activity, endothelial vasodilator function, and N-terminal pro-brain natriuretic peptide levels in chronic heart failure. J Cardiopulm Rehabil Prev 2008;28(2):99–106.

20. Laoutaris ID, Adamopoulos S, Manginas A, et al. Benefits of combined aerobic/resistance/inspiratory training in patients with chronic heart failure. A complete exercise model? A prospective randomised study. Int J Cardiol 2013;167(5):1967–72.

21. Dubach P, Myers J, Dziekan G, et al. Effect of high intensity exercise training on central hemodynamic responses to exercise in men with reduced left ventricular function. J Am Coll Cardiol 1997;29(7):1591–8.

22. Meyer T, Gorge G, Schwaab B, et al. An alternative approach for exercise prescription and efficacy testing in patients with chronic heart failure: a randomized controlled training study. Am Heart J 2005;149(5):e1–7.

23. Mezzani A, Agostoni P, Cohen-Solal A, et al. Standards for the use of cardiopulmonary exercise testing for the functional evaluation of cardiac patients: a report from the Exercise Physiology Section of the European Association for Cardiovascular Prevention and Rehabilitation. Eur J Cardiovasc Prev Rehabil 2009;16(3):249–67.

24. Dekerle J, Baron B, Dupont L, et al. Maximal lactate steady state, respiratory compensation threshold and critical power. Eur J Appl Physiol 2003;89(3–4):281–8.

25. Binder RK, Wonisch M, Corra U, et al. Methodological approach to the first and second lactate threshold in incremental cardiopulmonary exercise testing. Eur J Cardiovasc Prev Rehabil 2008;15(6):726–34.

26. De Maeyer C, Beckers P, Vrints CJ, et al. Exercise training in chronic heart failure. Ther Adv Chronic Dis 2013;4(3):105–17.

27. Page E, Cohen-Solal A, Jondeau G, et al. Comparison of treadmill and bicycle exercise in patients with chronic heart failure. Chest 1994;106(4):1002–6.

28. Beckers PJ, Possemiers NM, Van Craenenbroeck EM, et al. Impact of exercise testing mode on exercise parameters in patients with chronic heart failure. Eur J Prev Cardiol 2012;19(3):389–95.

29. Maeder MT, Wolber T, Ammann P, et al. Cardiopulmonary exercise testing in mild heart failure: impact of the mode of exercise on established prognostic predictors. Cardiology 2008;110(2):135–41.

30. Ismail H, McFarlane JR, Nojoumian AH, et al. Clinical outcomes and cardiovascular responses to different exercise training intensities in patients with heart failure: a systematic review and meta-analysis. JACC Heart Fail 2013;1(6):514–22.

31. Belardinelli R, Georgiou D, Cianci G, et al. Randomized, controlled trial of long-term moderate exercise training in chronic heart failure: effects on functional capacity, quality of life, and clinical outcome. Circulation 1999;99(9):1173–82.

32. Demopoulos L, Bijou R, Fergus I, et al. Exercise training in patients with severe congestive heart failure: enhancing peak aerobic capacity while minimizing the increase in ventricular wall stress. J Am Coll Cardiol 1997;29(3):597–603.

33. Mezzani A, Grassi B, Jones AM, et al. Speeding of pulmonary VO2 on-kinetics by light-to-moderate-intensity aerobic exercise training in chronic heart failure: clinical and pathophysiological correlates. Int J Cardiol 2013;167(5):2189–95.

34. Tjonna AE, Lee SJ, Rognmo O, et al. Aerobic interval training versus continuous moderate exercise as a treatment for the metabolic syndrome: a pilot study. Circulation 2008;118(4):346–54.

35. Rognmo O, Hetland E, Helgerud J, et al. High intensity aerobic interval exercise is superior to moderate

intensity exercise for increasing aerobic capacity in patients with coronary artery disease. Eur J Cardiovasc Prev Rehabil 2004;11(3):216–22.

36. Stoylen A, Conraads V, Halle M, et al. Controlled study of myocardial recovery after interval training in heart failure: SMARTEX-HF–rationale and design. Eur J Prev Cardiol 2012;19(4):813–21.

37. Schmid JP, Zurek M, Saner H. Chronotropic incompetence predicts impaired response to exercise training in heart failure patients with sinus rhythm. Eur J Prev Cardiol 2013;20(4):585–92.

38. Tabet JY, Meurin P, Beauvais F, et al. Absence of exercise capacity improvement after exercise training program: a strong prognostic factor in patients with chronic heart failure. Circ Heart Fail 2008;1(4): 220–6.

39. Conraads VM, Beckers P, Bosmans J, et al. Combined endurance/resistance training reduces plasma TNF-alpha receptor levels in patients with chronic heart failure and coronary artery disease. Eur Heart J 2002;23(23):1854–60.

40. Bjarnason-Wehrens B, Mayer-Berger W, Meister ER, et al. Recommendations for resistance exercise in cardiac rehabilitation. Recommendations of the German Federation for Cardiovascular Prevention and Rehabilitation. Eur J Cardiovasc Prev Rehabil 2004;11(4):352–61.

41. Meyer K. Resistance exercise in chronic heart failure–landmark studies and implications for practice. Clin Invest Med 2006;29(3):166–9.

42. Meyer FJ, Borst MM, Zugck C, et al. Respiratory muscle dysfunction in congestive heart failure: clinical correlation and prognostic significance. Circulation 2001;103(17):2153–8.

43. Wong YY, Ruiter G, Lubberink M, et al. Right ventricular failure in idiopathic pulmonary arterial hypertension is associated with inefficient myocardial oxygen utilization. Circ Heart Fail 2011;4(6):700–6.

44. Meyer FJ, Zugck C, Haass M, et al. Inefficient ventilation and reduced respiratory muscle capacity in congestive heart failure. Basic Res Cardiol 2000; 95(4):333–42.

45. Cahalin LP, Arena R, Guazzi M, et al. Inspiratory muscle training in heart disease and heart failure: a review of the literature with a focus on method of training and outcomes. Expert Rev Cardiovasc Ther 2013;11(2):161–77.

46. Dall'Ago P, Chiappa GR, Guths H, et al. Inspiratory muscle training in patients with heart failure and inspiratory muscle weakness: a randomized trial. J Am Coll Cardiol 2006;47(4):757–63.

47. Stein R, Chiappa GR, Guths H, et al. Inspiratory muscle training improves oxygen uptake efficiency slope in patients with chronic heart failure. J Cardiopulm Rehabil Prev 2009;29(6):392–5.

48. Smart NA, Giallauria F, Dieberg G. Efficacy of inspiratory muscle training in chronic heart failure patients: a systematic review and meta-analysis. Int J Cardiol 2013;167(4):1502–7.

49. Winkelmann ER, Chiappa GR, Lima CO, et al. Addition of inspiratory muscle training to aerobic training improves cardiorespiratory responses to exercise in patients with heart failure and inspiratory muscle weakness. Am Heart J 2009;158(5):768.e1–7.

Pharmacologic and Surgical Interventions to Improve Functional Capacity in Heart Failure

Antonio Abbate, MD, PhD[a],*,
Benjamin W. Van Tassell, PharmD[b], Justin M. Canada, CEP[c],
Dave L. Dixon, PharmD[b], Ross A. Arena, PhD, PT[d],
Giuseppe Biondi-Zoccai, MD[e]

KEYWORDS

- Heart failure • Functional capacity • Drugs • Treatments • Surgery • Device

KEY POINTS

- Heart failure is a clinical syndrome of breathlessness, lower extremity swelling, fatigue, and exercise intolerance affecting a large portion of the population worldwide, and associated with premature death.
- Exercise intolerance in heart failure results from, among other things, (1) impaired cardiac contractility, (2) impaired cardiac filling, and/or (3) inappropriate heart rate response.
- Heart failure therapies have multiple goals, including preventing death and hospitalizations and promoting improved symptom control and exercise tolerance.
- Therapies effective in reducing heart failure–related mortality have variable effects on exercise tolerance, with some causing an improvement and some providing no effect or transiently having a negative impact.
- Loop diuretics and aldosterone blockers, although not extensively studied, are routinely used to relieve congestion, improve cardiac filling, and improve exercise tolerance in heart failure.

INTRODUCTION

Heart Failure Syndrome

Heart failure (HF) is a clinical syndrome of breathlessness, lower extremity swelling, fatigue, and exercise intolerance that affects a significant portion of the global population.[1,2] The symptoms and limitations in patients with HF reflect the inability to maintain a cardiac output adequate to the individual's needs and/or the development of inappropriately high cardiac filling pressure leading to pulmonary and/or systemic congestion. Symptoms occurring at rest reflect a severely compromised condition referred to as decompensated HF, which requires urgent care. More often, patients with HF have symptoms occurring with

[a] VCU Pauley Heart Center, Virginia Commonwealth University, 1200 East Broad Street, Box 980281, Richmond, VA 23298, USA; [b] School of Pharmacy, Virginia Commonwealth University, 410 North 12th Street, Box 980533, Richmond, VA 23298, USA; [c] Department of Kinesiology and Health Sciences, College of Humanities and Sciences, Virginia Commonwealth University, 1200 East Marshall Street, Box 980419, Richmond, VA 23298, USA; [d] Department of Physical Therapy, College of Applied Health Sciences, University of Illinois at Chicago, 1919 West Taylor Street, 454 AHSB, Chicago, IL 60612, USA; [e] Department of Medical-Surgical Sciences and Biotechnologies, Sapienza University of Rome, Corso della Repubblica 79, Latina 04100, Italy
* Corresponding author.
E-mail address: aabbate@vcu.edu

Heart Failure Clin 11 (2015) 117–124
http://dx.doi.org/10.1016/j.hfc.2014.08.005
1551-7136/15/$ – see front matter © 2015 Elsevier Inc. All rights reserved.

exertion, reflecting a situation in which the needs are met when oxygen consumption (V_{O_2}) is at resting levels (ie, approximately 3.5 mL O_2/kg/min) but inadequate when the needs are increased by given level of exertion. Based on the relationship between symptoms and activity levels, the severity of HF is graded into different functional classes: no limitations (New York Heart Association [NYHA] class I), mild limitations (NYHA II), moderate limitations (NYHA III), or severe limitations or symptoms at rest (NYHA IV).[2] The greater the limitations, and the higher the NYHA class, the worse the quality of life and the prognosis in patients with HF. Understanding the determinants of functional limitations in HF is a necessary step to effectively treat HF and improve functional capacity.

Determinants of Functional Limitations in Heart Failure

HF is not synonymous with abnormal cardiac structure but reflects a cardiac function that is impaired or, at least, inadequate for the needs given the delicate balance required by the body to perform the required activities without untoward symptoms. According to the definition given earlier, an individual may have impaired cardiac function with a normal heart if the needs or demands are particularly increased (and outside of the physiologic range) as seen in high-output states, such as severe anemia. However, in most cases, HF is associated with abnormal cardiac structure. Three primary determinants of functional limitations in HF are cardiac contractility, diastolic filling, and heart rate (HR) (**Fig. 1**).

Left ventricular contractility

The primary central abnormality in HF is an impaired left ventricular (LV) contractility or contractile reserve. Patients with an LV ejection fraction (LVEF) less than 50% (or <40% depending on which definition is used) are referred to as having systolic HF or HF with reduced EF (HFrEF). An LVEF less than 50% is only observed in approximately 50% of patients diagnosed with HF, but the LVEF does not generally correlate with the severity of symptoms. This lack of correlation is expected because the cardiac output (CO) ultimately determines whether the metabolic demands are met, not the LVEF. CO is calculated as LV end-diastolic volume (LVEDV) × LVEF × HR. Therefore, a patient with LVEF of 30% may have the same CO as a patient with LVEF of 60%, if the LVEDV is double. What may be more important is the increase in CO with exertion, but the assessment of LVEF with exertion (contractile reserve) is rarely completed in patients with HF. The CO also depends on the performance of the right ventricle. An abnormal right ventricular (RV) systolic function represents another reason for an inappropriately low CO, even in the presence of normal LVEF.

Left ventricular diastole

The LVEDV is a critical determinant of both stroke volume (stroke volume = LVEDV × LVEF) and CO (LVEDV × LVEF × HR). Impaired LV filling during diastole may lead to an inappropriately small LVEDV and inadequate CO, even in the presence of normal LVEF. The most extreme example of this is the patient with hypovolemic shock in

CARDIAC FILLING   **CONTRACTILITY**   **FREQUENCY**

Overfilling
Underfilling

Frequency is the number of oscillations per second

LVEDV   ×   LVEF   ×   Heart Rate = C O

Impaired filling   *Systolic dysfunction*   *Bradycardia*

| Elevated filling pressures, Hypovolemia, Valvular Disease, Pulmonary Vascular Disease, RV failure, Tachyarrhythmia, AV dissociation | Ischemia, Infarction, Cardiomyopathy, Valvular Disease, Systemic HTN, Sepsis, Medications | Bradyarrhythmias, AV block, Chronotropic Incompetence |

Fig. 1. Cardiac determinants of impaired exercise capacity in HF. An overview of the cardiac determinants of impaired cardiac output (at rest or with exertion) and of impaired exercise capacity in HF. The heart is represented as a cylinder pump with a piston. The filling of the cylinder is important to determine the pump output. The most common conditions leading to impaired cardiac filling are listed. The cardiac contractility is represented by the power of the piston in the engine. If the piston loses power, the pump output is compromised. A list of common conditions leading to impaired systolic function is given. The frequency at which the piston runs determines the output per minute (cardiac output), the frequency may be inappropriately low at rest (bradycardia) or fail to increase with exertion (chronotropic incompetence). AV, atrioventricular; CO, cardiac output; HTN, hypertension; LVEDV, left ventricular end-diastolic volume; LVEF, left ventricular ejection fraction; RV, right ventricular.

whom a severe reduction in the circulating volume leads to inappropriate cardiac filling, inadequate CO, and shock. However, the impairment in LV filling in HF is not caused by an inadequate volume (except in the case of excessive diuretic use), but by the presence of structural abnormalities, as in atrioventricular valve stenosis, or more commonly by inappropriately high intracavitary pressures. The LV cavitary pressures depend on the preload (venous return to the heart), the afterload (obstacle to output; usually related to systemic vascular resistance and occasional aortic or pulmonary valve stenosis), and the intrinsic properties of the myocardium (diastolic function, which can be further divided into active relaxation and passive stiffness). An alteration in any of these factors can lead to inappropriately high intracavitary pressures and inadequate filling, and reduced CO. As an extreme example, a patient with severe mitral stenosis may have inadequate CO caused by impaired filling of the LV in the absence of abnormalities of the LV function.

Heart rate

HR is an important determinant in HF, because CO = LVEDV × LVEF × HR. An inappropriately low HR may lead to reduced CO, referred to as symptomatic bradycardia. Inappropriately high HR may also negatively affect CO but that is through an impairment of LV filling with each cycle,[3] referred to as symptomatic tachycardia.

Additional factors

Several additional factors may contribute to functional limitations in HF, but these factors generally lead to an abnormality in one of the determinants discussed earlier. For example, atrioventricular dissociation in atrial fibrillation may impair LV diastolic filling, or severe systemic or pulmonary hypertension may impair ejection and reduce LVEF. Moreover, functional limitations in HF may be associated with comorbidities often associated with HF but not necessarily leading to impaired CO, such as chronic pulmonary disease, obesity, and deconditioning.

Prognostic Factors in Heart Failure

Functional limitations and exercise intolerance are central to the HF syndrome. However, the adverse prognosis in patients with HF only partially depends on the impairment in functional capacity. Only one-half of HF deaths can be attributed to pump failure, whereas the remaining deaths are caused by arrhythmias or are related to other concomitant diseases (eg, ischemic heart disease).[4]

The increased risk of ventricular arrhythmias in HF is directly related to the presence of structural

heart disease and to the reduction in LVEF, with a significantly higher risk for patients with LVEF less than 30% to 40%.[5] Therefore, targeted treatments to prevent arrhythmia-related deaths are justified for patients with HF and a reduced LVEF.

Functional capacity is another important clinical prognostic factor in HF. Impaired functional capacity, measured by cardiopulmonary exercise testing or the 6-minute walk test, predicts increased mortality in patients with HF independently of LVEF.[6]

Coronary artery disease and hypertension are two of the most common causes of HF worldwide, and thus myocardial ischemia and target-organ hypertensive injury are common causes of morbidity and death in HF.

Therapeutic Approach in Heart Failure

Current guidelines recommend early identification and treatment of HF.[2] The American College of Cardiology/American Heart Association identify different stages of HF based on the presence/absence of structural heart abnormalities or dysfunction and presence/absence of symptoms.[2] Stage A describes patients without HF symptoms or structural heart disease but who are at risk of HF. Stage B is the presence of heart abnormalities in the absence of current or prior HF symptoms, whereas stage C refers to symptomatic HF in the presence of structural heart disease. Treatment with neurohormonal blockers and vasodilators is indicated in stages B and C to prevent the progression of cardiomyopathy and the incidence or worsening of symptoms.[2] Blockers of the renin-angiotensin-aldosterone and adrenergic systems prevent progression of cardiomyopathy (adverse remodeling), the incidence of HF symptoms, and HF-related mortality.[2] For patients with LVEF less than 30%, the implantable cardioverter-defibrillator (ICD) and the biventricular pacemaker for cardiac resynchronization have also been shown to improve survival in patients with HF.[2] Although the current treatment paradigm appropriately emphasizes prevention of HF-related mortality, it is important to remember that HF provides a significant burden to patients in terms of morbidity and disability. **Table 1** shows the effects of HF therapies on HF mortality and functional capacity.

Effects of Heart Failure Therapies on Functional Capacity

ICD therapy for prevention of arrhythmic death in HF provides a clear example of how a treatment effective in reducing HF mortality provides no improvement in HF symptoms or functional capacity.[7] Moreover, the ICD induces small injuries to the myocardium when the device fires during

Table 1
Effects of HF therapies on mortality and exercise capacity

	Mortality	Exercise Capacity	Notes
Angiotensin antagonists • ACE inhibitors • ARB	Decreased	Improved	Effects more pronounced in HFrEF or HFpEF with HTN
BAR blockers • β1 selective • Nonselective	Decreased	Reduced or Unaffected	Effects more pronounced in HFrEF
Aldosterone antagonists	Decreased	Improved	Effects more pronounced in HFrEF
Hydralazine/ISDN	Decreased	Improved	Effects more pronounced in HFrEF
Diuretics	Unknown	Unknown	No available data from randomized trials
Digoxin	Unaffected	Improved	Narrow therapeutic window
Ivabradine	Decreased	Improved	Not approved in the United States
PDE3 inhibitors	Increased	Improved	Favorable effects limited to the acute phase
PDE5 inhibitors	Unknown	Improved	Effects more pronounced in patients with PAH
CRT	Decreased	Improved	Effects seen in patients with HFrEF and LBBB
ICD	Decreased	Unaffected or Reduced	Limited to HFrEF
LVAD	Decreased	Improved	In selected patients with HFrEF
Ultrafiltration/renal replacement therapy	Unaffected	Improved	In selected patients

Abbreviations: ACE, angiotensin-converting enzyme; ARB, angiotensin receptor blocker; BAR, β-adrenergic receptor; CRT, cardiac resynchronization therapy; HFpEF, heart failure with preserved ejection fraction; HTN, systemic hypertension; ISDN, isosorbide dinitrate; LBBB, left bundle branch block; LVAD, LV assist device; PAH, pulmonary arterial hypertension; PDE, phosphodiesterase.

an arrhythmic event, and not only fails to improve HF symptoms but may worsen HF symptoms.[7] This apparent paradox clearly highlights the distinct goals of HF therapies. Many of the established therapies in HF offer nonsignificant improvements in functional capacity.

Vasodilators
Neurohormonal activation in HF is associated with increased systemic vascular resistance (SVR), which in turn opposes cardiac ejection and increases cardiac filling pressures. As such, vasodilators are a mainstay of HF therapy.[2] Inhibitors of the angiotensin system provide a reduction in SVR, which translates to an increase in CO with exercise tolerance.[8,9] This finding is particularly evident in hypertensive patients. The combination of hydralazine and isosorbide dinitrate provides a similar improvement in patients with HF.[10] However, the use of nifedipine, felodipine, or amlodipine in patients with HF was not associated with an improvement in exercise capacity,[11–14] suggesting that the mechanism by which vasodilation is obtained may be important.

β-Adrenergic blockers
β-Adrenergic receptor (BAR) blockers, once considered contraindicated in HF because of the

negative inotropic and chronotropic effects, are now an essential component of HF therapy because they have been found to significantly reduce associated mortality.[2] Initiation of BAR blockers may reduce peak Vo_2 in the short term, mostly because of blunting of the HR response and a reduction in peak HR.[15,16] Long-term treatment with BAR blockers, if treatment reverses the severity of the cardiomyopathy, improves cardiac metabolism and allows a similar exercise capacity to be maintained, but at a lower metabolic cost.[15–17] In a head-to-head study between a selective β1-adrenergic receptor (β1AR) blocker, metoprolol, and a nonselective α1β1β2AR blocker, carvedilol, a greater blunting of the chronotropic response with exercise, which is a marker of BAR responsiveness, with carvedilol was associated with a greater improvement in cardiac performance but also with a paradoxically lower peak Vo_2.[16] A decrease in peak HR with nebivolol, a β1AR antagonist with vasodilating properties, was similarly associated with a reduction in peak Vo_2.[18]

Aldosterone antagonists
Spironolactone, which has been shown to improve survival in patients with systolic HF, was also

shown to improve exercise capacity in a dose-dependent manner.[19]

Diuretics

Notwithstanding the lack of randomized controlled trials showing a favorable effect on HF survival, loop diuretics are the standard of care in HF because they relieve symptoms of congestion and improve quality of life. Although data from cohort studies found an association between high-dose loop diuretics and decreased survival,[20] this likely represents differences in the clinical condition of the patients studied. Formal studies on the effects of loop diuretics on exercise capacity in HF and evidence of congestion are lacking. In a small study of patients with systolic HF and no evidence of volume overload on physical examination, the addition of torsemide 5 mg once daily provided no benefit compared with placebo.[21] Thiazide diuretics are rarely used as first line for the treatment of volume overload but are occasionally used in combination with loop diuretics in patients who are refractory to loop diuretics.[2] For patients with severe renal impairment and/or who are refractory to diuretics, ultrafiltration or renal replacement therapy can be considered to improve exercise capacity.[22]

Digoxin

Digoxin is a Na+/K+ pump inhibitor that acts as a parasympathetic tone modulator and cardiac inotrope. Although digoxin is likely the oldest HF drug in use, clinical trials have failed to show an improvement in HF survival with digoxin.[23] Nevertheless, digoxin improved exercise capacity and reduced rates of hospitalizations for HF.[23–25] Routine use of digoxin is limited by several factors, including a variable ability to improve symptoms, narrow therapeutic window, association with significant drug-to-drug interactions, and increased risk of ventricular arrhythmias.[23–25]

Ivabradine

Ivabradine inhibits the intrinsic pacemaker activity of the sinoatrial node through funny current (I_f) K^+ channel inhibition, resulting in a reduced HR without adversely affecting systolic function.[26] Ivabradine also modulates LV diastolic function, independently of its effects on HF. In HF with reduced LVEF (HFrEF) and preserved LVEF (HFpEF), ivabradine improved exercise tolerance when given for 2 to 12 weeks.[27,28] Ivabradine is not approved for clinical use in the United Sates but it is widely used in Europe and the Asia-Pacific given the favorable results reported in the morbidity-mortality evaluation of the I_f inhibitor ivabradine in patients with coronary disease and left-ventricular dysfunction (BEAUTIFUL) and systolic heart failure treatment with the I_f inhibitor ivabradine trial (SHIFT) trials.[29,30]

Phosphodiesterase-3 inhibitors

Phosphodiesterase (PDE)-3 reduces cyclic adenosine monophosphate (cAMP) levels that regulate inotropic activity in cardiac cells. Intravenous PDE3 inhibitors are used in the setting of acute HF to improve cardiac contractility and output.[2] The use of an oral inhibitor, enoximone, provided an expected increase in exercise capacity, whereas the chronic use was fraught by a loss of benefit and an increase in arrhythmic death.[31]

Phosphodiesterase-5 inhibitors

PDE5 reduces cyclic guanosine monophosphate levels, which regulate vascular tone in smooth muscle cells. PDE5 inhibitors are used as vasodilators in patients with erectile dysfunction or pulmonary arterial hypertension. Sildenafil increased exercise capacity in patients with HF,[32,33] which was evident in patients with both HFrEF and HFpEF. This observation was largely mediated by a reduction in pulmonary arterial pressures (ie, RV afterload).[34] Dipyridamole, which functions by facilitating adenosine release and by inhibiting PDE5, also provided an improvement in cardiac performance and exercise capacity in patients with HFrEF.[35]

The long-term clinical benefits of PDE5 inhibitors in HFrEF and pulmonary hypertension remain unknown. Moreover, a recent study in patients with HFpEF failed to show any clear benefits with sildenafil on either exercise capacity or clinical status.[36]

Cardiac resynchronization therapy

The presence of a left bundle branch block leads to ventricular dyssynchrony, which promotes progression of cardiomyopathy and worsening HF. The use of a biventricular pacemaker, with 1 lead placed in the RV apex (standard location) and 1 placed through the coronary sinus in the posterolateral or anterolateral cardiac vein, provides simultaneous activation of the 2 ventricles, narrowing of the QRS, and reverse remodeling.[36] The use of a biventricular pacemaker is indicated for patients with symptomatic HF with severely reduced LVEF and prolonged QRS duration with left bundle branch morphology, and it is associated with improved exercise capacity and survival.[37]

Left ventricular mechanical support

In recent years, there has been a surge in the number of LV assist device (LVAD) implantations. The LVAD unloads the left ventricle, reduces filling pressures, and supports ejection, improving output and thus improving exercise capacity in patients with HF.[38] In patients with LVAD, exercise capacity is markedly improved depending on the pump speed and the underlying residual LV systolic function.[39,40] Patients with biventricular failure requiring mechanical support do poorly with LVAD alone and are treated with biventricular support with total artificial heart or heart transplant.[38] Patients with total artificial heart have a marked improvement in exercise capacity but are limited by a lack of HR response and blunted blood pressure response to exercise.[41]

Treatment of arrhythmias

As mentioned previously, arrhythmias may interfere with ventricular filling or contractility. Suppression of ventricular or atrial tachyarrhythmias may be necessary if they interfere with cardiac filling or systole. HF that is inappropriately low at rest or with exertion (chronotropic incompetence) may require the implantation of a pacemaker.[42]

Treatment of valvular disease

Stenosis of the atrioventricular valves leads to abnormal cardiac filling, whereas stenosis of the aortic or pulmonary valve leads to an impediment of cardiac ejection. Insufficiency of any of the cardiac valves translates into volume overload and an impediment in cardiac filling. Valve repair or replacement, when indicated, significantly improves exercise capacity in HF.[43]

Comorbid Conditions Affecting Exercise Capacity in Heart Failure

The epidemic of diabetes and obesity, in addition to an aging population, further burdens patients with HF because of the negative effects these comorbid conditions potentially have on exercise capacity. Pulmonary disease (obstructive or restrictive) impairs the increase in ventilation and oxygenation and further adds to the limitations seen in HF.[44] Anemia is also common in patients with HF, causing impaired oxygen delivering capacity and increased peripheral needs, which may be unmet if CO cannot appropriately increase.[45] In addition, patients with HF have a host of skeletal abnormalities, caused by the primary disease and compounded by a physically inactive lifestyle.[46] Comorbid conditions that are often associated with HF collectively contribute significantly to the functional limitations and reductions in exercise capacity that are often observed.

Practical Approach to Patients with Heart Failure and Exercise Intolerance

Improvement in exercise tolerance is a key goal of HF therapy. In the therapeutic approach, priority is given to treatments leading to improved survival in HF, such as angiotensin and aldosterone antagonists, BAR blockers, hydralazine/isosorbide, and cardiac resynchronization therapy (when indicated). Additional treatments should aim to improve LV filling by avoiding volume overload through the appropriate use of diuretics. Treatment of systemic or pulmonary hypertension should be considered. A careful analysis of intercurrent or concomitant illnesses is also important because a change in other factors may lead to destabilization in HF.

SUMMARY

HF is a clinical syndrome of breathlessness, fatigue, and exercise intolerance. Despite improvement in the management of HF, many patients remain unable to complete activities of daily living without experiencing symptoms. Although prevention of death in patients with HF is imperative, treatment of symptoms and improving functional capacity are equally important goals.

ACKNOWLEDGMENTS

Dr G. Biondi-Zoccai was, at the time of the preparation of this article, the Jack and Natalie Congdon Visiting Scholar at the VCU Pauley Heart Center, Virginia Commonwealth University.

REFERENCES

1. Braunwald E. Heart failure. JACC Heart Fail 2013; 1(1):1–20.
2. Writing Committee Members, Yancy CW, Jessup M, et al, American College of Cardiology Foundation/ American Heart Association Task Force on Practice Guidelines. 2013 ACCF/AHA guideline for the management of heart failure: a report of the American College of Cardiology Foundation/American Heart Association Task Force on Practice Guidelines. Circulation 2013;128(16):e240–327.
3. Hung J, Kelly DT, Hutton BF, et al. Influence of heart rate and atrial transport on left ventricular volume and function: relation to hemodynamic changes produced by supraventricular arrhythmia. Am J Cardiol 1981;48(4):632–8.
4. Orn S, Dickstein K. How do heart failure patients die? Eur Heart J 2002;4(Suppl):D59–65.
5. Huikuri HV, Castellanos A, Myerburg RJ. Sudden death due to cardiac arrhythmias. N Engl J Med 2001;345:1433–42.
6. Cahalin LP, Chase P, Arena R, et al. A meta-analysis of the prognostic significance of cardiopulmonary exercise testing in patients with heart failure. Heart Fail Rev 2013;18(1):79–94.

7. Moss AJ, Zareba W, Hall WJ, et al, Multicenter Automatic Defibrillator Implantation Trial II Investigators. Prophylactic implantation of a defibrillator in patients with myocardial infarction and reduced ejection fraction. N Engl J Med 2002;346(12):877–83.

8. Creager MA, Massie BM, Faxon DP, et al. Acute and long-term effects of enalapril on the cardiovascular response to exercise and exercise tolerance in patients with congestive heart failure. J Am Coll Cardiol 1985;6(1):163–73.

9. Lang RM, Elkayam U, Yellen LG, et al. Comparative effects of losartan and enalapril on exercise capacity and clinical status in patients with heart failure. The Losartan Pilot Exercise Study Investigators. J Am Coll Cardiol 1997;30(4):983–91.

10. Ziesche S, Cobb FR, Cohn JN, et al. Hydralazine and isosorbide dinitrate combination improves exercise tolerance in heart failure. Results from V-HeFT I and V-HeFT II. The V-HeFT VA Cooperative Studies Group. Circulation 1993;87(6 Suppl):VI56–64.

11. Magorien RD, Leier CV, Kolibash AJ, et al. Beneficial effects of nifedipine on rest and exercise myocardial energetics in patients with congestive heart failure. Circulation 1984;70(5):884–90.

12. Dunselman PH, Kuntze CE, van Bruggen A, et al. Efficacy of felodipine in congestive heart failure. Eur Heart J 1989;10(4):354–64.

13. Walsh JT, Andrews R, Curtis S, et al. Effects of amlodipine in patients with chronic heart failure. Am Heart J 1997;134(5 Pt 1):872–8.

14. Udelson JE, DeAbate CA, Berk M, et al. Effects of amlodipine on exercise tolerance, quality of life, and left ventricular function in patients with heart failure from left ventricular systolic dysfunction. Am Heart J 2000;139(3):503–10.

15. Metra M, Nardi M, Giubbini R, et al. Effects of short- and long-term carvedilol administration on rest and exercise hemodynamic variables, exercise capacity and clinical conditions in patients with idiopathic dilated cardiomyopathy. J Am Coll Cardiol 1994; 24(7):1678–87.

16. Metra M, Giubbini R, Nodari S, et al. Differential effects of beta-blockers in patients with heart failure: a prospective, randomized, double-blind comparison of the long-term effects of metoprolol versus carvedilol. Circulation 2000;102(5):546–51.

17. Effects of carvedilol, a vasodilator-beta-blocker, in patients with congestive heart failure due to ischemic heart disease. Australia-New Zealand Heart Failure Research Collaborative Group. Circulation 1995; 92(2):212–8.

18. Conraads VM, Metra M, Kamp O, et al. Effects of the long-term administration of nebivolol on the clinical symptoms, exercise capacity, and left ventricular function of patients with diastolic dysfunction: results of the ELANDD study. Eur J Heart Fail 2012;14(2): 219–25.

19. Cicoira M, Zanolla L, Rossi A, et al. Long-term, dose-dependent effects of spironolactone on left ventricular function and exercise tolerance in patients with chronic heart failure. J Am Coll Cardiol 2002;40(2):304–10.

20. Eshaghian S, Horwich TB, Fonarow GC. Relation of loop diuretic dose to mortality in advanced heart failure. Am J Cardiol 2006;97(12):1759–64.

21. Gupta S, Waywell C, Gandhi N, et al. The effects of adding torasemide to standard therapy on peak oxygen consumption, natriuretic peptides, and quality of life in patients with compensated left ventricular systolic dysfunction. Eur J Heart Fail 2010;12(7):746–52.

22. Agostoni PG, Marenzi GC, Pepi M, et al. Isolated ultrafiltration in moderate congestive heart failure. J Am Coll Cardiol 1993;21(2):424–31.

23. Digitalis Investigation Group. The effect of digoxin on mortality and morbidity in patients with heart failure. N Engl J Med 1997;336(8):525–33.

24. Sullivan M, Atwood JE, Myers J, et al. Increased exercise capacity after digoxin administration in patients with heart failure. J Am Coll Cardiol 1989; 13(5):1138–43.

25. Fleg JL, Rothfeld B, Gottlieb SH. Effect of maintenance digoxin therapy on aerobic performance and exercise left ventricular function in mild to moderate heart failure due to coronary artery disease: a randomized, placebo-controlled, crossover trial. J Am Coll Cardiol 1991;17(3):743–51.

26. Speranza L, Franceschelli S, Riccioni G. The biological effects of ivabradine in cardiovascular disease. Molecules 2012;17(5):4924–35.

27. Sarullo FM, Fazio G, Puccio D, et al. Impact of 'off-label' use of ivabradine on exercise capacity, gas exchange, functional class, quality of life, and neurohormonal modulation in patients with ischemic chronic heart failure. J Cardiovasc Pharmacol Ther 2010;15(4):349–55.

28. Kosmala W, Holland DJ, Rojek A, et al. Effect of I$_f$ channel inhibition on hemodynamic status and exercise tolerance in heart failure with preserved ejection fraction: a randomized trial. J Am Coll Cardiol 2013; 62(15):1330–8.

29. Fox K, Ford I, Steg PG, et al, BEAUTIFUL investigators. Heart rate as a prognostic risk factor in patients with coronary artery disease and left-ventricular systolic dysfunction (BEAUTIFUL): a subgroup analysis of a randomised controlled trial. Lancet 2008; 372(9641):817–21.

30. Swedberg K, Komajda M, Böhm M, et al, SHIFT Investigators. Ivabradine and outcomes in chronic heart failure (SHIFT): a randomised placebo-controlled study. Lancet 2010;376(9744):875–85. http://dx.doi.org/10.1016/S0140-6736(10)61198-1 [Erratum appears in Lancet 2010;376(9757):1988].

31. Uretsky BF, Jessup M, Konstam MA, et al. Multicenter trial of oral enoximone in patients with moderate to moderately severe congestive heart failure. Lack of

benefit compared with placebo. Enoximone Multicenter Trial Group. Circulation 1990;82(3):774–80.

32. Bocchi EA, Guimarães G, Mocelin A, et al. Sildenafil effects on exercise, neurohormonal activation, and erectile dysfunction in congestive heart failure: a double-blind, placebo-controlled, randomized study followed by a prospective treatment for erectile dysfunction. Circulation 2002;106(9):1097–103.

33. Guazzi M, Tumminello G, Di Marco F, et al. The effects of phosphodiesterase-5 inhibition with sildenafil on pulmonary hemodynamics and diffusion capacity, exercise ventilatory efficiency, and oxygen uptake kinetics in chronic heart failure. J Am Coll Cardiol 2004;44(12):2339–48.

34. Guazzi M, Myers J, Peberdy MA, et al. Ventilatory efficiency and dyspnea on exertion improvements are related to reduced pulmonary pressure in heart failure patients receiving Sildenafil. Int J Cardiol 2010; 144(3):410–2.

35. Sanada S, Asanuma H, Koretsune Y, et al. Long-term oral administration of dipyridamole improves both cardiac and physical status in patients with mild to moderate chronic heart failure: a prospective open-randomized study. Hypertens Res 2007; 30(10):913–9.

36. Redfield MM, Chen HH, Borlaug BA, et al, RELAX Trial. Effect of phosphodiesterase-5 inhibition on exercise capacity and clinical status in heart failure with preserved ejection fraction: a randomized clinical trial. JAMA 2013;309(12):1268–77.

37. Prinzen FW, Vernooy K, Auricchio A. Cardiac resynchronization therapy: state-of-the-art of current applications, guidelines, ongoing trials, and areas of controversy. Circulation 2013;128(22):2407–18.

38. Shah KB, Tang DG, Cooke RH, et al. Implantable mechanical circulatory support: demystifying patients with ventricular assist devices and artificial hearts. Clin Cardiol 2011;34(3):147–52.

39. Jung MH, Hansen PB, Sander K, et al. Effect of increasing pump speed during exercise on peak oxygen uptake in heart failure patients supported with a continuous-flow left ventricular assist device. A double-blind randomized study. Eur J Heart Fail 2014 [EPub ahead of print]. Accessed September 22, 2014.

40. Noor MR, Bowles C, Banner NR. Relationship between pump speed and exercise capacity during HeartMate II left ventricular assist device support: influence of residual left ventricular function. Eur J Heart Fail 2012;14:613–20.

41. Kohli HS, Canada J, Arena R, et al. Exercise blood pressure response during assisted circulatory support: comparison of the total artificial heart with a left ventricular assist device during rehabilitation. J Heart Lung Transplant 2011;30:1207–13.

42. Brubaker PH, Kitzman DW. Prevalence and management of chronotropic incompetence in heart failure. Curr Cardiol Rep 2007;9(3):229–35.

43. American College of Cardiology/American Heart Association Task Force on Practice Guidelines, Society of Cardiovascular Anesthesiologists, Society for Cardiovascular Angiography and Interventions, et al. ACC/AHA 2006 guidelines for the management of patients with valvular heart disease: a report of the American College of Cardiology/American Heart Association Task Force on Practice Guidelines (Writing Committee to Revise the 1998 Guidelines for the Management of Patients With Valvular Heart Disease): developed in collaboration with the Society of Cardiovascular Anesthesiologists: endorsed by the Society for Cardiovascular Angiography and Interventions and the Society of Thoracic Surgeons [review]. Circulation 2006;114(5):e84–231 [Erratum appears in Circulation 2007;115(15):e409; Circulation 2010;121(23):e443].

44. Guazzi M, Myers J, Vicenzi M, et al. Cardiopulmonary exercise testing characteristics in heart failure patients with and without concomitant chronic obstructive pulmonary disease. Am Heart J 2010; 160(5):900–5.

45. Okonko DO, Mandal AK, Missouris CG, et al. Disordered iron homeostasis in chronic heart failure: prevalence, predictors, and relation to anemia, exercise capacity, and survival. J Am Coll Cardiol 2011; 58(12):1241–51.

46. Nicoletti I, Cicoira M, Zanolla L, et al. Skeletal muscle abnormalities in chronic heart failure patients: relation to exercise capacity and therapeutic implications. Congest Heart Fail 2003;9(3):148–54.

Risks and Benefits of Weight Loss in Heart Failure

Carl J. Lavie, MD[a,b,c],*, Martin A. Alpert, MD[d],
Hector O. Ventura, MD[a]

KEYWORDS

- Obesity • Heart failure • Cardiovascular disease • Weight loss

KEY POINTS

- Obesity adversely affects many cardiovascular disease (CVD) risk factors and increases the risk of most CVD, including heart failure (HF).
- However, obese patients with HF have a better prognosis than lean patients with HF, which has been termed the *obesity paradox*.
- Current data support efforts at purposeful weight loss, particularly in individuals with more severe degrees of obesity (class III) and many with class II obesity.
- Incorporating physical activity, exercise training, and cardiorespiratory fitness into purposeful weight loss seems to be a particularly attractive option for patients with HF.

INTRODUCTION

Obesity is both a risk factor and a direct causal factor for the development of heart failure (HF), because of the variety of adverse hemodynamic changes in obesity that lead to adverse cardiac remodeling and ventricular dysfunction.[1–3] Overweight and obesity have been implicated as major risk factors for hypertension and coronary heart disease (CHD), which are 2 of the strongest risk factors related to the development of HF. Additionally, because obesity has adverse effects on cardiac structure and left ventricular (LV) systolic and, especially, diastolic function,[1–4] it is also a powerful risk factor for the development of HF.

However, despite the well-known strong association between overweight/obesity and major cardiovascular disease (CVD) risk factors for HF, numerous studies, including those in patients with established HF, have demonstrated an "obesity paradox," in that overweight and obese patients with HF have a more favorable clinical prognosis than do their leaner counterparts with the same degree of HF.[1]

This article reviews the adverse effects of weight gain and obesity on cardiac structure and function, and on the prevalence and functional classification of HF, and discusses the benefits and risks of weight loss in patients with established HF.

[a] Department of Cardiovascular Diseases, John Ochsner Heart and Vascular Institute, Ochsner Clinical School, The University of Queensland School of Medicine, 1514 Jefferson Highway, New Orleans, LA 70121-2483, USA; [b] Cardiac Rehabilitation, Exercise Laboratories, John Ochsner Heart and Vascular Institute, Ochsner Clinical School, The University of Queensland School of Medicine, 1514 Jefferson Highway, New Orleans, LA 70121-2483, USA; [c] Department of Preventive Medicine, Pennington Biomedical Research Center, Louisiana State University System, 6400 Perkins Road, Baton Rouge, LA 70808, USA; [d] Division of Cardiovascular Medicine, University of Missouri Health Sciences Center, 5 Hospital Drive Columbia, Room CE-338, Columbia, MO 65202, USA
* Corresponding author. Cardiac Rehabilitation, Exercise Laboratories, John Ochsner Heart and Vascular Institute, Ochsner Clinical School, The University of Queensland School of Medicine, 1514 Jefferson Highway, New Orleans, LA 70121-2483.
E-mail address: clavie@ochsner.org

Heart Failure Clin 11 (2015) 125–131
http://dx.doi.org/10.1016/j.hfc.2014.08.013
1551-7136/15/$ – see front matter © 2015 Elsevier Inc. All rights reserved.

Impact of Obesity on Hemodynamic Parameters

Considerable evidence demonstrates the adverse impact of weight gain and obesity on central and peripheral hemodynamics (**Box 1**, **Fig. 1**).[1–3] An early study by Alexander and colleagues[5] showed a positive correlation between degree of overweight on total blood volume, stroke volume (SV), and cardiac output (CO), all increasing with weight gain. Fat-free or nonosseous mass may have contributed to the alterations, because augmentation of total blood volume and CO cannot be accounted for by excess fat mass alone.[1–3] Typically, the heart rate in obese does not differ appreciably from that predicted for ideal body weight. In more severe obesity, oxygen consumption (Vo_2), CO, SV, right ventricular (RV) end-diastolic pressure, peripheral vascular resistance, mean pulmonary artery pressure, and mean arterial pressure exceeded that predicted for patients with normal weight. Conversely, systemic vascular resistance in obesity is lower than expected based on the level of arterial blood pressure (BP).[1–3] In patients with class III obesity (body mass index [BMI] $\geq$40 kg/m^2), exercise increased central blood volume and LV end-diastolic BP by 20% and 50%, respectively.[6]

Box 1
Effects of obesity on cardiac performance

A. Hemodynamics

   1. Increased blood volume

   2. Increased stroke volume

   3. Increased arterial pressure

   4. Increased LV wall stress

   5. Pulmonary artery hypertension

B. Cardiac structure

   1. LV concentric remodeling

   2. LV hypertrophy (eccentric and concentric)

   3. Left atrial enlargement

   4. RV hypertrophy

C. Cardiac function

   1. LV diastolic dysfunction

   2. LV systolic dysfunction

   3. RV Failure

D. Inflammation

   1. Increased C-reactive protein

   2. Overexpression of tumor necrosis factor

E. Neurohumoral

   1. Insulin resistance and hyperinsulinemia

   2. Leptin insensitivity and hyperleptinemia

   3. Reduced adiponectin

   4. Sympathetic nervous system activation

   5. Activation of renin-angiotensin-aldosterone system

   6. Overexpression of peroxisome proliferator-activator receptor

F. Cellular

   1. Hypertrophy

   2. Apoptosis

   3. Fibrosis

Abbreviations: LV, left ventricular; RV, right ventricular.

From Lavie CJ, Alpert MA, Arena R, et al. Impact of obesity and the obesity paradox on prevalence and prognosis in heart failure. JACC Heart Fail 2013;1:96; with permission.

Impact of Obesity on Cardiac Structure

The impact of obesity on LV structure and LV hypertrophy (LVH) is confounded by the inclusion of the effects of CHD and hypertension.[1–3] In class III obesity, heart weight, LV wall thickness, and LVH are all increased with variable effects on RV hypertrophy. However, even in normotensive class III obesity without known CHD, the obese had marked abnormalities in LV structure. In a Framingham Heart Study (n = 3922), Lauer and colleagues[7] found that BMI correlated positively with LV wall thickness, LV internal diastolic dimension, and LV mass, even after adjusting for BP and age. Virtually all of the studies assessing patients with different degrees of obesity demonstrate that LV internal diastolic dimension (or LV diastolic volume), LV wall thickness, and LV mass index were significantly greater in obese versus lean patients. Although early studies indicate that most obese patients have eccentric LVH, more recent studies indicate that obese patients, especially with elevated BP and hypertension, also have a high prevalence of concentric LVH or LV concentric remodeling.[1–4]

Obesity and Left Ventricular Function

The development of LVH in obesity, with or without elevated BP and hypertension, could predispose patients to LV diastolic dysfunction.[1–4] Thus, hemodynamic studies, especially in more severe obesity, have typically reported elevated levels of LV end-diastolic BP. In one Doppler echocardiographic study, LV diastolic dysfunction occurred in 12% of patients with class I obesity (BMI,

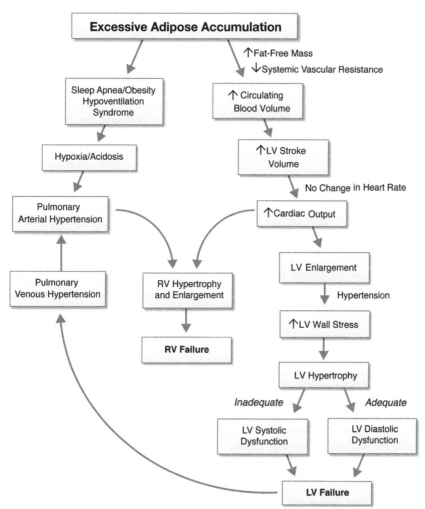

Fig. 1. The central hemodynamic, cardiac structural abnormalities and alterations in ventricular function that may occur in patients with severe obesity and predispose them to HF. LV hypertrophy in severe obesity may be eccentric or concentric. In uncomplicated (normotensive) severe obesity, eccentric LV hypertrophy predominates. In patients with severe obesity with long-standing systemic hypertension, concentric LV hypertrophy is frequently observed and may occur more commonly than eccentric LV hypertrophy. Whether and to what extent metabolic disturbances such as lipotoxicity, insulin resistance, leptin resistance, and alterations of the renin-angiotensin-aldosterone system contribute to obesity cardiomyopathy in humans is uncertain. RV, right ventricular. (*From* Lavie CJ, Alpert MA, Arena R, et al. Impact of obesity and the obesity paradox on prevalence and prognosis in heart failure. JACC Heart Fail 2013;1:95; with permission.)

30.0–34.9 kg/m^2), 35% with class II obesity (BMI, 35.0–39.9 kg/m^2), and 45% with class III, or "morbid," obesity.[8] Many other Doppler and radio-nuclide angiographic studies have confirmed the adverse effects of obesity on LV diastolic abnormalities.[1–4]

Most studies in obese subjects have shown no significant impact of excess adipose accumulation on systolic LV function.[1–3] If obese subjects had a lower LV systolic function than lean subjects, the differences were generally small, and LV ejection phase indices typically remain within the normal range. Recent studies that used tissue Doppler imaging of the mitral annulus indicate a progressive decline in peak myocardial systolic velocities with increasing degrees of obesity, with more abnormal myocardial strain and strain rate being detected more commonly in obese subjects.[9] Although early in obesity diastolic dysfunction seems to predominate over systolic dysfunction, severe obesity also demonstrates subtle abnormalities in systolic ventricular function.[1–4]

Mechanisms of Abnormal Cardiac Structure and Function in Obesity

The increased volume with uncomplicated obesity would be expected to produce eccentric LVH.[1-4] However, obese patients also have concentric LV remodeling and concentric LVH, which may be related with elevations in BP/hypertension, activation of the sympathetic nervous system (SNS) and renin angiotensin-aldosterone system (RAAS), and effects of growth factors, such as insulin-like growth factor.[2,3]

A variety of metabolic abnormalities may also contribute to the LV diastolic and/or systolic dysfunction, and to the LVH. Obese patients have evidence of lipotoxicity and lipoapoptosis, insulin resistance, hyperinsulinemia, and activation of the SNS and RAAS, and reduced levels of adiponectin. Although these abnormalities are clear in animal models of obesity, their relative and combined impact in humans remain uncertain and could be considered meager.[2,3]

Obesity and Heart Failure Prevalence

In a study of 74 morbidly obese patients by Alpert and colleagues,[10] nearly one-third had clinical evidence of HF, with the probability of HF markedly increasing with longer duration of morbid obesity, reaching prevalence rates exceeding 70% and 90% at 20 and 30 years of morbid obesity, respectively. In a study of 550 subjects without diabetes from Greece, however, BMI was not associated with HF risk, whereas metabolic syndrome was associated with a 2.5-fold higher risk of HF.[11] In contrast to patients of normal weight with metabolic syndrome, however, obese subjects without metabolic risk factors had a decreased risk of HF.

The best and probably largest study to assess the risk of obesity on future development of HF comes from the Framingham Heart Study participants.[12] This study of 5881 subjects demonstrated that for every 1 kg/m^2 increase in BMI, the risk of HF during a 14-year follow-up increased by 5% in men and 7% in women, respectively, with progressive increases in the risk of HF across all BMI categories.[12]

Obesity and Heart Failure Prognosis

Obesity adversely affects both systolic and, especially, diastolic ventricular function and increases the prevalence of HF. However, numerous studies and meta-analyses have shown that those who are overweight and obese with HF seem to have a better prognosis than do their leaner counterparts, a phenomenon termed the *obesity paradox*. This topic has been reviewed in detail elsewhere.[1]

Briefly, although generally this paradox has been demonstrated mostly with BMI criteria, which is potentially flawed because BMI assesses both fat mass and nonfat mass, including skeletal and muscle mass, the obesity paradox has also been demonstrated with body fat, and with central obesity/waist circumference (WC).[1,13-15] In a study of 209 patients with advanced systolic HF, Lavie and colleagues[13] showed that for every 1% increase in percent body fat, a 13% independent reduction in major cardiovascular events was seen. In a recent study that assessed WC, the patients with HF with both high BMI and WC had the best event-free survival.[14,15]

Perhaps the clearest example of the profound impact of the obesity paradox is seen in patients with frailty/cachexia in HF.[16] Frailty is defined as a biological syndrome characterized by declining overall function and loss of resistance to stressors, and this is known to be associated with considerable morbidity and mortality and high health care use and expenses, especially in older populations who have a high prevalence of HF. Cachexia is a particularly serious disorder of advanced HF, in which unintentional weight loss carries a greater burden of morbidity and mortality for most medical conditions, and reason exists to believe that this is the same case for advanced HF. Underweight patients often have the worst prognosis for many disorders, and this has been clearly noted in many studies describing the obesity paradox in HF.[16]

A limitation of most studies assessing obesity and prognosis in HF is the inability to control for nonpurposeful weight loss before study entry, which would be expected to be associated with a poor prognosis. In advanced HF, cachexia and wasting are independent predictors of higher mortality,[16,17] and to a certain extent, overweight and obesity in HF may represent the opposite of frailty/cachexia and, therefore, may actually be an example of reverse epidemiology.[18]

On the other hand, although an obesity paradox exists in HF, substantial evidence also suggests that the degree or severity of obesity also substantially influences prognosis.[1,19] The impact of morbid or class III obesity on HF prevalence and prognosis seems more concerning, particularly because recent statistics suggest that this severe obesity is increasing more so than in obesity in general.[1,19,20] Also, the level of obesity has deleterious effects on cardiovascular structure and function and markedly increases the prevalence and severity of HF.[1-3] Unlike in the overweight and mild degrees of obesity, wherein an obesity paradox generally exists, studies suggest that severe or class III obesity is associated with an ominous prognosis in HF.[18-20]

Evidence for Weight Loss in Heart Failure

Clinical guidelines from various societies in recent years have differed considerably regarding recommendations for weight loss. Currently none of the major societies have recommended weight loss for patients with HF who have a BMI less than 30 kg/m^2, with variable recommendations between the cutpoints of 30 to 40 kg/m^2, whereas most of the guidelines generally advocate weight loss for patients with a BMI of 40 kg/m^2 or greater.[1,19,20] Because of the lack of definitive large-scale clinical trials on the role of weight loss in HF on which to base firm recommendations, the most recent HF guidelines from the American College of Cardiology Foundation/American Heart Association do not provide firm recommendations for purposeful weight loss in HF.[21] Nevertheless, these HF guidelines recognize the poor prognosis in patients with more severe obesity, particularly those with morbid obesity. A recent study from Nagarajan and colleagues[22] from the Cleveland Clinic HF program confirms the obesity paradox in 501 patients in their advanced HF clinic, but their data indicate no obesity paradox and a poor prognosis in a small group of 21 patients with morbid obesity and HF.

Therefore, based on the constellation of data, recommendations for purposeful weight loss, as opposed to nonpurposeful weight loss and cachexia (which is associated with a poor clinical prognosis), is recommended for patients with HF and more severe obesity, and this seems particularly sound for those with a BMI of 40 kg/m^2 or greater and seems very reasonable for most patients with HF with a BMI of 35 kg/m^2 or greater.[1,16,19,20] In patients with HF and less severe degrees of obesity or those who are overweight, weight loss may be beneficial to improve symptoms and functional classification, but data on its impact on major clinical prognostic outcomes are lacking, with opposing data showing a better clinical prognosis in overweight and mildly obese patients with HF in the obesity paradox.[1–3,20]

Hemodynamic Effects of Weight Loss

In severe obesity, substantial weight loss reduces total and central blood volume, Vo$_2$, arterial venous oxygen differences, SV, CO, cardiac work, and LV work, with variable effects on systemic vascular resistance. Additionally, the impact of weight loss on LV filling pressures has also been variable, with reductions noted in some, but not all, patients with severe obesity.[2,3]

Weight Loss and Cardiac Structure

Weight loss has significantly produced reductions in LV diastolic chamber size, LV wall thickness, and overall LV mass and severity of LVH.[2,3] In a recent study, the prevalence of abnormal LV geometry (concentric remodeling or concentric or eccentric LVH) decreased from 71% to 43% with substantial weight loss.[23] Diet and exercise studies have generally demonstrated benefits of weight loss on cardiac structure, with the most dramatic effects being noted in patients who have undergone bariatric surgery and those with severe obesity.[2,3]

Weight Loss and Diastolic Function

Studies using various noninvasive cardiac technologies have consistently demonstrated improvements in LV diastolic filling with weight loss, generally noted across the entire spectrum of obesity.[1–3] The reason a relative lack of concordance is seen between the weight loss–related improvements in LV diastolic filling and the sometimes lack of change in LV end-diastolic BP is not clear.[2,3]

Effects of Weight Loss on Left Ventricular Systolic Function

Because most evidence indicates that obesity generally impacts diastolic dysfunction, as opposed to systolic dysfunction, most studies assessing LV systolic function before and after weight loss have, not surprisingly, noted impressive differences.[2,3] In one study, LV systolic function in patients with severe obesity improved after weight reduction, but predominantly in those with baseline LV systolic dysfunction.[24] Recent studies using tissue Doppler and speckle track imaging before and after weight loss have demonstrated improvements in systolic mitral annular velocities and reductions in myocardial deformation in all severities of obesity, even when LV ejection phase indices were in the normal range.[2,3,25–27] In a study by Kishi and colleagues,[28] increases in BMI over time, even when adjusted for other cardiovascular risk factors, were associated with adverse effects on systolic and diastolic function over 25 years, from adulthood to middle age.[28,29]

Impact of Weight Loss on Obesity Cardiomyopathy

Whether purposeful weight loss improves mortality in patients with class I and II obesity and HF remains uncertain. Although some studies have reported a worse prognosis with weight reduction,

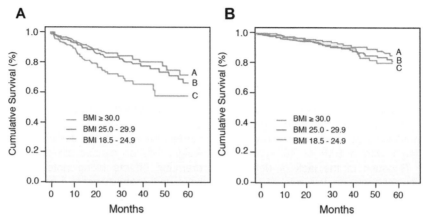

Fig. 2. Kaplan-Meier analyses according to BMI with the low CRF group (oxygen consumption <14 mL O$_2$/kg/min log rank 11.7; P = .003) and high CRF group (oxygen consumption ≥14 mL O$_2$/kg/min; log rank 1.72; P = .42) on the left and right, respectively. (*From* Lavie CJ, De Schutter A, Patel DA, et al. Does fitness completely explain the obesity paradox? Am Heart J 2013;166:3; with permission; *Adapted from* Lavie CJ, Cahalin LP, Chase P, et al. Impact of cardiorespiratory fitness on the obesity paradox in patients with heart failure. Mayo Clin Proc 2013;88:256.)

these studies generally did not exclude patients with nonpurposeful weight loss.[2,3,16,19] Furthermore, no large-scale studies have assessed the effects of purposeful weight loss on mortality even in patients with severe obesity. However, several small studies with dietary weight loss and bariatric surgery have noted improvements in functional class, quality of life, dyspnea, and edema after weight loss.[2,3,10,30]

Weight Loss with Exercise Training and Improved Cardiorespiratory Fitness

A full discussion of the benefits of exercise training and improved levels of cardiorespiratory fitness (CRF) is beyond the scope of this review[31]; this is addressed elsewhere in this issue. However, one of the strongest predictors of prognosis in HF and most CVD is CRF.[20] In fact, even when the obesity paradox is considered, CRF remains a critical predictor of prognosis[32,33]; HF patients with preserved CRF (defined as a peak Vo_2 of ≥14 mL O$_2$/kg/min) have a good prognosis and no obesity paradox is present.[32] However, in patients with HF and low CRF (defined as peak Vo_2 <14 mL O$_2$/kg/min) have a poor prognosis and a strong obesity paradox is present, wherein the lean patients with HF and low CRF have a particularly poor prognosis, having worse survival than overweight and, especially, obese patients with systolic HF (**Fig. 2**).[32,33]

Therefore, recommendations to increase physical activity are needed throughout the health care system,[34] because physical activity and formal exercise training are particularly beneficial in

HF.[31] Incorporating increasing physical activity and exercise training into a purposeful weight loss program seems to be especially attractive in efforts to reduce weight, improve symptoms and functional capacity, reduce hospitalizations, and improve survival in patients with HF.[20,31]

SUMMARY

Large-scale clinical trials are needed to better assess and define the risks and benefits of weight loss in HF. The constellation of current data supports efforts at purposeful weight loss, particularly in those with more severe degrees of obesity, including class III obesity and many with class II obesity. Incorporating the benefits of physical activity, exercise training, and CRF into purposeful weight loss in HF seems to be a particularly attractive option for these patients.

REFERENCES

1. Lavie CJ, Alpert MA, Arena R, et al. Impact of obesity and the obesity paradox on prevalence and prognosis in heart failure. JACC Heart Fail 2013;1:93–102.
2. Alpert MA, Omran J, Mehra A, et al. Impact of obesity and weight loss on cardiac performance and morphology in adults. Prog Cardiovasc Dis 2014;56:391–400.
3. Alpert MA, Lavie CJ, Agrawal H, et al. Obesity and heart failure: epidemiology, pathophysiology, clinical manifestations, and management. Transl Res 2014; 164:345–56.

4. Lavie CJ, Patel DA, Milani RV, et al. Impact of echocardiographic left ventricular geometry on clinical prognosis. Prog Cardiovasc Dis 2014;57:3–9.

5. Alexander JK, Dennis EW, Smith WG, et al. Blood volume, cardiac output and distribution of systemic blood flow in extreme obesity. Cardiovasc Res Cent Bull 1962;1:39–44.

6. Alexander JK. Obesity and cardiac performance. Am J Cardiol 1964;14:860–5.

7. Lauer MS, Anderson KM, Kannel WB, et al. The impact of obesity on left ventricular mass and geometry. The Framingham Heart Study. JAMA 1991;266: 231–6.

8. Pascual M, Pascual A, Soria F, et al. Effects of isolated obesity on systolic and diastolic left ventricular function. Heart 2003;89:1152–6.

9. Wong CY, O'Moore-Sullivan T, Leano R, et al. Alterations of left ventricular myocardial characteristics associated with obesity. Circulation 2004;110:3081–7.

10. Alpert MA, Terry BE, Mulekar M, et al. Cardiac morphology and left ventricular function in morbidly obese patients with and without congestive heart failure and effect of weight loss. Am J Cardiol 1997;80:736–40.

11. Voulgari C, Tentolouris N, Dilaveris P, et al. Increased heart failure risk in normal-weight people with metabolic syndrome compared with metabolically healthy obese individuals. J Am Coll Cardiol 2011; 58:1343–50.

12. Kenchaiah S, Evans JC, Levy D, et al. Obesity and the risk of heart failure. N Engl J Med 2002;347:305–13.

13. Lavie CJ, Osman AF, Milani RV, et al. Body composition and prognosis in chronic systolic heart failure: the obesity paradox. Am J Cardiol 2003;91:891–4.

14. Clark AL, Chyu J, Horwich TB. The obesity paradox in men versus women with systolic heart failure. Am J Cardiol 2012;110:77–82.

15. Clark AL, Fonarow GC, Horwich TB. Obesity and obesity paradox in heart failure. Prog Cardiovasc Dis 2014;56:409–14.

16. Lavie CJ, De Schutter A, Alpert MA, et al. Obesity paradox, cachexia, frailty and heart failure. Heart Fail Clin 2014;10:319–26.

17. Mehra MR. Fat, cachexia and the right ventricle in heart failure. J Am Coll Cardiol 2013;62:1671–3.

18. Lavie CJ, Mehra MR, Milani RV. Obesity and heart failure prognosis: paradox or reverse epidemiology? Eur Heart J 2005;26:5–7.

19. Lavie CJ, Ventura HO. Analyzing the weight of evidence on the obesity paradox and heart failure: is there a limit to the madness? Congest Heart Fail 2013;19:158–9.

20. Lavie CJ, McAuley PA, Church TS, et al. Obesity and cardiovascular diseases: implications regarding fitness, fatness, and severity in the obesity paradox. J Am Coll Cardiol 2014;63:1345–54.

21. Writing Committee Members, Yancy CW, Jessup M, Bozkurt B, et al. 2013 ACCF/AHA guideline for the management of heart failure: a report of the American College of Cardiology Foundation/American Heart Association Task Force on practice guidelines. Circulation 2013;128:e240–319.

22. Nagarajan V, Cauthen CA, Starling RC, et al. Prognosis of morbid obesity patients with advance heart failure. Congest Heart Fail 2013;19:160–4.

23. Haufe S, Utz W, Engeli S, et al. Left ventricular mass and function with reduced-fat or reduced-carbohydrate hypocaloric diets in overweight and obese subjects. Hypertension 2012;59:70–5.

24. Alpert MA, Terry BE, Lambert CR, et al. Factors influencing left ventricular systolic function in non-hypertensive morbidly obese patients and effect of weight loss induced by gastroplasty. Am J Cardiol 1993;75:773–7.

25. Wong C, Marwick TH. Obesity cardiomyopathy: pathogenesis and pathophysiology. Nat Clin Pract Cardiovasc Med 2007;4:436–43.

26. Kossaify A, Nicolais N. Impact of overweight and obesity on left ventricular diastolic function and value of tissue Doppler echocardiography. Clin Med Insights Cardiol 2013;7:43–50.

27. Grapsa J, Tan TL, Paschou SA, et al. The effect of bariatric surgery on echocardiographic indices: a review of the literature. Eur J Clin Invest 2013;43: 1224–30.

28. Kishi S, Armstrong AC, Gidding SS, et al. Association of obesity in early adulthood and middle age with incipient left ventricular dysfunction and structural remodeling: the CARDIA Study (Coronary Artery Risk Development in Young Adults). JACC Heart Fail 2014. [Epub ahead of print].

29. Lavie CJ, Milani RV, Ventura HO. Effects of obesity and weight changes on cardiac and vascular structure and function: does the clinical impact carry any weight? JACC Heart Fail 2014. [Epub ahead of print].

30. Miranda WR, Batsis JA, Sarr MG, et al. Impact of bariatric surgery on quality of life, functional capacity and symptoms in patients with heart failure. Obes Surg 2013;23:1101–5.

31. Lavie CJ, Berra K, Arena R. Formal cardiac rehabilitation and exercise training programs in heart failure. J Cardiopulm Rehabil Prev 2013;33:209–11.

32. Lavie CJ, Cahalin LP, Chase P, et al. Impact of cardiorespiratory fitness on the obesity paradox in patients with heart failure. Mayo Clin Proc 2013;88: 251–8.

33. Lavie CJ, De Schutter A, Patel DA, et al. Does fitness completely explain the obesity paradox? Am Heart J 2013;166:1–3.

34. Vuori IM, Lavie CJ, Blair SN. Physical activity promotion in the health care system. Mayo Clin Proc 2013; 88:1446–61.

Much Potential but Many Unanswered Questions for High-Intensity Intermittent Exercise Training for Patients with Heart Failure

CrossMark

Sherry O. Pinkstaff, PhD, PT

KEYWORDS

- Heart failure • Exercise • High intensity • Intermittent • Interval

KEY POINTS

- Moderate-intensity continuous exercise (MICE) has been the clinical standard for patients with heart failure (HF) but evidence is mounting for the effectiveness of high-intensity intermittent exercise (HIIE).
- HIIE is associated with clinically significant improvements in peak oxygen consumption (Vo_{2peak}) as well as many other variables associated with exercise capacity and cardiovascular function.
- The number of studies in which HIIE was used to treat patients with HF remains small, representing fewer than 200 patients.
- HIIE has not been associated with adverse events in the studies conducted to date.
- More research is needed before HIIE can become the clinical standard for patients with HF.

INTRODUCTION

There is a robust trove of scientific studies that support the positive physical and mental health benefits associated with aerobic exercise for apparently healthy individuals. This evidence underlies the government-backed physical activity guidelines, which suggest 30 minutes of moderate-intensity exercise on most if not all days of the week.[1,2] These recommendations also suggest that more vigorous exercise can be performed on fewer days for the same benefit, a recommendation that reflects the inverse dose-response relationship between physical activity and disease.[3–5] Those benefits include significant reductions in the risk factors associated with cardiovascular disease (CVD). There is also ample evidence for the use of aerobic exercise in CVD patient populations to improve numerous health-related outcomes.

Aerobic exercise was once contraindicated for patients with HF. In the early days of its use in this patient population, no greater than moderate-intensity training was recommended. Current guidelines recommend that patients with clinically stable HF perform aerobic MICE training (ie, 50%–80% of peak capacity) for up to 45 minutes on most days of the week.[6,7] Since the 1980s, many studies have demonstrated the safety and effectiveness of aerobic MICE in patients with HF.[8] Despite these positive results, a recent large, multicenter, randomized clinical trial, Heart Failure: A Controlled Trial Investigating Outcomes of

Disclosures: This author has no conflicts of interest to disclose.
Physical Therapy Program, Department of Clinical and Applied Movement Sciences, University of North Florida, 1 UNF Drive, Jacksonville, FL 32224, USA
E-mail address: s.pinkstaff@unf.edu

Heart Failure Clin 11 (2015) 133–148
http://dx.doi.org/10.1016/j.hfc.2014.08.008
1551-7136/15/$ – see front matter © 2015 Elsevier Inc. All rights reserved.

Exercise Training (HF-ACTION), demonstrated no overall improvement in all-cause mortality and hospitalization.[9] Importantly, after adjusting for highly prognostic clinical values for the same endpoints, exercise training did result in a modest prognostic improvement. Nonetheless, to many investigators, this remains a disappointing result.

Recently clinicians and researchers have begun to investigate HIIE training as an intervention for this patient population. This type of training has been used extensively in healthy populations, in the context of athletic performance. A vast majority of the studies investigating the effect have been done in these populations. Although many fewer studies have been conducted in a patient population representing a much smaller number of patients, the results are promising. HIIE training seems safe and improves physiology, quality of life, and functional capacity.[10–14] Many unanswered questions, however, remain.

Therefore, the objective of this review is to define HIIE, discuss its physiologic benefit for patients with HF, outline the studies that have been conducted to date, and discuss the issues that need to be resolved before this exercise intervention is more widely embraced by the clinical community.

PRINCIPLES OF HIGH-INTENSITY INTERMITTENT EXERCISE

HIIE involves the use of short periods of exercise interspersed with rest periods. The duration and intensity of the exercise and rest can be varied in numerous ways. The American College of Sports Medicine defines intensity as a percentage of heart rate (HR) reserve or Vo_2 reserve (Vo_2R). These are relative values that must be individually prescribed. Hard or very hard intensity is 60% to less than 85% and 85% to less than 100%, respectively. Exercise training at greater than 100% HR reserve (HRR) or Vo_2R has been used primarily for athletic training and is not considered for this review. For comparison, moderate intensity is defined as 40% to less than 60% HR reserve or Vo_2R. The rationale for HIIE is that the short periods of exercise followed by rest periods allow for greater time spent at a higher intensity of exercise (compared with continuous exercise).[15] This greater intensity requires different energy production pathways to be used as well as additional muscle fiber recruitment. Together, these provide an increased potential for both central and peripheral adaptation. In a study of more than 5000 apparently healthy men and women, relative exercise training intensity was more important than duration in reducing the risk of all-cause and coronary heart disease mortality.[15]

There seems to be a mechanistic basis for this exercise intensity dependence. HF is characterized on the cellular level by dysfunctional cardiomyocyte activity. Aerobic exercise can repair or reverse some of these pathologic changes, especially when that exercise is high intensity (>90% of Vo_{2peak}). In animal studies, the physiologic adaptations to chronic exercise training are explained by changes to cardiomyocyte function. In rats and mice, improvement in cardiac pump function, as a result of positive changes to the cardiomyocyte, is achieved by high-intensity exercise.[16] Furthermore, it has been suggested that for patient populations, high-intensity exercise training may be required for positive central adaptations, such as cardiac dilatation, ejection fraction, stroke volume, or other systolic parameters.[17]

EFFICACY/PHYSIOLOGIC BENEFITS OF HIIE TRAINING
Acute Effects

Recent studies have evaluated the acute effects of HIIE training in patients with HF (**Table 1**). In the most recent, a total of 13 patients with systolic HF were randomized to perform a single bout of high HIIE or MICE during which gas exchange and central hemodynamic factors were measured.[18] The HIIE bout resulted in similar cardiac output (CO), stroke volume, and oxygen extraction compared with MICE. Importantly, the hemodynamic response to HIIE was stable throughout the training session. This stability is consistent with the lack of adverse events in this cohort, a finding that is similar to other published accounts of this type of training. Participants also tended to rate the perceived exertion lower and were more likely to be able to complete the bout of HIIE. This study complements an earlier study that demonstrated that when compared with steady state exercise, HIIE resulted in comparable increases in left ventricular (LV) ejection fraction, stroke volume, CO, ratings of leg fatigue, and dyspnea.[19] The investigators also concluded that these results spoke to the safety of HIIE training.

Tomczak and colleagues[20] used MRI to assess the changes in biventricular function after a single bout of HIIE. The major finding was that biventricular function improved with a decrease in end-systolic volume and an increase in LV ejection fraction. The investigators suggested this improvement may be related to reduced systemic peripheral resistance or alternatively to improved cardiomyocyte contractility. Diastolic function was also improved as demonstrated by an increased peak untwisting rate, resulting in improved LV suction and diastolic filling.

Chronic Adaptations

Most of the studies evaluating the effects of HIIE have been chronic training studies using various protocols, with some making comparisons to MICE and others with nonexercise standard care. All these studies find benefit from HIIE. The major benefits fall into several categories: exercise capacity, ventilatory efficiency, ventilatory threshold (VT)/anaerobic threshold (AT), cardiac and vascular function, and quality of life. The following discussion is a synopsis of the main outcomes assessed. See **Table 1** for an overview of the main findings of each study.

Exercise capacity

The importance of exercise capacity in terms of prognosis in the context of health and disease cannot be overstated. Small improvements in exercise capacity, as measured by changes in Vo_{2peak}, can have a profound impact on the risk of all-cause and cardiovascular morbidity and mortality.[21] It follows that the major goal of aerobic exercise training is to improve cardiorespiratory fitness. There is also a dose-response relationship where greater improvements in aerobic capacity are associated with greater reductions in risk.

Wisløff and colleagues[10] showed that 12 weeks of exercise training resulted in a 46% increase in Vo_{2peak} for those performing HIIE compared with a 14% increase for those performing MICE. Freyssin and colleagues[12] used an 8-week HIIE program, which resulted in a 27% increase in Vo_{2peak}. In a study by Fu and colleagues,[13] patients with HF undergoing an HIIE program for 12 weeks had a 22% increase in Vo_{2peak}. Similarly, in a 16-week program comparing HIIE to MICE training, Smart and Steele[22] reported a significant increase (21%) only in the former group. Finally, in a recent study, Chrysohoou and colleagues[11] looked at the effect of 12 weeks of HIIE training and demonstrated a 31% improvement in Vo_{2peak}. In all of these studies, with the exception of that by Smart and Steele[22], the absolute increase in Vo_2 was greater than 1 metabolic equivalent (MET), a clinically relevant increase. A systematic review of 33 studies representing more than 100,000 apparently healthy subjects demonstrated 13% and 15% risk reductions for all-cause and cardiovascular-related mortality for each 1 MET in aerobic capacity, respectively.[21]

Six-minute walk test (6MWT) distance has been shown to correlate moderately well with Vo_{2peak} in patients with HF.[23] It has been used in many studies as a surrogate for Vo_{2peak} and to measure changes in exercise capacity after aerobic training. Similarly, total exercise time during an exercise test and peak work rate (WR_{peak}) also correlated with exercise capacity. Nilsson and colleagues[24] showed that following 16 weeks of HIIE training, patients increased their walking distance and exercise time significantly. The exercise training group was compared with a standard care nonexercising group. In the same group of patients, the long-term effects of exercise training were investigated. After 12 months, the gains in measures of exercise capacity were still significant.[25] Freyssin and colleagues[12] also used 6MWT distance and exercise time to measure change in functional capacity after an 8-week training protocol. This study showed a 47% increase in exercise time for the HIIE group versus a 12% increase for the MICE group. Similarly, 6MWT distance increased 12% and 6%, respectively, for the HIIE and MICE groups. Chrysohoou and colleagues[11] demonstrated a 13% improvement in 6MWT distance and a 25% improvement in WR_{peak}.

The chronotropic response to exercise is related to the health of the autonomic nervous system and has been found impaired in patients with HF.[26] Specifically, HRR is slowed in patients with HF and is hastened in the highly fit.[27] HRR can be improved with chronic MICE training.[28] Only one study has considered this variable in an investigation using HIIE. Dimopoulos and colleagues[29] found that although 16 weeks of MICE and HIIE training both improved Vo_{2peak}, only MICE training resulted in a significant improvement in HRR in the first minute of recovery.

Ventilatory efficiency

Measures of ventilatory efficiency describe how much ventilation is required for a given Vo_2 or carbon dioxide production. The slope of the ratio of minute ventilation to carbon dioxide elimination (V_E/Vco_2) has been shown highly prognostic for morbidity and mortality in patients with HF.[30] The oxygen uptake efficiency slope (OUES) is a mathematically derived variable based on the slope of Vo_2 (Y axis) and the log transformation of V_E (X axis). This variable has also been shown important in the assessment of patients with HF.[31] The findings for the effects of HIIE training are more mixed for these variables. For example, in the study by Fu and colleagues,[13] both of these variables were significantly improved (higher OUES and lower V_E/Vco_2 slope) in the HIIE group but not in the MICE or control groups. Smart and Steele[22] also confirm a reduction in V_E/Vco_2 slope after 16 weeks of HIIE training. In contrast, there was no significant improvement in the V_E/Vco_2 slope for the

Table 1
Patient demographics, intervention parameters, main outcomes, and adverse events for chronic and acute training studies

Citation	HF Inclusion Criteria	Intervention Parameters	Main Outcomes	Adverse Events and Dropouts
Chronic Training Studies				
Chrysohoou et al,[11] 2014	Stable systolic dilated or ischemic HF, NYHA class II–IV, LVEF ≤50%	• HIIE (n = 33, 29 men): alternating intervals of 30 s exercise at 100% WR_{peak} and 30 s of passive rest; total exercise time = 45 min • Control (n = 39, 28 men): physician monitoring only • 3 d/wk × 12 wk • Exercise mode: cycling (BE)	• HIIE group had a significantly improved QOL • 6MWT distance, Vo_{2peak}, Vco_2, and PPO were significantly greater for HIIE vs control	• No adverse events • 17 Discontinued HIIE group (0 for cardiac causes) • 11 Discontinued control group (2 for cardiac causes)
Iellamo et al,[42] 2013	Stable ischemic HF (last MI >6 mo prior), NYHA class II or III, LVEF <40%	• Used TRIMPi method to ensure equal total training load between groups • HIIE group (n = 8, 8 men): 4-min intervals at 75%–80% HRR with active pauses of 3 min at 45%–50% HRR • MICE group (n = 8, 8 men): 45%–60% of HRR for 30–45 min • 12 wk (2 d/wk for first 3 wk, 3 d/wk for 2nd 3 wk, 4 d/wk for 3rd 3 wk, 5 d/wk for final 3 wk) • Exercise mode: walking (TM)	• Vo_{2peak} significantly increased within both groups without significant difference between the groups • AT increased more in the MICE group • Resting CO, SV, and LV ejection fraction were not significantly changed in either group	• No adverse events • 2 Subjects discontinued the HIIE group • 2 Subjects discontinued the MICE group • 1 Subject discontinued due to atrial fibrillation (not reported which group); 3 subjects discontinued not due to medical reasons

| Fu et al,[13] 2013 | Stable HF, NYHA class II and III, LV ejection fraction ≤40% or >40% with pulmonary edema of cardiac origin | • HIIE (n = 14, 9 men): 3-min intervals at 80% VO_{2peak}; 3 min active rest at 40% VO_{2peak}
• MICE (n = 13, 8 men): 60% VO_{2peak} for 30 min
• Control (n = 13, 9 men): general advice about home-based physical activity
• 3 d/wk for 12 wk
• Exercise mode: cycling (BE) | • HIIE group experienced improvements in V_E, VO_2, VCO_2, work rate; no changes in the same for the MICE or control groups
• HIIE group had higher OUES and lower V_E/VCO_2 slope compared with MICE
• HIIE resulted in increased CO, decreased TPR, and increased LVEF; these values remained unchanged in MICE and declined for the control group (except LVEF, which remained unchanged)
• HIIE enhanced cerebral/muscular blood flow and muscular O_2 utilization during exercise
• HIIE significantly reduced markers of inflammation/oxidative stress
• HIIE significantly decreased MLWHF and increased the score for SF-36 physical and mental subclass
• No significant changes in measures of fitness or ventilatory efficiency occurred in the MICE or the control group
• MICE significantly decreased only the disease-specific QOL score | • 1 Subject each discontinued in HIIE and control group
• 2 Subjects discontinued in MICE group
• No reason given for subject dropouts |

(continued on next page)

Table 1
(continued)

Citation	HF Inclusion Criteria	Intervention Parameters	Main Outcomes	Adverse Events and Dropouts
Freyssin et al,[12] 2012	Stable chronic HF, LV ejection fraction <40%	• HIIE (n = 12, 6 men): 3 sets of 12 repetitions of 30 s of exercise followed by 60 s of passive rest. Exercise intensity was 50% (first 4 wk) and 80% (last 4 wk). ○ Exercise mode: cycling (BE) • MICE (n = 14, 7 men): walking or cycling for 45 min; intensity was set as equal to the HR at the VT_1 (determined by the baseline exercise test) • Both groups also performed water aerobics, strengthening exercises, stretching, and relaxation • 5 d/wk × 8 wk	• HIIE: Vo_{2peak} duration of the exercise test, oxygen pulse, Vo_2 at the VT_1, and 6MWT distance all increased significantly • MICE: time at VT_1 and 6MWT distance increased significantly. The improvement in the time at the VT_1 was significantly higher for the HIIE group than for the MICE group • Both groups similarly improved scores of depression and anxiety	• No adverse events • No dropouts
Smart & Steele,[22] 2012	Stable chronic HF, LVEF <35% and 2 minor and 1 major Framingham criteria, NYHA class II and III	• HIIE (n = 13, 13 men): intervals of 60 s exercise (70% Vo_{2peak}) and 60 s passive rest × 60 min • MICE (n = 10, 8 men): 30 min of continuous exercise at 70% Vo_{2peak} • Frequency: 3×/wk × 16 wk • Exercise mode: cycling (BE)	• HIIE: significant increase in Vo_{2peak}, VT, and significant improvement (decrease) in the Ve/Vco_2 slope • MICE: significant increase in VT • No significant improvements for either group in measures of cardiovascular function, such as systolic and diastolic volumes and LVEF	• No adverse events • No dropouts

Source	Population	Protocol	Results	Adverse Events
Nilsson et al,[24,25] 2008	Ischemic, dilated or hypertensive stable HF, NYHA class II–IIIB, LVEF <40% or ≥40% with symptoms of HF	• HIIE (n = 38, 31 men): 3-min intervals of high-intensity and 2-min intervals of moderate-intensity exercise (rated using Borg scale) with each interval lasting 5–10 min for a total of 50 min • 2×/wk × 16 wk • Exercise mode: aerobic dance • Control (n = 38, 32 men): No supervised exercise; not discouraged from regular physical activity	• HIIE: 6MWT distance, exercise time, workload, and QOL all significantly improved; no improvement in the same for MICE or control group • After 12 mo, improvements in 6MWT distance, exercise time, workload, and QOL remained significant	• No adverse events • 2 Subjects in each group discontinued; 1 subject died (control), 1 subject did not like group assignment (control), 1 subject had a stroke (HIIE), 1 subject dropped out without explanation (HIIE)
Wisløff et al,[10] 2007	Stable postinfarction HF, LVEF <40%	• HIIE (n = 9, 7 men): 4-min intervals at 90%–95% HR_{peak}; intervals separated with active (50%–70% HR_{peak}) pauses of 3 min. Total exercise time = 48 min • MICE (n = 8, 7 men): 70% HR_{peak} for 47 min • HIIE and MICE: 3×/wk (2 supervised, 1 independent) × 12 wk • Control (n = 9, 6 men): supervised exercise (47 min of continuous walking) plus advice about exercise ○ Frequency: Once every 3 wk • Exercise mode: walking (TM)	• HIIE resulted in significantly greater improvements in VO_{2peak}, AT, work economy, exercise intensity, inclination of treadmill, lactate as a % of HR_{peak}, systolic and diastolic function, levels of proBNP, FMD, and QOL vs MICE and control • MICE resulted in significantly greater improvement in AT as a % of VO_{2peak} vs HIIE and control • MICE resulted in significant improvement from baseline in VO_{2peak} • MICE resulted in significantly greater improvement in FMD vs control	• No adverse events • 1 Subject died of cardiac causes not during exercise (in MICE group)

(continued on next page)

Table 1
(continued)

Citation	HF Inclusion Criteria	Intervention Parameters	Main Outcomes	Adverse Events and Dropouts
Roditis et al,[32] 2007	Stable dilated or ischemic HF, NYHA class I–III	• HIIE (n = 11,10 men): alternating intervals of 30 s exercise at 100% WR_{peak} and 30 s of passive rest × 40 min; intensity was increased 10% every month • MICE (n = 10, 9 men): 50% WR_{peak} × 40 min; intensity was increased 5% every month • Frequency: 3×/wk × 12 wk • Exercise mode: cycling (BE)	• Phase I oxygen uptake kinetics significantly improved in both groups equally with the difference between groups not statistically significant • Phase II oxygen uptake kinetics improved significantly only in the MICE group • Vo_{2peak} improved significantly in both groups with no statistically significant difference between groups • AT improved significantly only in the MICE group	• No adverse event data reported • 5 Subjects dropped out due to orthopedic problems or scheduling • 3 Subjects who completed all assessments were excluded due to data analysis difficulties
Dimopoulos et al,[29] 2006	Stable dilated or ischemic HF, NYHA class I–III	• HIIE (n = 10, 9 men): alternating intervals of 30 s exercise at 100% WR_{peak} and 30 s of passive rest × 40 min; intensity was increased 10% every month • MICE: 50% WR_{peak} × 40 min; intensity was increased 5% every month • Frequency: 3×/wk × 12 wk • Exercise mode: cycling (BE)	• HIIE group: significant improvement in peal Vo_2, WR_{peak} and Vo_2/t-slope • MICE group: significant improvement in CR, HRR_1, Vo_{2peak} AT, WR_{peak} and Vo_2/t-slope	• No adverse event data reported • 5 Subjects dropped out due to orthopedic problems or scheduling conflicts

Acute Studies

Gayda et al,[18] 2012	Stable systolic HF with reduced ejection fraction, LVEF <40%, NYHA class I–III	• HIIE (n = 13, 13 men): 2 sets of 8-min intervals at 100% of PPO. Each interval was composed of repeated bouts of 30 s at 100% of PPO interspersed by 30 s of passive recovery; 4 min of passive recovery between the sets • MICE: 60% of PPO × 22 min	• Mean VO_2, % VO_{2peak}, and V_E were higher during MICE • Mean hemodynamic variables (SV, CO, and $C_{(a-v)}O_2$ and oxygen kinetics) were not different during MICE and HIIE • Investigators concluded the hemodynamic response during HIIE was stable	• No adverse events • No dropouts

Tomczak et al,[20] 2011	Nonischemic stable HF, NYHA class I or II, LVEF <50%	• HIIE (n = 9, 6 men)
		• 4 Intervals of
		  ○ 95% HR_{peak} × 4 min
		  ○ 3 min active recovery (no intensity reported)
			• Postexercise decrease in ESV and improved diastolic function
			• Increase in LVEF 30 min postexercise
				• No adverse events
				• 3 Recruited subjects did not complete the study; no reason reported

Abbreviations: BE, bicycle ergometer; BNP, brain natriuretic peptide; $C_{(a-v)}O_2$, concentration of O2 in the arteries minus the veins (ie, oxygen extraction); CR, chronotropic response; ESV, end-systolic volume; FMD, flow-mediated dilation; HR_{peak}, heart rate peak; HRR_1, HR recovery in the first minute of recovery; HRR, HR reserve; LVEF, LV ejection fraction; MI, myocardial infarction; NYHA, New York Heart Association; PPO, peak power output; SF-36, short form 36 health survey; SV, stroke volume; TRIMPi, training impulses; TM, treadmill; TPR, total peripheral resistance; VT_1, first VT.

patients performing HIIE (or MICE) in either the Dimopoulos and colleagues,[29] or Roditis and colleagues[32] investigations.

Ventilatory threshold and lactate

Minute ventilation increases linearly with Vo_2 up to a particular workload at which point there is a dislinear break. This inflection point is called the VT and is believed primarily related to an increased production of CO_2. This point is sometimes called the AT. This point has been shown clinically relevant in patients with HF. For example, an early AT (as a percentage of Vo_{2peak}) is prognostic for early death in patients with HF.[33] Concurrently, as exercise continues, lactate accumulation outpaces removal and, when plotted against workload, a clear upward inflection of the slope can be seen. This point is called the lactate threshold. Lactate accumulation is a key factor underlying the hyperventilatory response in HF.[34] Increases in the VT (or AT) are associated with better aerobic fitness. Fu and colleagues[13] demonstrated a 27% and 22% improvement in the Vo_2 and Ve at the VT, respectively, in a group of patients undertaking HIIE training. For both, this was a significantly better improvement in these variables than was experienced by those participating in a MICE program. Subjects in the study by Freyssin and colleagues[12] made a similar 22% improvement in Vo_2 at VT. This study also measured the time at which the VT was reached and this improved in both MICE and HIIE groups, although more so in the latter. Wisløff and colleagues[10] measured lactate ion concentration, which was 59% lower at a given submaximal walking speed, an improvement that indicates improved fitness. MICE in this cohort did not result in a significant improvement in this variable.

Cardiac and vascular function

Improvements in Vo_2 can be the result of improvements of any component along the oxygen transport chain. According to the Fick equation, the major components are CO and oxygen extraction. The individual contribution from the central (ie, CO) and peripheral (O_2 extraction) components has been demonstrated in healthy populations.[35,36] In the HF patient population, there has been some debate over which adaptation, central or peripheral, is primarily responsible for the change in Vo_2 seen after chronic exercise training.[37–39] In one of the few studies that evaluated cardiac function in patients with HF after HIIE, Wisløff and colleagues[10] demonstrated that all measures of LV systolic and diastolic function were significantly improved after HIIE but not MICE. This study further showed significant improvements in peripheral function. Specifically, for both MICE and HIIE training groups, endothelial function, as measured by flow-mediated dilation, improved; gains were greater in the HIIE group.

In a comprehensive study on the topic of the effect of HIIE training on cardiovascular hemodynamics and peripheral oxygen metabolism, Fu and colleagues investigated changes in CO, peripheral oxygen extraction, and LV ejection fraction. Changes in hemoglobin concentrations were used to evaluate cerebral and muscular hemodynamics. Only the group participating in HIIE had significant improvements in these parameters. Specifically, CO as well as LV ejection fraction were increased. The improvement in CO was provided by an increase in stroke volume and a decrease in total peripheral resistance. Also, the HIIE training program led to improvements in cerebral and muscular blood flow and peripheral (ie, muscle) oxygen extraction. Contrasting these positive results, Smart and Steele[22] reported no significant improvements for patients performing 16 weeks of HIIE or MICE training in variables, such as resting and postexercise LV ejection fraction, end-systolic and end-diastolic volume, and systolic and diastolic velocities.

Quality of life

Patients with HF rate their quality of life (QOL) across many domains as substantially lower than their healthy peers. Specifically, their self-assessment of their physical function and ability to perform physical tasks related to work or other daily activities is similar to those with other chronic illnesses, such as kidney failure, depression, and hepatitis.[40] Low QOL independently predicts morbidity and mortality in patients with HF.[41] QOL is frequently assessed in training studies. The study by Chrysohoou and colleagues[11] primarily addressed changes in QOL after an intervention of HIIE training and showed a 66% reduction (a positive improvement) in Minnesota Living with Heart Failure (MLWHF) questionnaire score. This improvement in QOL was attributed to the significant improvement in aerobic capacity, enabling patients to perform and participate in daily and recreational activities with greater ease. Nilsson and colleagues[24,25] demonstrated a 50% improvement in MLWHF score, which was maintained 12 months after the conclusion of the training intervention. In contrast, Smart and Steele[22] failed to find significant improvements in QOL using the MLWHF questionnaire total score after HIIE training. Using the Hare-Davis Cardiac Depression Scale, QOL improved significantly and more so for those performing MICE. Using the MacNew global score for QOL in CVD, the study by Wisløff and colleagues[10] showed an improvement in this variable for both MICE and HIIE groups although the improvement was significantly greater for the latter.

A study that deserves consideration apart from these investigations is one by Iellamo and colleagues[42] In this study, a method to quantify the training stimulus from the total duration, intensity, and individual HR was used to precisely match the dose of exercise for 2 groups, 1 performing MICE and the other HIIE. The investigators argue that this is necessary because the same relative HR or Vo_2 values can result in different physiologic responses, possibly due to differences in individual internal training load. The results indicated improvements in Vo_{2peak} were achieved in both groups without significant differences between groups. In contrast to most of the other studies, there were similar (and significant) improvements in many exercise variables for both groups.

HIIE PRESCRIPTION CONSIDERATIONS

A significant issue when discussing the studies that have been conducted on HIIE training is that of the differences in protocols used. Programming for continuous exercise is straightforward compared with that of interval training. The duration of on (exercise) versus off (rest) time as well as the total number of intervals can be varied in countless permutations. Moreover, the rest periods can be either active or passive, adding another variable that can be manipulated.

As seen in **Table 2**, there are few similarities between the protocols that have been used thus far. For the 8 chronic training studies, weekly frequency was 2 or 3 days per week and total number of weeks as few as 8 and as many as 16. Total exercise time varied from 30 to 60 minutes. Common modes of exercise were cycling (bicycle ergometer) and walking (treadmill). Three of the 8 studies used 30 seconds of high-intensity exercise and brief (1 minute or less) passive rest periods. Of the remaining 5 studies, 2 used 3- or 4-minute exercise bouts with active rest periods of 3 minutes and 1 used a 60-second exercise bout with an equal passive rest. The final 2 studies had the most unique approach, using a significantly longer exercise duration and active rest as well as a nontraditional mode of exercise (aerobic dance). This heterogeneity means that only broad generalizations can be made about the effect of HIIE training. It is unclear which parameter is the most important in producing the positive physiologic adaptations. Finally, these differences in protocol may underlie the sometimes conflicting results seen between studies.

Only 1 investigation in a patient population has attempted to determine the optimal mix of these variables.[43] In this study, 4 protocols were compared: 2 protocols used active recovery and 2 used passive recovery. These were each paired with either a short (30-second) or long (90-second) duration of exercise and rest. Therefore, 4 protocols were compared: (1) 30-second on/off with passive recovery; (2) 30-second on/off with active recovery; (3) 90-second on/off with passive recovery; and (4) 90-second on/off with active recovery. Total exercise time for each was 30 minutes or until the patient could no longer continue. The intensity was set at 100% of peak power output, determined by a baseline exercise test. The investigators sought to determine which protocol resulted in the greatest time spent near Vo_{2peak} and which would be better tolerated. The results indicated that the time spent at greater than 90%, greater than 95%, and greater than 100% of Vo_{2peak} was significantly lower for the short duration protocol with passive rest. The difference was less than 3 minutes, however, which, the investigators argue, may not be clinically significant. Also, the exercise time at greater than 80% and greater than 85% of Vo_{2peak}, a high-intensity stimulus, was not different between protocols. By several measures, this short-duration/passive rest protocol was better tolerated and may have been especially appropriate for those with the lowest exercise capacity. The investigators concluded that short durations of exercise and passive rest provided the best stimulus for patients with HF undergoing HIIE training. The investigators were not attempting to determine which protocol resulted in the best physiologic adaptations.

Ultimately, the issue of protocol selection must be resolved to allow for effective comparisons between studies. Greater clarity will also aid clinicians who are prescribing and supervising exercise training. Specific guidelines may also improve the clinical acceptability of this mode of exercise, giving clinicians more confidence in the potential outcome and safety of HIIE. As succinctly stated elsewhere, "A similar approach to the study of the dose-response relationships, as would be utilized in the evaluation of new drugs that are tested for efficacy and safety before they enter any market, should be employed."[16] Protocols may need to be tailored based on some clinical signs/symptoms. For example, severity of disease may be one way to group patients. It is likely there is a range of values for intensity and duration of rest and exercise below which the effects of HIIE are similar to MICE.

Table 2
Protocols used in chronic and acute training studies

	Chronic Training Studies								Acute Training Studies	
	Chrysohoou[11]	Fu[13]	Freyssin[12]	Smart[22]	Nilsson[24,25]	Wisløff[10]	Roditis[32]	Dimopoulos[29]	Gayda[18]	Tomczak[20]
Duration of exercise	30 s	3 min	30 s	60 s	5–10 min	4 min	30 s	30 s	30 s	4 min
Intensity of exercise	100% WR$_{peak}$	80% VO$_{2peak}$ (~80% HR reserve)	50% of PPO first 4 wk, 80% of PPO second 4 wk	70% VO$_{2peak}$	High, Borg scale 15–18	90%–95% HR$_{peak}$	100%–120% WR$_{peak}$	100% WR$_{peak}$	100% PPO	~95% HR$_{peak}$
Duration of rest	30 s	3 min	60 s Between intervals; 5 min between sets	60 s	2 min	3 min	30 s	30 s	30 s Between intervals; 4 min between sets	3 min
Active vs passive rest (intensity, if active)	Passive	Active, 40% VO$_{2peak}$	Passive	Passive	Active, moderate intensity (Borg scale 11–13)	Active, 50%–70% HR$_{peak}$	Passive	Passive	Passive	Active, intensity not reported
No. of intervals	—	5	3 Sets of 12 intervals	—	5	4	—	—	2 Sets of 8-min intervals	4 Intervals
Total exercise time	45 min	30 min	54 min (not counting rest between sets)	60 min	50 min	48 min	40 min	40 min	16 min (not counting rest between sets)	48 min
Frequency	3 d/wk × 12 wk	3 d/wk × 12 wk	8 wk	3 d/wk × 16 wk	2 d/wk × 16 wk	3 d/wk (2 Supervised in clinic, 1 independent at home) × 12 wk	3 d/wk × 12 wk	3 d/wk × 12 wk	1 Time	1 Time
Mode	Cycle	Cycle	Cycle	Cycle	Aerobic dance	Treadmill	Cycle	Cycle	Cycle	Treadmill

Abbreviation: PPO, peak power output.

SUMMARY/DISCUSSION

In summary, several studies have now been conducted using HIIE as a chronic training stimulus. In many of those investigations, comparisons have been made to MICE training. In almost all, significant improvements have been demonstrated in many important markers associated with cardiorespiratory fitness. Additionally, improvements in cardiovascular and endothelial function and reductions in systemic inflammation have been shown. Along with no adverse events reported in the training studies, 2 additional investigations into the acute effects of HIIE add to the evidence to support the safety of this type of training. The major limitation of the studies that have been conducted to date, however, is small sample size, resulting in fewer than 200 patients on which to base all of these conclusions. Beyond this, several additional questions remain related to safety, compliance, and feasibility.

First, are the positive physiologic changes associated with HIIE training clinically important? Briefly, the answer seems to be yes. The results of the studies included in this review indicate that HIIE training results in significant improvements in Vo_{2peak}. This is clinically important because cardiorespiratory fitness is one of the strongest predictors of all-cause and cardiac-related morbidity and mortality.[21] Numerous studies confirm the importance of Vo_{2peak} in the prognosis of patients with HF.[44,45] In the studies included in this review, when comparisons were made between HIIE and MICE, the former was often superior in eliciting changes in Vo_{2peak}. In most of the studies, MICE failed to significantly improve Vo_{2peak}, a finding in contrast to numerous other studies representing thousands of patients.[8] Despite this inconsistency, it has been shown that a lack of improvement in exercise capacity after a MICE training program confers a poor prognosis for patients with HF.[46] Once larger studies are conducted, it will be interesting to note if there is still a fraction of patients who are nonresponders.

Much work has been done over the past 15 years to demonstrate the importance of other exercise testing variables, in particular the Ve/Vco_2 slope. For patients with HF, this measure of ventilatory efficiency has been shown a better prognostic indicator than Vo_{2peak}.[30] The ability of HIIE training to have a positive impact on this variable is more in question. Although 1 study found HIEE training significantly improved the Ve/Vco_2 slope, another found that only MICE training did.

Finally, there are not yet any data on morbidity and mortality outcomes after HIIE training, an area of clinical importance. Producing this data will take many more subjects followed over much longer periods of time. This remains an unanswered question for MICE as well, as demonstrated by the HF-ACTION results.[9]

To date, only 1 study has looked at the long-term effects of HIIE training. Nilsson and colleagues[25] followed subjects for 12 months after the conclusion of training and the positive adaptations remained significant at follow-up, which is encouraging. If it is true that HIIE training can induce changes in cardiomyocyte function and reverse pathologic LV remodeling, it may be that these changes can be maintained for an extended period. As with any exercise training program, however, the effects begin to reverse with detraining. If the effects of HIIE are more long lasting than MICE, the former mode of training will clearly be a more attractive option in appropriate patients.

The next question that remains unanswered relates to the safety of HIIE: Does this approach increase risk of adverse events during training? The major concern related to the use of HIIE training lies in the increased risk for acute cardiovascular events, which is highest for individuals with the lowest exercise capacity without a history of regular physical activity. Moreover, the risk is training intensity dependent.[47] Despite this, no adverse events were reported in any of the studies that have been conducted to date (see **Table 1** for a list of all adverse events and dropouts that have been reported). The total number of patients, however, included in these studies who engaged in HIIE training, less than 200, is small. Moreover, most of the included patients had well-preserved systolic function. It is fair to say that the total research population assessed using HIIE training to this point does not yet reflect the characteristics of the heterogeneous HF patient population as a whole.

What is the effect of HIIE on exercise compliance? Achieving high compliance represents one of the major challenges to all exercise interventions. In the HF-ACTION, only 30% to 40% of patients followed the training recommendations after 3 months.[9] Of the studies included in this review, none of them reported patient dropouts due to displeasure with the training stimulus. In one of the acute training effect studies, it was observed that there was a tendency for a lower rating of perceived exertion for HIIE versus MICE.[18] Although this result did not reach statistical significance, it is nonetheless interesting and somewhat counterintuitive. On the other hand, in a study investigating protocol optimization, it was found that active rest was associated with a greater percentage of subjects unable to complete the planned 30-minute bout of exercise.[43] This was an important outcome. It led to the conclusion that patients were able to exercise for a longer duration at a higher percentage of V_{O_2} but fewer were able to complete the entire exercise bout. This has implications for protocol selection but may also have an impact on long-term adherence with the exercise prescription.

The issues of clinical benefit, safety, and compliance are interrelated. Is the additional benefit from HIIE training clinically relevant? If it is, what is the tradeoff with risk of adverse events in a true clinical rehabilitation setting? And, what is the tradeoff between intensity and compliance? Is compliance improved or further diminished by the additional intensity? Finally, if HIIE training provides a greater clinical benefit, is safe, and is at least as good as MICE in terms of compliance, then the final question to answer is one of feasibility. The issue of feasibility cuts across multiple dimensions. First, there are logistical and institutional considerations. For instance, there will be a need for greater supervision because of the increased risk associated with high-intensity exercise. This may result in increasing staff-to-patient ratios and a less favorable financial model for cardiac rehabilitation. The feasibility question also is relevant when considering how this might be applied in a much more heterogeneous patient population. Compared with the research population, the clinical HF population is older and sicker and presents with more comorbid conditions. Determining who is most appropriate for this type of exercise and who will benefit the most will be a major challenge for studies that have yet to be conducted.

These are all questions that can be answered with appropriately designed studies. If the answers all favor HIIE training, then perhaps it should replace MICE as the clinical standard.

REFERENCES

1. Haskell WL, Lee IM, Pate RR, et al. Physical activity and public health: updated recommendation for adults from the American College of Sports Medicine and the American Heart Association. Circulation 2007;116(9):1081–93. http://dx.doi.org/10.1161/CIRCULATIONAHA.107.185649.
2. U.S. Department of Health and Human Services 2008 Physical Activity Guidelines. Available at: http://www.health.gov/paguidelines/guidelines/. Accessed July 22, 2014.
3. Tanasescu M, Leitzmann MF, Rimm EB, et al. Exercise type and intensity in relation to coronary heart disease in men. JAMA 2002;288(16):1994–2000. Available at: http://www.ncbi.nlm.nih.gov/pubmed/12387651. Accessed July 30, 2014.
4. Yu S, Yarnell JW, Sweetnam PM, et al. What level of physical activity protects against premature cardiovascular death? The Caerphilly study. Heart 2003;89(5):502–6. Available at: http://www.pubmed-central.nih.gov/articlerender.fcgi?artid=1767647&tool=pmcentrez&rendertype=abstract. Accessed July 30, 2014.
5. O'Donovan G, Owen A, Bird SR, et al. Changes in cardiorespiratory fitness and coronary heart disease risk factors following 24 wk of moderate- or high-intensity exercise of equal energy cost. J Appl Physiol (1985) 2005;98(5):1619–25. http://dx.doi.org/10.1152/japplphysiol.01310.2004.
6. Hunt SA, Abraham WT, Chin MH, et al. 2009 focused update incorporated into the ACC/AHA 2005 Guidelines for the Diagnosis and Management of Heart Failure in Adults: a report of the American College of Cardiology Foundation/American Heart Association Task Force on Practice Guidelines: developed in collaboration with the International Society for Heart and Lung Transplantation. Circulation 2009;119(14):e391–479. http://dx.doi.org/10.1161/CIRCULATIONAHA.109.192065.
7. Piña IL, Apstein CS, Balady GJ, et al. Exercise and heart failure: a statement from the American Heart Association Committee on exercise, rehabilitation, and prevention. Circulation 2003;107(8):1210–25. Available at: http://www.ncbi.nlm.nih.gov/pubmed/12615804. Accessed July 22, 2014.
8. Taylor RS, Sagar VA, Davies EJ, et al. Exercise-based rehabilitation for heart failure. Cochrane Database Syst Rev 2014;(4):CD003331. http://dx.doi.org/10.1002/14651858.CD003331.pub4.
9. O'Connor CM, Whellan DJ, Lee KL, et al. Efficacy and safety of exercise training in patients with chronic heart failure: HF-ACTION randomized controlled trial. JAMA 2009;301(14):1439–50. http://dx.doi.org/10.1001/jama.2009.454.
10. Wisløff U, Støylen A, Loennechen JP, et al. Superior cardiovascular effect of aerobic interval training versus moderate continuous training in heart failure patients: a randomized study. Circulation 2007;115(24):3086–94. http://dx.doi.org/10.1161/CIRCULATIONAHA.106.675041.
11. Chrysohoou C, Tsitsinakis G, Vogiatzis I, et al. High intensity, interval exercise improves quality of life of patients with chronic heart failure: a randomized controlled trial. QJM 2014;107(1):25–32. http://dx.doi.org/10.1093/qjmed/hct194.
12. Freyssin C, Verkindt C, Prieur F, et al. Cardiac rehabilitation in chronic heart failure: effect of an 8-week, high-intensity interval training versus continuous training. Arch Phys Med Rehabil 2012;93(8):1359–64. http://dx.doi.org/10.1016/j.apmr.2012.03.007.
13. Fu TC, Wang CH, Lin PS, et al. Aerobic interval training improves oxygen uptake efficiency by enhancing cerebral and muscular hemodynamics

in patients with heart failure. Int J Cardiol 2013; 167(1):41–50. http://dx.doi.org/10.1016/j.ijcard. 2011.11.086.

14. Smart NA, Dieberg G, Giallauria F. Intermittent versus continuous exercise training in chronic heart failure: a meta-analysis. Int J Cardiol 2013;166(2):352–8. http://dx.doi.org/10.1016/j.ijcard.2011.10.075.

15. Schnohr P, Marott JL, Jensen JS, et al. Intensity versus duration of cycling, impact on all-cause and coronary heart disease mortality: the Copenhagen City Heart study. Eur J Prev Cardiol 2012;19(1):73–80. http://dx.doi.org/10.1177/1741826710393196.

16. Kemi OJ, Wisloff U. High-intensity aerobic exercise training improves the heart in health and disease. J Cardiopulm Rehabil Prev 2010;30(1):2–11. http://dx.doi.org/10.1097/HCR.0b013e3181c56b89.

17. Rognmo Ø, Hetland E, Helgerud J, et al. High intensity aerobic interval exercise is superior to moderate intensity exercise for increasing aerobic capacity in patients with coronary artery disease. Eur J Cardiovasc Prev Rehabil 2004;11(3):216–22. Available at: http://www.ncbi.nlm.nih.gov/pubmed/15179103. Accessed July 14, 2014.

18. Gayda M, Normandin E, Meyer P, et al. Central hemodynamic responses during acute high-intensity interval exercise and moderate continuous exercise in patients with heart failure. Appl Physiol Nutr Metab 2012;37(6):1171–8. http://dx.doi.org/10.1139/h2012-109.

19. Meyer K, Foster C, Georgakopoulos N, et al. Comparison of left ventricular function during interval versus steady-state exercise training in patients with chronic congestive heart failure. Am J Cardiol 1998;82(11):1382–7. Available at: http://www.ncbi.nlm.nih.gov/pubmed/9856924. Accessed July 2, 2014.

20. Tomczak CR, Thompson RB, Paterson I, et al. Effect of acute high-intensity interval exercise on postexercise biventricular function in mild heart failure. J Appl Physiol 2011;110(2):398–406. http://dx.doi.org/10.1152/japplphysiol.01114.2010.

21. Kodama S, Saito K, Tanaka S, et al. Cardiorespiratory fitness as a quantitative predictor of all-cause mortality and cardiovascular events in healthy men and women: a meta-analysis. JAMA 2009;301(19): 2024–35. http://dx.doi.org/10.1001/jama.2009.681.

22. Smart NA, Steele M. A comparison of 16 weeks of continuous vs intermittent exercise training in chronic heart failure patients. Congest Heart Fail 2012;18(4):205–11. http://dx.doi.org/10.1111/j.1751-7133.2011.00274.x.

23. Cahalin LP. The six-minute walk test predicts peak oxygen uptake and survival in patients with advanced heart failure. Chest 1996;110(2):325. http://dx.doi.org/10.1378/chest.110.2.325.

24. Nilsson BB, Westheim A, Risberg MA. Effects of group-based high-intensity aerobic interval training in patients with chronic heart failure. Am J Cardiol 2008;102(10):1361–5. http://dx.doi.org/10.1016/j.amjcard.2008.07.016.

25. Nilsson BB, Westheim A, Risberg MA. Long-term effects of a group-based high-intensity aerobic interval-training program in patients with chronic heart failure. Am J Cardiol 2008;102(9):1220–4. http://dx.doi.org/10.1016/j.amjcard.2008.06.046.

26. Packer M. The neurohormonal hypothesis: a theory to explain the mechanism of disease progression in heart failure. J Am Coll Cardiol 1992;20(1):248–54. Available at: http://www.ncbi.nlm.nih.gov/pubmed/1351488. Accessed July 30, 2014.

27. Imai K, Sato H, Hori M, et al. Vagally mediated heart rate recovery after exercise is accelerated in athletes but blunted in patients with chronic heart failure. J Am Coll Cardiol 1994;24(6):1529–35. Available at: http://www.ncbi.nlm.nih.gov/pubmed/7930286. Accessed July 30, 2014.

28. Keteyian SJ, Brawner CA, Schairer JR, et al. Effects of exercise training on chronotropic incompetence in patients with heart failure. Am Heart J 1999;138(2 Pt 1):233–40. Available at: http://www.ncbi.nlm.nih.gov/pubmed/10426833. Accessed July 30, 2014.

29. Dimopoulos S, Anastasiou-Nana M, Sakellariou D, et al. Effects of exercise rehabilitation program on heart rate recovery in patients with chronic heart failure. Eur J Cardiovasc Prev Rehabil 2006;13(1):67–73. Available at: http://www.ncbi.nlm.nih.gov/pubmed/16449866. Accessed July 30, 2014.

30. Arena R, Myers J, Hsu L, et al. The minute ventilation/carbon dioxide production slope is prognostically superior to the oxygen uptake efficiency slope. J Card Fail 2007;13(6):462–9. Available at: http://www.ncbi.nlm.nih.gov/pubmed/17675060.

31. Arena R, Arrowood JA, Fei DY, et al. Maximal aerobic capacity and the oxygen uptake efficiency slope as predictors of large artery stiffness in apparently healthy subjects. J Cardiopulm Rehabil Prev 2009;29(4):248–54. http://dx.doi.org/10.1097/HCR.0b013e3181a3338c.

32. Roditis P, Dimopoulos S, Sakellariou D, et al. The effects of exercise training on the kinetics of oxygen uptake in patients with chronic heart failure. Eur J Cardiovasc Prev Rehabil 2007;14(2):304–11. http://dx.doi.org/10.1097/HJR.0b013e32808621a3.

33. Gitt AK. Exercise anaerobic threshold and ventilatory efficiency identify heart failure patients for high risk of early death. Circulation 2002;106(24):3079–84. http://dx.doi.org/10.1161/01.CIR.0000041428.99427.06.

34. Arena R, Myers J, Forman DE, et al. Should high-intensity-aerobic interval training become the clinical standard in heart failure? Heart Fail Rev 2013;18(1):95–105. http://dx.doi.org/10.1007/s10741-012-9333-z.

35. Saltin B, Blomqvist G, Mitchell JH, et al. Response to exercise after bed rest and after training. Circulation

1968;38(Suppl 5):VII1–78. Available at: http://www.ncbi.nlm.nih.gov/pubmed/5696236. Accessed July 21, 2014.

36. Hawley JA. Adaptations of skeletal muscle to prolonged, intense endurance training. Clin Exp Pharmacol Physiol 2002;29(3):218–22. Available at: http://www.ncbi.nlm.nih.gov/pubmed/11906487. Accessed July 21, 2014.

37. Hambrecht R. Effects of exercise training on left ventricular function and peripheral resistance in patients with chronic heart failure. JAMA 2000;283(23):3095. http://dx.doi.org/10.1001/jama.283.23.3095.

38. Clark AL, Poole-Wilson PA, Coats AJ. Exercise limitation in chronic heart failure: central role of the periphery. J Am Coll Cardiol 1996;28(5):1092–102. http://dx.doi.org/10.1016/S0735-1097(96)00323-3.

39. Mezzani A, Corrà U, Giannuzzi P. Central adaptations to exercise training in patients with chronic heart failure. Heart Fail Rev 2008;13(1):13–20. http://dx.doi.org/10.1007/s10741-007-9053-y.

40. Juenger J, Schellberg D, Kraemer S, et al. Health related quality of life in patients with congestive heart failure: comparison with other chronic diseases and relation to functional variables. Heart 2002;87(3):235–41. Available at: http://www.pubmedcentral.nih.gov/articlerender.fcgi?artid=1767036&tool=pmcentrez&rendertype=abstract. Accessed July 21, 2014.

41. Konstam V, Salem D, Pouleur H, et al. Baseline quality of life as a predictor of mortality and hospitalization in 5,025 patients with congestive heart failure. SOLVD Investigations. Studies of Left Ventricular Dysfunction Investigators. Am J Cardiol 1996;78(8):890–5. Available at: http://www.ncbi.nlm.nih.gov/pubmed/8888661. Accessed July 18, 2014.

42. Iellamo F, Manzi V, Caminiti G, et al. Matched dose interval and continuous exercise training induce similar cardiorespiratory and metabolic adaptations in patients with heart failure. Int J Cardiol 2013;167(6):2561–5. http://dx.doi.org/10.1016/j.ijcard.2012.06.057.

43. Meyer P, Normandin E, Gayda M, et al. High-intensity interval exercise in chronic heart failure: protocol optimization. J Card Fail 2012;18(2):126–33. http://dx.doi.org/10.1016/j.cardfail.2011.10.010.

44. Mancini DM, Eisen H, Kussmaul W, et al. Value of peak exercise oxygen consumption for optimal timing of cardiac transplantation in ambulatory patients with heart failure. Circulation 1991;83(3):778–86. Available at: http://www.ncbi.nlm.nih.gov/pubmed/1999029. Accessed November 29, 2013.

45. O'Neill JO, Young JB, Pothier CE, et al. Peak oxygen consumption as a predictor of death in patients with heart failure receiving beta-blockers. Circulation 2005;111(18):2313–8. http://dx.doi.org/10.1161/01.CIR.0000164270.72123.18.

46. Tabet JY, Meurin P, Beauvais F, et al. Absence of exercise capacity improvement after exercise training program: a strong prognostic factor in patients with chronic heart failure. Circ Heart Fail 2008;1(4):220–6. http://dx.doi.org/10.1161/CIRCHEARTFAILURE.108.775460.

47. Thompson PD, Franklin BA, Balady GJ, et al. Exercise and acute cardiovascular events placing the risks into perspective: a scientific statement from the American Heart Association Council on Nutrition, Physical Activity, and Metabolism and the Council on Clinical Cardiology. Circulation 2007;115(17):2358–68. http://dx.doi.org/10.1161/CIRCULATIONAHA.107.181485.

Breathing Exercises and Inspiratory Muscle Training in Heart Failure

Lawrence P. Cahalin, PhD, PT, CCS[a],*,
Ross A. Arena, PhD, PT[b]

KEYWORDS

- Functional capacity • Respiratory muscle weakness • Rehabilitation • Exercise training

KEY POINTS

- Because of the intimate and linked functional and compensatory relationships it is often difficult to identify the primary determinant limiting exercise in heart failure (HF).
- Respiratory contributions have been shown to limit exercise in patients with HF due to abnormalities in ventilation, perfusion, or both ventilation and perfusion.
- Breathing exercises and inspiratory muscle training seem to have substantial potential to improve exercise and functional performance in HF and should be considered as key components of a rehabilitation program in this patient population.

INTRODUCTION

Respiratory contributions have been shown to limit exercise in patients with heart failure (HF). The manner by which the respiratory system limits exercise is due to abnormalities in ventilation, perfusion, or both ventilation and perfusion.[1–16] The key factors limiting ventilation in HF include pulmonary edema, loss of elastic recoil of the lungs, ascites, and inspiratory muscle weakness.[1–7] Thus, the abnormalities in ventilation in HF are mostly restrictive in origin, producing a ventilatory response during exercise in HF that is characterized by: (1) decreased tidal volume, end-tidal carbon dioxide, peak oxygen consumption (Vo_2), and tidal volume to ventilation ratio (VT/VE); and (2) increased respiratory rate, VE, peak dead space ventilation to tidal volume ratio (VD/VT), ventilation to Vo_2 ratio (VE/Vo_2), and the VE/carbon dioxide consumption (VE/Vco_2) slope.[7–9] The key factors limiting perfusion in HF include poor right ventricular performance, elevated pulmonary artery pressure, and

elevated pulmonary vascular resistance (PVR).[2,8,9,14] Ventilation-perfusion abnormalities in HF are due to these factors in addition to several other potential factors, including ventricular asynchrony, cardiac arrhythmias, and loss of viable and elastic lung tissue, as in advanced HF. All of these factors contribute to a ventilation-perfusion mismatch of varying degrees.[1–15] The purpose of this article is to demonstrate how breathing exercises (BE) and inspiratory muscle training (IMT) have the potential to improve many of these abnormalities in ventilation, perfusion, and ventilation-perfusion matching. The rationale for BE and IMT in HF is provided, followed by an extensive review of the literature of BE and IMT in HF. The role of BE and IMT in HF is expanded to patients with pulmonary hypertension (PH) to highlight (1) the manner by which the pulmonary vasculature affects respiratory performance, and (2) the potential that both BE and IMT have on improving the pulmonary vasculature and pathophysiology of HF.

[a] Department of Physical Therapy, Leonard M. Miller School of Medicine, University of Miami, Miami, 5915 Ponce de Leon Boulevard, Coral Gables, FL 33146-2435, USA; [b] Department of Physical Therapy, College of Applied Health Sciences, University of Illinois at Chicago, 1919 West Taylor Street, Room 459, Chicago, IL 60612, USA
* Corresponding author. Department of Physical Therapy, Leonard M. Miller School of Medicine, University of Miami, 5915 Ponce de Leon Boulevard, Fifth Floor, Coral Gables, FL 33146-2435.
E-mail address: l.cahalin@miami.edu

Heart Failure Clin 11 (2015) 149–172
http://dx.doi.org/10.1016/j.hfc.2014.09.002
1551-7136/15/$ – see front matter © 2015 Elsevier Inc. All rights reserved.

RESPIRATORY MUSCLE WEAKNESS IN HEART FAILURE
Inspiratory Muscle Weakness

Inspiratory muscle weakness is a key factor responsible for abnormal ventilation in HF.[3–6] A substantial body of literature has identified the relationship that inspiratory muscle weakness has with symptoms, exercise intolerance, inefficient ventilation, and abnormal cardiopulmonary exercise testing (CPX) results.[3–7] Inspiratory muscle strength has been found to be significantly correlated to peak Vo_2, and is an independent predictor of survival in patients with HF that is comparable to peak Vo_2.[17] Inspiratory muscle strength also seems to be related to type of HF, as patients with dilated cardiomyopathy were observed to have significantly lower strength than patients with ischemic cardiomyopathy.[18] In addition, patients with HF preserved ejection fraction (HFpEF) have been observed to have significantly poorer inspiratory muscle strength in comparison with apparently healthy normal subjects.[19]

Inspiratory muscle weakness was also found to be a significant independent risk factor for myocardial infarction (MI) and cardiovascular disease (CVD) and a nearly significant independent risk factor for stroke in a large study of almost 4000 apparently healthy subjects aged 65 years and older.[20] Poor inspiratory muscle strength remained a significant independent risk factor even after controlling for age, gender, smoking status, anthropometric indices, left ventricular mass, lipids, and systolic blood pressure, with a hazard ratio of 1.5 for both MI and CVD. However, adjustment for forced vital capacity (FVC) lessened the significance of inspiratory muscle strength to a nearly significant predictor of MI, CVD, and stroke, but there was no interaction effect with obstructive lung disease.[20] In this same study, cross-sectional analyses revealed that inspiratory muscle strength was significantly correlated to C-reactive protein (CRP), fibrinogen, and white blood cell count in a negative direction while it was directly related to serum albumin.[20] The investigators concluded that inspiratory muscle weakness may be a marker of an underlying pathophysiologic process mediated through mechanisms that are mechanical, metabolic, or related to oxidative stress.[20]

Furthermore, in a large cohort of patients (N = 532) with HF reduced ejection fraction (HFrEF) of whom 65% demonstrated evidence of PH, inspiratory muscle strength was found to be significantly different between New York Heart Association (NYHA) functional classes, with NYHA class I patients having significantly greater strength than those in all other NYHA classes, and NYHA class IV patients having significantly poorer strength than those in all other NYHA classes.[21] The same study examined the mouth occlusion pressure at 0.1 second of inspiration ($P_{0.1}$) in relation to maximal inspiratory pressure (MIP), and found that the $P_{0.1}$/MIP, a measure assumed to reflect the load imposed on the inspiratory muscles, increased in parallel with NYHA functional class and was significantly different among all classes (**Table 1**).[21] Moreover, MIP was found to be significantly related to pulmonary artery pressure (PAP), cardiac output, and PVR, and $P_{0.1}$/MIP was found to be significantly related to PAP, pulmonary capillary wedge pressure (PCWP), and the transpulmonary gradient (**Fig. 1**).[21] In another study, the inspiratory capacity of patients with PH was

Table 1
Inspiratory performance and pulmonary vascular measures among New York Heart Association (NYHA) classification levels I to IV in patients with heart failure

	NYHA I (n = 32)	NYHA II (n = 121)	NYHA III (n = 239)	NYHA IV (n = 80)
Pi_{max}, % predicted	89.4 ± 5.6	72.9 ± 4.3 n.s.	56.6 ± 7.3 $P = .0034$	37.2 ± 3.4 $P = .0026$
PAPm, mm Hg	30 ± 12.5	34 ± 10.6 n.s.	40.4 ± 8.6 $P = .0041$	50.3 ± 13.2 $P = .0037$
PVR, Wood units	13 ± 0.8	1.8 ± 1.1 n.s.	3.6 ± 2.2 $P = .0039$	6.1 ± 2.2 $P = .0046$
TPG, mm Hg	4 ± 2.1	4.6 ± 3.1 n.s.	8.4 ± 5.3 $P = .0037$	14.1 ± 7.1 $P = .0029$

Abbreviations: n.s., not significant; PAPm, mean pulmonary artery pressure; Pi_{max}, maximal inspiratory pressure; PVR, pulmonary vascular resistance; TPG, transpulmonary pressure gradient.

From Filusch A, Ewert R, Altesellmeier M, et al. Respiratory muscle dysfunction in congestive heart failure—the role of pulmonary hypertension. Int J Cardiol 2011;150:182–5; with permission.

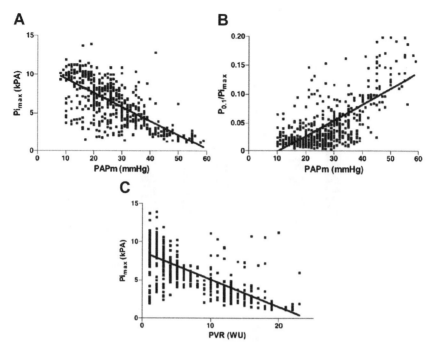

Fig. 1. Relationship between pulmonary artery pressure and (*A*) maximum inspiratory pressure (MIP) and (*B*) $P_{0.1}$/MIP, and (*C*) the relationship between pulmonary vascular resistance (PVR) and MIP. $P_{0.1}$, mouth occlusion pressure at 0.1 second of inspiration; PAPm, mean pulmonary artery pressure; Pi_{max}, maximal inspiratory pressure. (*From* Filusch A, Ewert R, Altesellmeier M, et al. Respiratory muscle dysfunction in congestive heart failure—the role of pulmonary hypertension. Int J Cardiol 2011;150:182–5; with permission.)

found to be an independent predictor of survival.[22] Thus, inspiratory performance appears to be significantly impaired with greater severity of PH, and is related to exercise and functional status, many indices of the pulmonary vasculature, CVD, and survival.[3–7,17–22]

Reasons for inspiratory muscle weakness in HF include the aforementioned factors (mechanisms that are mechanical, metabolic, or related to oxidative stress) in addition to skeletal muscle myopathy, deconditioning, and altered inspiratory muscle fiber type as a result of chronic HF.[3–6,16–23] In fact, Tukinov and colleagues[23] found a significantly lower percentage of type II and type IIa muscle fibers and a greater percentage of type I muscle fibers in the costal diaphragm of patients with HF in comparison with healthy individuals. A greater percentage of type I fibers appears to be a disease-induced adaptation derived from the pathophysiologic effects of HF yielding greater levels of inspiratory endurance, at the cost of poorer inspiratory strength and power.[23] Identical changes have been observed in patients with chronic obstructive pulmonary disease, which were reversed by IMT performed using a Threshold-loading device at 60% of MIP, 30 minutes per day, 5 days per

week, for 5 weeks (**Fig. 2**).[24] In addition to IMT improving skeletal muscle fiber type, the significant improvements in MIP, maximal expiratory pressure (MEP), maximal sustainable inspiratory pressure during progressive inspiratory loading (Pthmax), and elapsed time breathing at 80% of MIP (Tth80) are noteworthy and clinically important (see **Fig. 2**). In view of the foregoing discussion, inspiratory muscle weakness is an important pathophysiologic manifestation of HF with substantial diagnostic and prognostic significance, highlighting the interrelatedness of the cardiac and respiratory systems as well as the potential role improving inspiratory strength may have in HF.[3–6,16–23]

Expiratory Muscle Weakness

Expiratory muscle weakness has also been found in patients with both HFpEF and HFrEF.[3,4,7,19] In patients with HFrEF it has been found to be related to the dyspnea of HF.[3,4] However, little literature has examined the relationship of expiratory muscle strength to exercise intolerance, inefficient ventilation, or abnormal CPX results.[3,4,7] Thus, further examination of expiratory muscle strength in patients with HF is warranted.

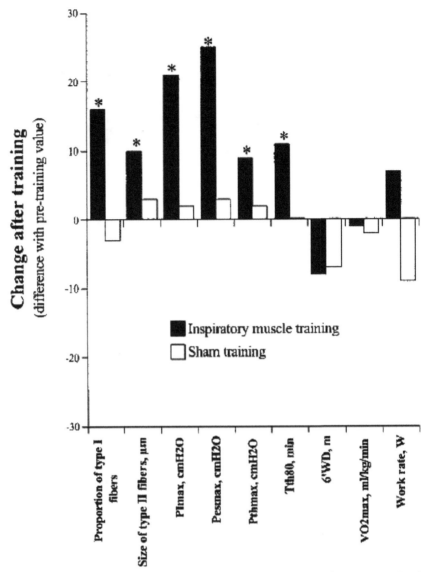

Fig. 2. The effect of chronic obstructive pulmonary disease and inspiratory muscle training on inspiratory muscle fiber type, respiratory performance, and functional capacity. 6'WD, 6-minute walking distance; Pesmax, maximum esophageal pressure; Pthmax, maximal sustainable inspiratory pressure during progressive inspiratory loading; Tth80, elapsed time breathing at 80% of MIP. (*From* Ramirez-Sarmiento A, Orozco-Levi M, Guell R, et al. Inspiratory muscle training in patients with chronic obstructive pulmonary disease: structural adaptation and physiologic outcomes. Am J Respir Crit Care Med 2002;166:1491–7; with permission.)

RESPIRATORY MUSCLE ENDURANCE IN HEART FAILURE
Inspiratory Muscle Endurance

Inspiratory muscle endurance (IME) has been observed to be decreased in patients with HF.[5,7,25] However, it appears that only 2 studies have examined IME in patients with HF in comparison with healthy individuals.[5,25] Inspiratory muscle endurance was examined using an incremental threshold load yielding several obtained outcome measures during the IME test including the MIP achieved, the maximal pressure achieved during the IME test as a proportion of the MIP, and the duration that the IME test was performed in seconds.[5,25] The IME results demonstrated that all indices were significantly lower in patients with HF when compared with apparently healthy adults in both studies.[5,25] Furthermore, poorer inspiratory muscle endurance in HF seems to be due to a significantly greater inspiratory muscle load to capacity ratio, which led to a maladaptive breathing pattern characterized by a shorter expiratory time and prolonged ratio of inspiratory time to total breath time (Ti/Ttot).[25] Improving the maladaptive breathing pattern by simply slowing the respiratory rate (via prolonged exhalation and altering the Ti/Ttot) in patients with HF has the potential to significantly improve many pathophysiologic manifestations of HF.[26–29]

One particular reason why altering the Ti/Ttot seems to be intimately related to IME is because muscle sympathetic nerve activity (MSNA) has been observed to vary within the respiratory cycle, with substantially greater MSNA being modulated during expiration.[30] Furthermore, deep, slow breathing produced almost complete sympathoinhibition in a group of healthy subjects, which was observed to occur from mid-inspiration to mid-expiration.[30] Moreover, altering the Ti/Ttot appeared to shift the sympathoinhibition such that slow inspiration produced a later inhibition and fast inspiration produced an earlier inhibition during the inspiratory phase.[30] Thus, altering the Ti/Ttot via different breathing strategies has the potential to favorably alter the autonomic nervous system in both health and disease as well as IME.[26–30]

No studies have specifically examined the relationship of IME with exercise intolerance, inefficient ventilation, and abnormal CPX results in patients with HF. However, 2 possible surrogate measures of IME have been previously studied in HF, namely maximal voluntary ventilation (MVV) and maximal sustainable ventilatory capacity (MSVC).[31] The MSVC was defined as the highest workload achieved during a progressive respiratory muscle exercise test beginning at 20% of MVV and increasing the workload by 20% increments every 3 minutes to a maximal tolerated level, during which end-tidal CO_2 was measured and excess CO_2 removed or added depending on measured values.[31] The MSVC was found to be significantly correlated with submaximal dyspnea, peak CPX VE, MIP, MEP, forced expiratory volume in 1 second (FEV_1), and MVV.[31] Of note, both at rest and at MSVC, patients with HF were observed to have diminished inspiratory and expiratory flow and an unchanged Ti/Ttot ratio compared with apparently healthy subjects (**Fig. 3**).[31] Lastly, it is surprising the IME is compromised given the greater percentage of type 1 muscle fibers in the costal diaphragm of HF patients,[23] but the diminished inspiratory and expiratory flow, unchanged Ti/Ttot ratio, and excessive VE for a given level of CO_2 associated with HF may be key factors in compromising IME in addition to exercise and functional performance.[5,25,30,31] Nonetheless, further investigation of IME in HF is warranted.

Expiratory Muscle Endurance

Expiratory muscle endurance (EME) does not appear to have been investigated in patients with HF. However, EME has been examined in healthy individuals using a protocol similar to that for IME testing via an incremental threshold loading test.[32–34] The EME in apparently healthy individuals was observed to correlate with dyspnea, which was significantly improved after 4 weeks of expiratory muscle training (EMT).[32,33] The improvement in dyspnea after EMT was associated with a significant increase in MEP and expiratory time, a decrease in both VE and respiratory rate during submaximal exercise, and increased VE at peak exercise.[32–34]

Although EME has not been investigated in patients with HF, EME testing to fatigue in apparently healthy subjects has been found to elicit a respiratory muscle metaboreflex similar to that observed with fatiguing contractions of the diaphragm.[35] Thus, examination of EME and the associated cardiorespiratory response would seem to be warranted in patients with HF. Furthermore, EMT is likely to attenuate the respiratory muscle metaboreflex and to improve exercise and functional performance.

BREATHING EXERCISES IN HEART FAILURE: REVIEW OF THE LITERATURE

A growing body of literature has documented the role of basic to advanced BE in the management of patients with HF.[7,36–59] **Table 2** shows the studies that have examined the effects of BE and IMT in patients with HF.[36–59] **Table 3** presents the studies examining the effects of slowed BE in patients with HF.[26–29] **Table 4** lists studies that have examined the effects of BE in patients with PH.[28,60–62] The specific outcome measures and results of BE on the outcome measures are summarized in **Tables 2–4** and are discussed here.

Inspiratory Muscle Training

A substantial body of literature has examined the role of IMT in HF.[7,37–50,52–59,63–67] In fact there have been 5 systematic reviews covering this topic, and the results of each review have been favorable regarding many of the pathophysiologic manifestations of HF.[63–67] **Table 2** summarizes the studies examining the effects of IMT in patients with HF and the effects on various outcome measures. Although most IMT studies have been in patients with HFrEF,[36–56,58,59] one study found IMT to be beneficial for patients with HFpEF.[57]

Twenty-two studies to date have examined the effects of IMT in persons with heart disease and

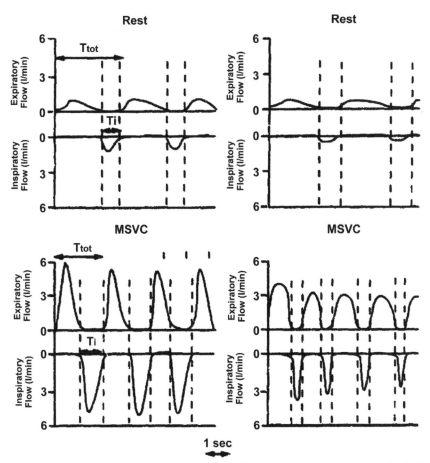

Fig. 3. Inspiratory and expiratory flow at rest and at maximal sustainable ventilatory capacity (MSVC) in apparently healthy subjects (*left panel*) and patients with heart failure (*right panel*). (*From* Mancini DM, Henson D, LaManca J, et al. Evidence of reduced respiratory muscle endurance in patients with heart failure. J Am Coll Cardiol 1994;24(4):972–81; with permission.)

HF (see **Table 2**).[37–50,52–59] Four of the studies included patients with heart disease who partially or fully met HF diagnostic criteria (eg, ejection fraction [EF] <50%, NYHA class III–IV symptoms).[36,40,45,51] Eighteen of the studies were randomized controlled trials[39,41–48,50–59] and the remaining 4 were quasi-experimental studies.[37,38,40,49] The sample size for most studies was small except for one (n = 276) that administered IMT to patients with ischemic heart disease before coronary artery bypass grafting (CABG) surgery.[45] The mode of IMT in most studies (n = 15) was the Threshold inspiratory muscle trainer (Philips Respironics, Andover, MA, USA) at an intensity of approximately 30% of MIP, and the average duration was 30 minutes for 12 weeks, 7 days per week.[37–39,41–43,45,46,49–55,57] The duration and progression of IMT varied in each study that utilized the Threshold inspiratory muscle training device, but usually maintained the same duration or increased it slightly, and maintained the training intensity at 30% to 40% of MIP by weekly reassessment of MIP.[37–39,41–43,45,46,49–55,57] One study administered a variety of BE (isocapnic hyperpnea, inspiratory strength training, and breathing calisthenics) in addition to Threshold IMT,[37] and one study administered combined Threshold IMT and Threshold EMT.[43] Five studies performed by the same investigators administered IMT using the Test of Incremental Respiratory Endurance (TIRE) via the TRAINAIR device (Project Electronics Ltd, Kent, UK) at 60% of MIP/sustained MIP (SMIP) with an increasing work to rest ratio for 20 to 30 minutes, 3 times per week.[44,47,48,56,59] TRAINAIR IMT was performed to the point of exhaustion,[44,47,48,56,59] and was combined with both aerobic and resistance training in one of the studies[56] and with aerobic training in another study.[59]

All but 1 of the 22 studies found IMT to improve 1 or more pathophysiologic manifestations of HF.[39] The one study not observing such an improvement had a small number of subjects in each group (n = 8) and administered IMT for only 15 minutes, twice daily for 8 weeks at 30% of the MIP.[39] The manifestations of HF that were significantly improved by IMT in 1 or more of the studies included dyspnea, quality of life, balance, peripheral muscle strength and blood flow, peripheral muscle sympathetic nervous activity, heart rate, respiratory rate, peak Vo_2, 6-minute walk test distance, ventilation, VE/Vco$_2$ slope, oxygen uptake efficiency, circulatory power, recovery oxygen kinetics, and several indices of cardiac performance (see **Table 2**).[36–38,40–59]

Expiratory Muscle Training

The effect of EMT in patients with HF has been examined in 2 studies, both of which incorporated EMT with IMT (see **Table 2**).[37,43] In one study, EMT was performed at 5% to 15% of MEP for 12 weeks for 15 to 20 minutes, 5 days per week.[43] In this combined IMT and EMT study the Threshold inspiratory muscle trainer was used for both IMT and EMT, with EMT performed by using the Threshold trainer in reverse and exhaling through a flanged mouthpiece at the distal end of the trainer.[43] IMT was performed using the standard mouthpiece included with the Threshold trainer.[43]

In the other study EMT included isocapnic hyperpnea, expiratory strength training, and breathing calisthenics performed for approximately 45 minutes, 3 days per week for 12 weeks.[37] Expiratory strength training was performed via a 2-way valve connected to a pressure gauge through which a patient exhaled at MEP to residual volume. Ten repetitions at MEP were performed, and each repetition was held for 10 seconds with a 15-second rest period between each of the 10 repetitions.[37] Breathing calisthenics included 8 repetitions of 4 different BE aimed at strengthening the abdominal muscles in the supine and seated positions, but focused on contraction of the abdominal muscles during exhalation.[37] The role of EMT in HF has received limited investigation despite the facts that expiratory muscle strength and endurance are poor in HF and expiratory muscle strength is related to dyspnea in HF.[3–7,31–35] Furthermore, that the expiratory muscles contribute to the respiratory muscle metaboreflex suggests that EMT may be warranted in the management of patients with HF. Nonetheless, despite limited investigation of EMT in HF, preliminary findings on improving breathing, exercise, and functional performance hold promise.[7,32–34,37,43]

Diaphragmatic Breathing Exercises

Two studies examined the influence of diaphragmatic BE in patients with heart disease (see **Table 2**).[36,51] Both studies included HF patients, but the percentage of patients with HF was reported in only one of the studies (17%).[36] One of the studies examined the effects of relaxation training combined with aerobic exercise versus aerobic exercise alone on cardiac events (hospital readmission for unstable angina, coronary artery bypass graft surgery, recurrent myocardial infarction as well as cardiac death) two years after an acute myocardial infarction.[36] Relaxation training was performed via diaphragmatic BE with electromyographic biofeedback. Diaphragmatic BE were administered once per week for 5 weeks via 6 individual sessions of 1 hour each, and were described as follows:

The patient learns to achieve a shift in the respiratory pattern, such that inspiration expands both the lower abdomen and costal margin, without movement in the shoulder region; exhalation is moderated and slow. Consequently, tidal volume increases and respiration rate slows down; respiration becomes more full, involving the trunk as a whole, and requiring less effort.[36]

Patients practiced diaphragmatic BE in supine, sitting, and standing positions, and were instructed to perform diaphragmatic BE as described on a daily basis and when experiencing chest discomfort.[36]

Aerobic exercise consisted of 5 weeks of daily bicycling at 70% to 80% of the maximal heart rate achieved during exercise testing.[36] The results showed a reduction in cardiac events and decreased hospital readmissions in the combined relaxation and aerobic exercise training group in comparison with aerobic exercise alone. The greatest difference between the combined versus single intervention was in hospital readmission (8 vs 22, respectively), with readmission for unstable angina being most influenced by the combined intervention of diaphragmatic BE and aerobic exercise (3 vs 12, respectively).[36] The investigators attributed these findings to learned relaxation techniques to enable better coping during episodes of anginal pain.[36] The possibility of favorable changes in neurohumeral activity may also be responsible for the findings observed in this study.[26,27] Similar learned relaxation techniques to control breathing in patients with HF who suffer from dyspnea would be very valuable.

The other study of diaphragmatic BE examined the effect of diaphragmatic BE on heart rate

Table 2
Studies of breathing exercises and inspiratory muscle training in heart failure

Authors,[Ref.] Year	N	Mode of BE or IMT	Study Measurements	Study Outcomes
van Dixhoorn et al,[36] 1987	Exp = 43 Con = 47	Diaphragmatic BE for 60 min 1×/wk for 6 wk combined with AE	Cardiac events and hospital readmission	Reduction of cardiac events and decreased hospital readmissions
Mancini et al,[37] 1995	Exp = 8 Con = 6	Threshold @ 30% of MIP + a variety of BE for 12 wk (90 min, 3×/wk)	MIP, MEP, IME, 6MWT, exercise duration, peak V_{O_2}, HR, BP, RR, TV, VE, dyspnea	Improved MIP, MEP, IME, 6MWT, exercise duration, peak V_{O_2}, VE, and dyspnea
Cahalin et al,[38] 1997	8	Threshold @ 20% of MIP for 8 wk (5–15 min, 3×/d, 7×/wk)	MIP, MEP, dyspnea	Improved MIP, MEP, and dyspnea
Johnson et al,[39] 1998	Exp = 8 Con = 8	Threshold @ 30% of MIP for 8 wk (15 min, 2×/d, 7×/wk)	MIP, MEP, exercise duration, 100 m walk test, QOL	Improved MIP and MEP, but no significant change in other measures
Darnley et al,[40] 1999[a]	9	Hans-Rudolph valve attached to tubing with a progressive increase in the length of tubing each week of a 4-wk study (4, 5 min BE/60 min session, 3×/wk)	Exercise duration, PFTs, HR, diaphragmatic excursion and velocity	Improved exercise duration and diaphragmatic velocity
Weiner et al,[41] 1999	Exp = 10 Con = 10	Threshold @ 60% of MIP for 12 wk (30 min, 6×/wk)	MIP, MEP, IME, PFTs, peak V_{O_2}, 12MWT, dyspnea	Improved MIP, MEP, IME, PFTs, 12MWT, and dyspnea
Martinez et al,[42] 2001[b]	Exp = 11 Con = 9	Threshold @ 30% of MIP for 6 wk (15 min, 2×/d, 6×/wk)	MIP, IME, peak V_{O_2}, 6MWT, dyspnea	Improved MIP, IME, peak V_{O_2}, 6MWT, and dyspnea
Cahalin et al,[43] 2001	Exp = 6 Con = 6 Cross-over	Threshold IMT @ 40% of MIP and Threshold EMT @ 5%–15% of MEP for 12 wk (30–40 min, 5×/wk)	MIP, MEP, IME, PFTs, peak V_{O_2}, 6MWT, cycling endurance, dyspnea, QOL	Improved MIP, MEP, IME, PFTs, peak V_{O_2}, 6MWT, dyspnea, and QOL
Laoutaris et al,[44] 2004	Exp = 20 Con = 15	TIRE @ 60% of MIP/SMIP for 10 wk (3×/wk for an uncertain duration)	MIP, SMIP, peak V_{O_2}, VE, HR, 6MWT, dyspnea, QOL	Improved MIP, SMIP, peak V_{O_2}, HR, 6MWT, dyspnea, and QOL
Hulzebos et al,[45] 2006[c]	Exp = 139 Con = 137	Threshold @ 30% of MIP for 14–90 d (mean = 30) before CABG surgery (20 min, 7×/wk)	MIP, MEP, IME, postoperative pulmonary complications	Improved MIP, IME, and postoperative pulmonary complications
Dall'Ago et al,[46] 2006	Exp = 16 Con = 16	Threshold @ 30% of MIP for 12 wk (30 min, 7×/wk)	MIP, MEP, IME, peak V_{O_2}, VE, VE/$V_{E_{CO_2}}$ slope, recovery O_2, 6MWT, dyspnea, QOL	Improved MIP, MEP, IME, peak V_{O_2}, VE, VE/$V_{E_{CO_2}}$ slope, recovery O_2, 6MWT, dyspnea, and QOL

Study	Sample	Protocol	Variables Measured	Results
Laoutaris et al,[47] 2007	Exp = 15, Con = 23	TIRE @ 60% of MIP/SMIP for 10 wk (3×/wk for an uncertain duration)	MIP, SMIP, PFTs, peak VO_2, VE, 6MWT, dyspnea, TNF-α, TNF receptor I, interleukin-6, CRP, Fas, Fas ligand	Improved MIP, SMIP, PFTs, peak VO_2, 6MWT, dyspnea, and TNF receptor I change
Laoutaris et al,[48] 2008	Exp = 14, Con = 9	TIRE @ 60% of MIP/SMIP for 10 wk (3×/wk for an uncertain duration)	MIP, SMIP, peak VO_2, dyspnea, VE, VE/VCO_2 slope, HRV, NT-proBNP, endothelial vasodilation	Improved MIP, SMIP, peak VO_2, and dyspnea
Chiappa et al,[49] 2008	18	Threshold @ 30% of MIP for 4 wk (30 min, 7×/wk)	MIP, MEP, diaphragm thickness, resting & exercise calf and forearm blood flow	Improved MIP, MEP, diaphragm thickness, and resting & exercise calf and forearm blood flow
Padula et al,[50] 2009[d]	Exp = 15, Con = 17	Threshold @ 30% of MIP for 12 wk (10–20 min, 7×/wk)	MIP, RR, dyspnea, self-efficacy, QOL	Improved MIP, RR, and dyspnea
Kulur et al,[51] 2009	Exp = 145, Con = 60	Diaphragmatic BE	HRV, hemoglobin A_{1C}, blood glucose	Improved HRV, hemoglobin A_{1C}, and glucose
Stein et al,[52] 2009	Exp = 16, Con = 16	Threshold @ 30% of MIP for 12 wk (30 min, 7×/wk)	MIP, OUES	Improved MIP and OUES
Winkelmann et al,[53] 2009	Exp = 12, Con = 12	Threshold @ 30% of MIP for 12 wk (30 min, 7×/wk)	MIP, MEP, IME, OUES, peak VO_2, VE, VE/VCO_2 slope, VE oscillation, recovery O_2 kinetics, 6MWT, QOL	Improved MIP, MEP, IME, OUES, peak VO_2, VE, VE/VCO_2 slope, VE oscillation, recovery O_2 kinetics, and QOL
Bosnak-Guclu et al,[54] 2011	Exp = 16, Con = 14	Threshold @ 40% of MIP for 6 wk (30 min, 7×/wk)	MIP, MEP, 6MWT, balance, quadriceps isometric strength, dyspnea, fatigue, PFTs, depression, QOL	Improved MIP, MEP, PFTs, 6MWT, balance, quadriceps isometric strength, dyspnea, depression, and QOL
Mello et al,[55] 2012	Exp = 15, Con = 12	Threshold @ 30% of MIP for 12 wk (10 min, 3×/day, 7×/wk); mostly home-based	MIP, peak VO_2, VE/VCO_2, VE/VCO_2 slope, HRV, MSNA, QOL	Improved MIP, peak VO_2, VE/VCO_2 slope, HRV, MSNA, and QOL
Laoutaris et al,[56] 2013	Exp = 13, Con = 14	TIRE @ 60% of MIP/SMIP for 12 wk (20 min, 3×/wk)	MIP, SMIP, peak VO_2, dyspnea, VE, VE/VCO_2 slope, VT, CP, quadriceps isometric strength & endurance, LVEF, LVESD, LVEDD, QOL	Improved dyspnea, MIP, SMIP, peak VO_2, VE/VCO_2 slope, VT, CP, quadriceps isometric strength & endurance, LVEF, LVESD, LVEDD, and QOL
Palau et al,[57] 2013	Exp = 13, Con = 13	Threshold @ % of MIP for 12 wk (min, ×/d, ×/wk)	MIP, MEP, IME, peak VO_2, VE, VE/VCO_2 slope, VT, 6MWT, diastolic function, prognostic biomarkers, QOL	Improved MIP, MEP, IME, peak VO_2, VE, VE/VCO_2 slope, 6MWT, and QOL

(continued on next page)

Table 2
(continued)

Authors,[Ref.] Year	N	Mode of BE or IMT	Study Measurements	Study Outcomes
Marco et al,[58] 2013	Exp = 11 Con = 11	Oxygen dual-valve prototype through which 10 daily maximal consecutive inspirations were performed for 4 wk	MIP, MEP, IME	Improved MIP, MEP, and IME
Adamopoulos et al,[59] 2014	Exp = 21 Con = 22	TIRE @ 60% of MIP/SMIP for 12 wk (30 min, 3×/wk)	MIP, SMIP, PFTs, peak V_{O_2}, dyspnea, VE, VE/V$_{CO_2}$ slope, VT, CRP, NT-proBNP, LVEF, LVESD, LVEDD, QOL	Improved SMIP, dyspnea, CRP, NT-ProBNP, LVEF, and QOL

Abbreviations: 6MWT, 6-minute walk test; 12MWT, 12-minute walk test; BE, breathing exercises; Con, control group; CP, circulatory power (peak V_{O_2} × peak systolic blood pressure); CRP, C-reactive protein; EMT, expiratory muscle training; Exp, experimental group; HR, heart rate; HRV, heart rate variability; IME, inspiratory muscle endurance; IMT, inspiratory muscle training; LVEDD, left ventricular end-diastolic diameter; LVEF, left ventricular ejection fraction; LVESD, left ventricular end-systolic diameter; MEP, maximal expiratory pressure; MIP, maximal inspiratory pressure; MSNA, muscle sympathetic nervous activity; NT-proBNP, N-terminal prohormone of B-type natriuretic peptide; O_2, oxygen; OUES, oxygen uptake efficiency slope; PFTs, pulmonary function tests; PW, peak workload; QOL, quality of life; RR, respiratory rate; SMIP, sustained maximal inspiratory pressure; TNF, tumor necrosis factor; TV, tidal volume; VE, ventilation; VE/V$_{CO_2}$, ventilation to carbon dioxide ratio; V_{O_2}, oxygen consumption; VT, ventilatory threshold.

[a] All but 1 of the 9 subjects with ischemic heart disease had a left ventricular ejection fraction ≤50%; the 1 other subject had a left ventricular ejection fraction of 52% (mean left ventricular ejection fraction = 46.6% ± 4%).

[b] The control group performed IMT in the same manner as the experimental group except that the IMT workload was less (10% of MIP), which may have been responsible for the improvement in dyspnea, MIP, IME, and peak V_{O_2} in the control group. Only the experimental group had a significant improvement in the 6MWT distance ambulated.

[c] Approximately 40% of the subjects had a left ventricular ejection fraction less than 50%; 63% of the IMT group and 76.5% of the Usual Care group experienced NYHA class III symptoms and approximately 2% of the IMT group and Usual Care group experienced NYHA class IV symptoms.

[d] The control group consisted of patient education, which included information on basic anatomy and physiology of the heart, diet, medication regimen, sleep, rest, and activity patterns, and what and when to report to the doctor.

Data from Refs.[36–59]

Table 3
Studies of slowed breathing exercises in heart failure

Authors,[Ref.] Year	N	Mode of IMT	Study Measurements	Study Outcomes
Bernardi et al,[26] 1998	Exp = 50 Con = 11	Acute and chronic (4 wk) controlled breathing @ a frequency of 6 breaths/min for 60 min daily focusing on thoracic expansion and DBE	RR, SaO_2, Exercise Duration, peak VO_2, VE, dyspnea	Improved RR, SaO_2, exercise duration, peak VO_2, VE, and dyspnea
Bernardi et al,[27] 2002	Exp = 81 Con = 21	Acute controlled breathing @ a frequency of 6 breaths/min for 4 min	RR, baroreflex sensitivity, R-R wave interval, SBP, DBP	Improved RR, baroreflex sensitivity, R-R wave interval, SBP, and DBP
Parati et al,[28] 2008	Exp = 12 Con = 12	Device-guided paced BE for 10 wk (18 min 2×/d at an RR <10 breaths/min) performed in the home	RR, LVEF, PAP, FEV_1, NYHA classification, VE/VCO_2, QOL	Improved RR, LVEF, PAP, FEV_1, NYHA classification, VE/VCO_2, and QOL
Ekman et al,[29] 2011	Exp = 30 Con = 35	Device-guided paced BE for 4 wk (20 min 2×/d at an RR <10 breaths/min) while increasing exhalation time relative to inhalation time	RR, dyspnea, NYHA Classification	Improved RR, dyspnea, and NYHA classification in responders (patients who were able to reduce their average RR and increase the exhalation time relative to inhalation time >0.2)

Abbreviations: Con, control; DBP, diastolic blood pressure; Exp, experimental; FEV_1, forced expiratory volume in 1 second; LVEF, left ventricular ejection fraction; NYHA, New York Heart Association; PAP, pulmonary artery pressure; QOL, quality of life; RR, respiratory rate; SBP, systolic blood pressure; SpO_2, arterial oxygen saturation; VE, minute ventilation; VE/VCO_2, minute ventilation/carbon dioxide production; VO_2, oxygen consumption.
Data from Refs.[26–29]

Table 4
Studies of breathing exercises in pulmonary hypertension

Authors,[Ref.] Year	N	Mode of IMT	Study Measurements	Study Outcomes
Mereles et al,[60] 2006	Exp = 15 Con = 15	BE for 15–30 min, 5×/wk for the first 3 wk after which they were performed every other day for 12 more weeks and included stretching, yoga, PLB, and "strengthening of respiratory muscles" combined with (1) RT performed for 15–30 min, 5×/wk for the first 3 wk after which they were performed every other day for 12 more weeks, (2) biking for 10–30 min daily at 60%–80% peak HR for the first 3 wk after which biking was performed 5×/wk for 12 more weeks, and (3) walking for 60 min, 5×/wk for the first 3 wk after which they walked 2×/wk for 12 more weeks	6MWT, PW, peak VO_2, VO_2 at AT, HR, BP, RR, TV, VE, dyspnea, QOL, WHO functional class, PASP	Improved 6MWT, PW, peak VO_2, VO_2 at AT, HR, BP, RR, TV, VE, dyspnea, QOL, WHO functional class, and PASP
Parati et al,[28] 2008	Exp = 12 Con = 12	Device-guided paced BE for 10 wk (18 min 2×/d at an RR <10 breaths/min) performed in the home	RR, LVEF, PAP, FEV$_1$, NYHA classification, VE/V$_{CO_2}$, QOL	Improved RR, LVEF, PAP, FEV$_1$, NYHA classification, VE/V$_{CO_2}$, and QOL

Study	N	Intervention	Outcomes	Results
Grunig et al,[61] 2011	58	BE for 15–30 min, 5×/wk for the first 3 wk after which they were performed every other day for an average of 24 ± 12 mo and included stretching, yoga, PLB, and "strengthening of respiratory muscles" combined with the same exercises administered by Mereles et al[60]	Time to clinical worsening, survival, adverse events, 6MWT, PW, peak VO_2, VO_2 at AT, HR, BP, RR, TV, VE, dyspnea, QOL, WHO functional class	Improved 6MWT, PW, peak VO_2, VO_2 at AT, HR, BP, RR, TV, VE, QOL, WHO functional class. Survival at 12 and 24 mo was 100% and 95%, respectively (1 death due to PH). One patient listed for lung transplantation was removed from the waiting list. Nine patients were administered new PH treatment, 3 patients had a deterioration in WHO functional class and 6MWT, 1 patient was hospitalized, and 1 patient underwent lung transplantation
Kabitz et al,[62] 2014	7	BE for 15–30 min, 5×/wk for the first 3 wk after which they were performed every other day for 12 more weeks and included stretching, yoga, PLB, and "strengthening of respiratory muscles" combined with the same exercises administered by Mereles et al[60]	6MWT, MIP, MEP, $P_{0.1}$/MIP, sniff MIP, and twitch mouth pressure via supramaximal bilateral anterior magnetic phrenic nerve stimulation	Improved 6MWT, MEP, sniff MIP, and twitch mouth pressure with a near significant increase in MIP ($P = .08$)

Breathing exercises were combined with aerobic and resistance exercise in all but one of the studies (Parati and colleagues[28]).

All but one of the studies (Kabitz and colleagues[62]) enrolled patients with heart failure. Kabitz and colleagues enrolled patients with invasively confirmed PAH, but excluded patients with "left heart disease."

Abbreviations: 6MWT, 6-minute walk test; AT, anaerobic threshold; BE, breathing exercises; BP, blood pressure; Con, control; Exp, experimental; FEV_1, forced expiratory volume in 1 second; HR, heart rate; LVEF, left ventricular ejection fraction; MEP, maximum expiratory pressure; MIP, maximum inspiratory pressure; NYHA, New York Heart Association; $P_{0.1}$, mouth occlusion pressure at 0.1 second of inspiration; PAP, pulmonary artery pressure; PASP, pulmonary artery systolic pressure; PLB, pursed lip breathing; PW, peak work; QOL, quality of life; RR, respiratory rate; RT, resistance training; TV, tidal volume; VE, minute ventilation; VE/VCO_2, minute ventilation/carbon dioxide production; VO_2, oxygen consumption; WHO, World Health Organization.

Data from Refs.[28,60–62]

variability (HRV), glycosylated hemoglobin (HbA_{1C}), and blood glucose in 145 randomly selected male patients with ischemic heart disease (IHD), of whom 52 had IHD and diabetes and 48 had IHD and diabetic neuropathy.[51] Diaphragmatic BE were performed in the supine position, and patients were instructed to take "ten slow full diaphragmatic breathing exercises at a time" with a 30- to 60-second rest period between each set of 10 diaphragmatic BE for a total of 10 to 15 minutes twice per day for 12 months.[51] Patients were also instructed "to inhale slowly and deeply through the nose into the bottom of the lungs" and "after taking a full breath, the patients were asked to hold it for a moment and then to exhale slowly through controlled expiration".[51] Monthly outpatient visits took place during which patient adherence as well as examination, further instruction, and motivation in diaphragmatic BE was performed.[51] The results of the study found that diaphragmatic BE significantly improved HRV, HbA_{1C}, and blood glucose in compliant subjects, and significantly improved HRV alone in noncompliant subjects after 12 months.[51] Despite both studies finding significant improvements from diaphragmatic BE, the results should be cautiously interpreted and applied to patients with HF, as HF patients represented a small percentage of the subjects enrolled in both studies.[36,51]

Slowed Breathing Exercises

The effect of slowed breathing in patients with HF has been examined in 4 studies (see **Table 3**),[26–29] 2 of which were performed by the same investigators.[26,27] In 2 of the slowed BE studies breathing was slowed via implementation of complete yoga breathing techniques, during which patients were instructed to focus on thoracic expansion and diaphragmatic breathing and to lower the respiratory rate to 6 breaths per minute.[26,27,68]

In the 2 other studies device-guided paced breathing (RESPeRATE; InterCure Ltd, Lod, Israel) was used to slow breathing via the introduction of low- and high-frequency tones to entrain exhalation and inhalation, respectively.[28,29] Low- and high-frequency tones were introduced to patients via headphones while a belt-type respiration sensor worn around the chest or upper abdomen measured the respiratory cycle. During the first 3 minutes of use the device measured spontaneous breathing, after which exhalation was lengthened via prolonged low-frequency tones, resulting in a respiratory rate less than 10 breaths per minute.[28,29] The end of exhalation was signaled by the introduction of a high-frequency tone, at which

time patients inhaled. Thus, Ti/Ttot was automatically altered via the introduction of low- and high-frequency sounds. Device-guided BE was performed for approximately 20 minutes twice per day for 10 weeks in one study and for 4 weeks in the other study.[28,29]

Slow breathing in patients with HF has been observed to decrease chemoreflex activity to hypoxia and hypercapnia and to increase baroreflex activity by improving vagal tone.[26–28] Moreover, the increase in baroreflex activity from slowed breathing was found to be positively correlated to baseline baroreflex activity during spontaneous breathing and, despite not being significantly different, patients with greater baseline baroreflex activity had less severe HF reflected by lower NYHA classification. Thus, patients with less severe HF may be most responsive to slowed breathing and, despite being statistically significant, the correlation between baseline baroreflex activity and the increase in baroreflex activity from slowed breathing was rather low ($r = 0.20$; $P<.04$).

Slowed breathing via device-guided paced BE in patients with HF and pulmonary arterial hypertension (PAH) significantly improved left ventricular EF, PAP, systolic blood pressure, peak Vo_2, Vo_2 at the anaerobic threshold, O_2 pulse, VE/Vco_2, FEV_1, NYHA classification, and quality of life.[28] A second study examining the effects of device-guided slowed breathing in patients with HF and persistent dyspnea (a level of 2/5 at rest was required for enrollment) despite optimal medical management found significant improvements in dyspnea, respiratory rate, and NYHA classification in responders to slowed BE. Responders to slowed breathing were defined as patients having the ability to reduce respiratory rate and increase exhalation time relative to inhalation time greater than 0.2. Thus, alteration of the Ti/Ttot ratio seems to be an important factor in achieving successful results from slowed BE, and the identification of a threshold value around 0.2 is clinically important.

In view of the aforementioned results, slowed BE appears to have substantial potential to improve key pathophysiologic manifestations of HF. Of note is that manipulation of breathing by frequent practice seems to have the potential to maintain low respiratory rates because the resting respiratory rates of regular hata yoga practitioners has been observed to be approximately 6 breaths per minute, which was significantly lower than a matched control group not practicing hata yoga.[69] In view of these findings, further examination of the effects of slowed BE and maintenance of slowed BE is warranted. Perhaps the combination of slowed BE with IMT or EMT would produce even greater improvements in the pathophysiologic manifestations of HF. Also, further investigation of a threshold value to better direct BE for patients with HF is warranted. Furthermore, examination of optimal methods to provide complete yoga breathing techniques to patients with HF who are breathless is needed, as achieving a reduction in the respiratory rate and altering the Ti/Ttot ratio in such patients may be clinically difficult. Finally, despite there being a statistically significant correlation between baseline baroreflex activity and the increase in baroreflex activity from slowed breathing, the correlation was modest at best, and although slowed breathing may be most efficacious at improving baroreflex activity in patients with less severe HF, it is possible that slowed breathing may be just as effective in patients with more severe HF. Further investigation of slowed breathing on baroreflex activity and other measures in patients with different levels of HF severity is warranted.

Breathing Exercises in Pulmonary Hypertension

Four studies have examined the effects of BE in patients with PH, which are shown in **Table 4**. All but 1 of the studies[28] was performed by the same group of investigators.[60–62] The 3 studies performed by the same group administered BE with resistance training, cycling exercise, and walking. The BE in these 3 studies included stretching, yoga, pursed-lips breathing, and "strengthening of respiratory muscles" via unreported methods for 15 to 30 minutes, 5 days per week for the first 3 weeks, after which they were performed every other day for 12 more weeks.[60–62] The results of combined BE and additional exercises produced favorable results including improvements in many CPX measures, World Health Organization (WHO) functional class, dyspnea, quality of life, and, importantly, pulmonary artery systolic pressure. Results of the other 2 studies by this group were also favorable, including improvements in many CPX measures and both volitional and nonvolitional tests of respiratory performance in addition to excellent 1-year and 2-year survival (100% and 95%, respectively) despite the patients having severe chronic PH.[60–62]

The other study of BE in patients with PH is reported earlier in this article and consisted of slowed BE via device-guided paced BE, which significantly improved many CPX indices in addition to left ventricular EF and PAP.[28] Thus, BE alone and combined with a variety of exercises in patients with PH seem to have substantial promise in altering the pulmonary vasculature and in many pathophysiologic manifestations of HF.[28,60–62] Further investigation of BE alone and combined with other forms of exercise in patients with PH is warranted.

RATIONALE AND FURTHER SUPPORT FOR BREATHING EXERCISES AND INSPIRATORY MUSCLE TRAINING IN HEART FAILURE AND PULMONARY ARTERIAL HYPERTENSION
Improving Alveolar Gas Diffusion Abnormalities

The likelihood of alveolar gas diffusion abnormalities limiting exercise tolerance in HF and altering cardiorespiratory performance has been reported.[1] In fact, several important significant relationships have been found to support the role of alveolar gas diffusion abnormalities in limiting exercise and functional performance in HF despite a lack of significant arterial oxygen desaturation during exercise, including: (1) baseline diffusion capacity for carbon monoxide (DLCO); (2) peak Vo_2; (3) alveolar-capillary membrane conductance; and (4) VE/Vco_2.[2] These significant relationships highlight the role that alveolar-capillary function has in exercise and breathing, and the ability of the alveolar-capillary interface to accommodate to imposed demands and maintain arterial oxygenation despite inefficient ventilation and impaired ventilation-perfusion matching in patients with HF.[2]

The most likely reason for the lack of arterial oxygen desaturation during exercise in patients with HF lies in the recruitment of alveolar-capillary membrane conductance areas to compensate for decreased pulmonary perfusion.[2] Such recruitment suggests that the alveolar-capillary membrane is pliable, at least in less advanced HF, and accommodates to imposed demands, which is important in regard to therapeutic efforts to improve exercise tolerance in HF patients and, in particular, to BE.[1,2] Therapeutic efforts that promote such recruitment may improve arterial oxygenation despite poor pulmonary perfusion.[2]

It is likely that slowed breathing and alteration of the Ti/Ttot ratio promotes such recruitment in view of the results outlined in the previous section.[26–29,36,51,60,62] In fact, perhaps slow, deep breathing facilitates not only baroreflex activity and arterial oxygenation but also improves lung and chest wall compliance by decreasing the restrictive characteristics associated with HF via several related mechanisms, including: (1) increasing chest wall mobility and motion; (2) attenuating airway and lung tissue hypersensitivity and sympathetic nervous system activity; and (3) increasing oxygen availability.[70] Similar changes have been observed with β-adrenergic blockers in patients with HF,[71] and similar mechanisms to improve lung tissue repair in left heart disease have been proposed.[72] Future studies of the role that BE and IMT may have in improving alveolar gas diffusion abnormalities and the restrictive characteristics of HF are needed.

In fact, a previous article investigated the influence of pulmonary edema and its restrictive characteristics on exercise tolerance, and revealed that even subclinical fluid retention can significantly impair exercise ability. Diuresis alone significantly increased exercise tolerance (9.2 ± 4.2 to 12.5 ± 4.7 minutes) and was associated with significant improvement in symptoms, ventilation, and lactate levels.[1] Of note is that at matched peak workloads ventilation decreased from 45 ± 12 to 35 ± 9 L/min. Subclinical fluid retention and pulmonary edema pose significant problems for breathing and HF management, and a recent study found that inspiratory muscle testing and training provided valuable information regarding an acute HF exacerbation, subclinical fluid retention, and pulmonary edema.[73]

Assessing Inspiratory Performance to Manage Heart Failure Exacerbations

Acute HF exacerbations are common and have become a key metric in the hospitalization of HF patients in the United States.[74] Hospitals in the United States are penalized when HF-related readmission rates are high and are awarded when they are low or reduced.[74] A recent observation during IMT in a patient with HFpEF revealed key changes in measures of inspiratory performance that appeared to precede clinical signs and symptoms of an acute HF exacerbation.[73] **Fig. 4** shows several measures of inspiratory performance obtained during IMT via the TIRE including the MIP, SMIP, inspiratory duration, and inspiratory endurance measured as the accumulated area (summation of SMIP values throughout IMT). The MIP, SMIP, inspiratory duration, and accumulated area were observed to be 79 cm H_2O (76% of predicted), 8.2 J, 9.8 seconds, and 2355 pressure-time units (PTU), respectively (see **Fig. 4**).[73] After three 50-minute sessions of IMT the patient demonstrated a similar MIP and SMIP, improved inspiratory duration and accumulated area (17% and 287%, respectively), and improved dyspnea, fatigue, and sleep. However, 2 days later TIRE testing revealed a reduction in MIP, SMIP, and accumulated area (38%, 33%, and 7%, respectively), increased oscillation during inspiration,

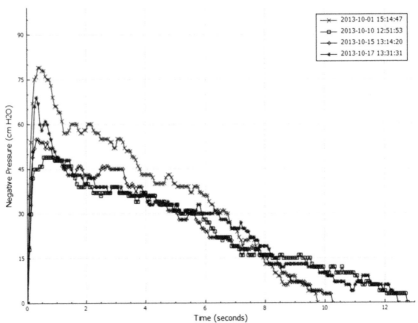

Date & Time	MIP (cmH20)		SMIP (J)		Area		Time (sec)		Max Level	Acc Area	
» 2013-10-01 15:14:47	79.00	0%	8.17	0%	376.69	0%	9.81	0%	A6	2355.69	0%
2013-10-03 13:22:58	81.00	2%	7.98	-2%	359.56	-4%	10.19	3%	D4	7487.94	217%
2013-10-08 13:21:17	69.00	-12%	6.17	-24%	319.25	-15%	11.56	17%	E6	9117.44	287%
» 2013-10-10 12:51:53	49.00	-37%	5.44	-33%	312.25	-17%	12.81	30%	E4	8499.25	260%
» 2013-10-15 13:14:20	55.00	-30%	5.56	-32%	296.62	-21%	10.31	5%	D6	6201.25	163%
» 2013-10-17 13:31:31	69.00	-12%	6.06	-25%	331.50	-11%	12.50	27%	F6	9794.44	315%

Fig. 4. Test of incremental respiratory endurance testing and training results in a heart failure patient experiencing an acute exacerbation of heart failure.

increased inspiratory duration, and a less steep SMIP slope. Examination of the patient revealed the same body weight and no signs of HF exacerbation. Surprisingly, 5 days later the patient's body weight increased 2.7 kg, with signs of an acute HF exacerbation and similar reductions in inspiratory performance. Five days following the start of pharmacologic management of the HF exacerbation, body weight decreased and inspiratory performance improved, with the most notable improvement in inspiratory endurance (19% gain).

This case study demonstrates the effects of an acute HF exacerbation on inspiratory performance, with many novel findings, including the beneficial effects of IMT on inspiratory performance and symptoms in a patient with HFpEF in addition to the role of TIRE testing in identifying the onset of an acute HF exacerbation before it was clinically evident. The reduction in inspiratory performance, increased inspiratory oscillation, and a less steep SMIP slope highlight altered inspiratory mechanics associated with an acute HF exacerbation that improved after pharmacologic treatment. Oscillatory ventilation is an ominous finding in HF and appears to be detectable via TIRE testing.[2,7,8] The decrease in the steepness of the SMIP slope is also a novel finding that highlights a reduction in the generation of inspiratory force and lengthened SMIP duration, which may be an attempt to optimize cardiorespiratory function by altering the Ti/Ttot, inspiratory work, and neurohumeral activity. IMT and serial examination of inspiratory performance in HF may improve inspiratory performance and lead to better management of acute HF exacerbations, but requires further investigation.

The serial examination of inspiratory performance is required to administer optimal IMT prescriptions. Thus, an IMT prescription enables inspiratory performance to be measured at least 2 days per week and at most daily. Although not all IMT prescriptions require or provide the examination of inspiratory performance, several IMT devices require that it be measured before each IMT session. In fact, TIRE testing and IMT, available through the RT2 (DeVilbiss Healthcare, Wollaston, UK), TRAINAIR (Project Electronics Ltd), or PrO_2 (PrO_2, Smithfield, RI, USA) IMT devices require inspiratory performance to be measured before beginning each IMT session. An example of the TIRE testing and training template is shown in **Fig. 4**, in which MIP, SMIP, and inspiratory duration have been previously reviewed in a patient with an acute HF exacerbation.

The MIP is the highest pressure measured during inspiration and is measured at residual volume (RV) or functional residual capacity (FRC), the unit of measure being centimeters of water (cm H_2O). Recall that the MIP shown in **Fig. 4** is 79 cm H_2O. The standardized methods that are used to measure MIP encourage subjects to inspire deeply and to generate as much pressure as possible within 1 to 2 seconds of inspiration. The SMIP, on the other hand, is measured from residual volume/functional residual capacity (RV/FRC) to total lung capacity (TLC) and represents the work under the curve that is generated from the start of inspiration to MIP to the end of inspiration, at 9.8 seconds on the x-axis of **Fig. 4**. The SMIP unit of measure can be described in both joules and the area under the curve, with the area under the curve unit of measure being PTU (see **Fig. 4**). In view of this, the SMIP has been described as single breath inspiratory work capacity, and represents single breath work/endurance. The SMIP presented in **Fig. 4** represents 8.17 J and 376.69 PTU.

All of the aforementioned measurements can be used to serially examine inspiratory performance in HF patients in a variety of settings, including the home. The PrO_2 IMT device enables inspiratory muscle testing and IMT data to be uploaded to a cloud, to be shared with other users and health care providers. The capacity for data sharing is particularly important for HF patients confined to the home in need of serial assessment and IMT. Further investigation of the serial examination of inspiratory performance and IMT using such devices in HF patients is needed, but preliminary data[73] and previous findings highlighting the prognostic significance of inspiratory performance in HF[3–7,17–29] make this an important method to better manage patients with HF.

Improving Pulmonary Perfusion

It is possible that many of the beneficial effects of IMT and BE seen in patients with HF are due to improvements in pulmonary perfusion. Direct and indirect evidence strongly suggests that BE and IMT improve pulmonary perfusion in view of improvements in PAP and PVR,[28,60] consistent improvement in peak VE/Vco$_2$ and the VE/Vco$_2$ slope in every study of BE and IMT that has examined this parameter of ventilation-perfusion matching (N = 6),[28,46,53,55–57] and the finding that the VE/Vco$_2$ slope is significantly correlated with right ventricular oxidative metabolism ($r = 0.61$; $P = .003$), which was significantly greater in patients with a VE/Vco$_2$ slope of 34 or greater in comparison to patients with a VE/Vco$_2$ slope of less than 34 (0.93 ± 0.16 vs 0.77 ± 0.16; $P = .04$).[14] Thus, PVR may be a major determinant of ventilatory inefficiency in patients with HF that appears to be favorably altered via BE and IMT.[14,28,46,53,55–57,60]

It is possible that the favorable effects of BE on the pulmonary vasculature and pulmonary perfusion may be even greater with targeted BE, IMT, and EMT during which alteration of the Ti/Ttot ratio and MSNA is optimized.[14,28,30,46,53,55–57,60]

In fact, although the pathophysiologic mechanisms leading to exercise oscillatory ventilation (EOV) are not completely understood, IMT has the potential to decrease EOV, based on (1) stabilizing the feedback systems that control ventilation and improving the circulation time; (2) decreasing the chemosensitivity to $PaCO_2$ and PaO_2; (3) repairing baroreflex activity; and (4) decreasing pulmonary pressures and improving right ventricle to pulmonary circulation coupling.[2,7,8] Only one IMT study has examined EOV, which was found to significantly improve after 12 weeks of Threshold IMT combined with aerobic exercise training.[53] At the very least, BE and IMT favorably alter right ventricle to pulmonary circulation coupling, producing many of the aforesaid improvements.[15]

Improving Muscle Sympathetic Nerve Activity and the Autonomic Nervous System

As briefly discussed previously, MSNA has been observed to vary within the respiratory cycle, with substantially greater MSNA being modulated during expiration, and deep, slow breathing producing almost complete sympathoinhibition in a group of healthy subjects, which was observed to occur from mid-inspiration to mid-expiration.[30] Two studies have keenly demonstrated that sympathoinhibition is also present in some patients with HF,[75,76] and that it seems to be closely related to both resting tidal volume and the lung inflation reflex because patients demonstrating sympathoinhibition had significantly greater tidal volume and a significantly lower respiratory rate during spontaneous breathing when compared with patients not demonstrating sympathoinhibition.[75] Furthermore, patients without sympathoinhibition required a greater tidal volume to induce sympathoinhibition.[75] Thus, methods to improve tidal volume and induce the lung inflation reflex are likely to facilitate sympathoinhibition. Targeted IMT and deep, slowed BE are likely to induce sympathoinhibition.

However, not all HF patients are capable of inducing sympathoinhibition because only approximately half of the patients in both studies were observed to demonstrate sympathoinhibition.[75,76] Of importance is that in HF patients demonstrating sympathoinhibition, deep, slow breathing was observed to significantly decrease steady-state MSNA acutely in HF patients with high levels of resting sympathetic tone.[76] Device-guided breathing (RESPeRATE) resulted in a significant reduction in respiratory rate (16.4 ± 3.9 to 6.7 ± 2.8/min), significant increase in tidal volume (499 ± 206 to 1177 ± 497 mL), and 31% reduction in steady-state MSNA.[76]

The finding that approximately half of the HF patients examined in these studies were capable of inducing sympathoinhibition is important and worthy of further investigation,[75,76] because no significant difference in patient characteristics was observed between those with and without sympathoinhibition,[75,76] and because BE may be more specifically prescribed to patients with HF if sympathoinhibition is present or absent. In fact it may be that slow, deep breathing may be a sufficient intervention for patients observed to induce sympathoinhibition, whereas other therapeutic interventions such as IMT, EMT, or both may be necessary to facilitate sympathoinhibition in patients unable to induce a reduction in MSNA during baseline examination. Thus, identifying particular characteristics in patients with and without sympathoinhibition may improve the implementation and prescription of BE in patients with HF.

IMPLEMENTATION OF BREATHING EXERCISES AND INSPIRATORY MUSCLE TRAINING IN HEART FAILURE

Implementation of BE and IMT in patients with HF can be basic or very advanced, and depends on availability of equipment and time constraints of the health care professionals, among many other factors. Basic BE and IMT methods are provided in **Box 1**. Proper implementation of BE requires a baseline measure of at least MIP and MEP in addition to IME.[36–59] The methods used to measure these outcomes are described in **Box 1**. Furthermore, a comparison of observed MIP and MEP values should be made to determine the percentage of predicted value for MIP and MEP.[77] The methods to perform such a comparison are outlined in **Box 1**.[77] Finally, the methods used to implement IME, strength, and power training, as well as EMT, are described in **Box 1**.[7,78,79]

Several additional aspects of IMT and EMT are also included in **Box 1**, such as utilization of a nasal sniff in testing and training the inspiratory muscles.[80] Although the nasal sniff has not been specifically studied in patients with HF, the available literature suggests that it is likely to provide important prognostic information in addition to therapeutic effects.[80] Utilization of the sniff reflex has the potential to optimize diaphragmatic contraction, which may help to promote greater IMT effects.[80] Furthermore, inspiratory and expiratory airway reflexes have the potential to improve

Box 1
Methods to implement breathing exercises and inspiratory and expiratory muscle training

Measurement of respiratory muscle strength: During the measurement of breathing muscle strength the patient should wear a nose clip and be seated with the trunk at a 90° angle to the hips. Maximum inspiratory pressure (MIP), maximum expiratory pressure (MEP), and endurance can be measured with commercially available devices or with a standard sphygmomanometer used to measure blood pressure, and the tubing from the manometer can be attached to a mouthpiece. However, the unit of measure will be mm Hg and can be converted to cm H_2O (the standard unit of measure for MIP and MEP) by multiplying mm Hg by 1.36.

Procedure:

1. MIP

    a. Have patient expire fully (near residual volume).

    b. Motivate patient to inspire as forcefully as possible.

    c. Document the MIP and repeat the above until a stable baseline is observed.

MIP (cm H_2O) _____ _____ _____ _____ _____ _____ _____

2. MEP

    a. Have patient inspire fully (total lung capacity).

    b. Motivate patient to exhale as forcefully as possible.

    c. Document the MEP and repeat the above until a stable baseline is observed.

MEP (cm H_2O) _____ _____ _____ _____ _____ _____ _____

3. Comparing measured MIP and MEP with previously published "normal" values

    Prediction equations from Black and Hyatt.[77]

    Men 20–54 years of age:

    MIP = 129 − (Age × 0.13)

    MEP = 229 + (Age × 0.08)

    Men 55–80 years of age:

    MIP = 120 − (Age × 0.25)

    MEP = 353 − (Age × 2.33)

    Women 20–54 years of age:

    MIP = 100 − (Age × 0.39)

    MEP = 158 − (Age × 0.18)

    Women 55–86 years of age:

    MIP = 122 − (Age × 0.79)

    MEP = 210 − (Age × 1.14)

4. Measurement of inspiratory muscle endurance: Ask the patient to inhale at a level that is greater than 50% of MIP with a constant rate of inspiration using a metronome or timer while monitoring each inspiratory effort (with commercially available devices or a standard sphygmomanometer as described above). Record the number of inspirations or the amount of time the patient is able to continue inspiring at a level that is greater than 50% of MIP. The endurance test is terminated when the patient is unable to achieve an inspiratory force that is greater than 50% of MIP on 2 to 3 consecutive attempts.

5. Inspiratory muscle endurance training: Inspiratory muscle endurance training is accomplished using low to moderate inspiratory flow against low to moderate levels of resistance for an inspiratory time period of 12 to 20 seconds, but repeated for 15 to 30 minutes per session.

6. Inspiratory muscle strength training: Inspiratory muscle strength training is accomplished using moderate inspiratory flow against moderate to high levels of resistance for an inspiratory duration of 8 to 12 seconds for 5 to 15 minutes per session.

7. Inspiratory muscle power training: Inspiratory muscle power training (IMT) is accomplished using rapid inspiratory flow against different levels of resistance during a short inspiratory duration (4–8 seconds) and for a short period of time (2–5 minutes). A leak larger than the standard 2 mm size seems to facilitate such power IMT.

8. Expiratory muscle training: Expiratory muscle training (EMT) can be provided as for IMT and can focus on endurance, strength, or power capacity using the principles outlined above. EMT can be best administered via a flanged mouthpiece to prevent air from leaking around nonflanged mouthpieces. EMT in heart failure has previously been performed in 2 ways. (1) A variety of exercises including isocapnic hyperpnea, expiratory strength training, and breathing calisthenics performed for approximately 45 minutes, 3 days per week.[37] Expiratory strength training was performed via a 2-way valve connected to a pressure gauge through which a patient exhaled at MEP to total lung capacity. Ten repetitions at MEP were performed and each repetition was held for 10 seconds with a 15-second rest period between each of the 10 repetitions.[37] Breathing calisthenics included 8 repetitions of 4 different breathing exercises (BE) aimed at strengthening the abdominal muscles in the supine and seated positions, but focused on contraction of the abdominal muscles during exhalation.[37] (2) Use of the Threshold IMT device (with a flanged mouthpiece) at 5% to 15% of MEP for 15 to 20 minutes, 5 days per week, combined with IMT.[43]

9. Slowed breathing exercises: Slowed BE can be administered via yoga BE or device-guided methods with an apparent goal breathing frequency rate of 6 breaths per minute.

10. Diaphragmatic breathing exercises: Diaphragmatic BE can be implemented with all of the above BE (including EMT, but reversing diaphragmatic action in addition to abdominal and lateral costal motion) and should focus on expanding the lower abdomen and lateral costal area without shoulder movement during inspiration while exhalation should be controlled and slow.[36] Patients typically practice diaphragmatic BE in supine or semisupine position initially, followed by sitting and standing using the methods described above.

vagal tone and should therefore be incorporated into BE, IMT, and EMT research efforts.[80] However, specific methods to incorporate such reflexes with BE and the effects on HF outcomes are in need of investigation.

It is possible that IMT combined with EMT, slowed breathing, and additional efforts to alter the Ti/Ttot ratio will produce favorable effects on breathing, exercise tolerance, and functional performance in addition to the pathophysiologic manifestations of HF. However, further examination of such combinations of respiratory muscle training is needed.

Novel Methods to Provide Breathing Exercises and Inspiratory Muscle Training

Several novel methods of providing BE and IMT have been described, and include yoga BE,[26,27] slowed BE via device-guided techniques,[28,29] and TIRE IMT.[44,47,48,56,59] Although diaphragmatic BE are not novel,[36,51] novel methods to examine the effects of such BE are needed. Yoga BE have been described in detail, and further attempts to easily examine complete yoga breathing techniques, during which patients are instructed to focus on thoracic expansion and diaphragmatic breathing to lower the respiratory rate to 6 breaths per minute, are needed.[26,27,68] Nonetheless, yoga BE have a long history, and many of the methods used to administer diaphragmatic BE can be incorporated with yoga BE to provide optimal BE to patients with HF.[26,27,36,51,68]

Device-guided BE provides substantial ease in the administration of BE and effectiveness in improving a variety of pathophysiologic manifestations of HF.[28,29] Further use and examination of the effects of device-guided BE in HF are needed, but the available data appear very promising.[28,29] Finally, TIRE IMT provides isokinetic-like IMT via inspiratory flow resistive loading (IFRL), which depends on the velocity or flow of inspiration. A faster airflow correlates with greater inspiratory muscle power and pressure generation capability throughout inspiration with biofeedback, which enables efforts to be targeted at different locations throughout inspiration.[7] **Fig. 4** shows how IMT efforts could be targeted at $^1/_4$, $^1/_2$, $^3/_4$, and the very terminal portion of the SMIP and, because the velocity of flow can be altered, provides a platform from which to perform power IMT [rapid inspiratory flow against high levels of resistance during a short inspiratory duration (4–8 seconds) and for a short period of time (2–5 minutes); possibly using a larger leak in the IMT mouthpiece], strength IMT (moderate inspiratory flow against moderate to high levels of resistance for an inspiratory duration of 8–12 seconds for 5–15 minutes), and endurance IMT (low to moderate inspiratory flow against low to moderate levels of resistance for an inspiratory duration of 12–20 seconds for 15–30 minutes) (see **Box 1**).[78,79] Of note is that IMT targeted at the terminal portion of the SMIP appears to substantially lengthen the inspiratory duration, thus optimally altering the Ti/Ttot ratio and facilitating endurance IMT.[7] Because resistance with IFRL depends on the velocity or flow of inspiration, a faster airflow correlates with greater inspiratory muscle power and pressure generation, whereas a slower airflow correlates with less inspiratory muscle power and pressure generation, yielding a greater capacity to alter the Ti/Ttot ratio and the IMT prescription.

SUMMARY

The function and compensatory mechanisms of the heart and lungs are intimately related and linked because they both supply oxygen to the body. Because of the intimate and linked functional and compensatory relationships, BE and IMT have substantial potential to improve exercise and functional performance in HF. Slowed BE have substantial potential to improve key pathophysiologic manifestations of HF. In view of the beneficial effects of altering the Ti/Ttot ratio, further examination of the effects of different BE and combined BE with IMT or EMT is needed. For example, perhaps a greater focus should be placed on EMT and different methods to administer EMT in patients with HF. In addition, perhaps IMT and EMT should be performed with different speeds of inspiration and expiration, respectively, and targeted at different locations of both, to alter the Ti/Ttot and facilitate not only greater inspiratory endurance but greater inspiratory strength and power. In conclusion, BE are gaining a new level of importance in managing both health and disease, and the results of this review reveal that BE and IMT can improve functional and exercise performance in addition to many pathophysiologic manifestations of HF.

REFERENCES

1. Chomsky DB, Lang CC, Rayos G, et al. Treatment of subclinical fluid retention in patients with symptomatic heart failure: effect on exercise performance. J Heart Lung Transplant 1997;16(8):846–53.
2. Guazzi M. Alveolar gas diffusion abnormalities in heart failure. J Card Fail 2008;14:695–702.
3. Hammond MD, Bauer KA, Sharp JT, et al. Respiratory muscle strength in congestive heart failure. Chest 1990;98(5):1091–4.
4. McParland C, Krishnan B, Wang Y, et al. Inspiratory muscle weakness and dyspnea in congestive heart failure. Am Rev Respir Dis 1992;146:467.
5. Walsh JT, Andrews R, Johnson P, et al. Inspiratory muscle endurance in patients with chronic heart failure. Heart 1996;76(4):332–6.
6. Meyer FJ, Zugck C, Haass M, et al. Inefficient ventilation and reduced respiratory muscle capacity in congestive heart failure. Basic Res Cardiol 2000; 95(4):333–42.
7. Cahalin LP, Arena R, Guazzi M, et al. Inspiratory muscle training in heart disease and heart failure—a review of the literature with a focus on method of training and outcomes. Expert Rev Cardiovasc Ther 2013;11(2):161–77.
8. Arena R, Guazzi M, Myers J. Ventilatory abnormalities during exercise in heart failure: a mini review. Curr Respir Med Rev 2007;3:179–87.
9. Wasserman K, Zhang YY, Gitt A, et al. Lung function and exercise gas exchange in chronic heart failure. Circulation 1997;96:2221–7.
10. Waxman AB. Pulmonary function test abnormalities in pulmonary vascular disease and chronic heart failure. Clin Chest Med 2001;22(4):751–8.
11. Hawkins NM, Petrie MC, Jhund PS, et al. Heart failure and chronic obstructive pulmonary disease: diagnostic pitfalls and epidemiology. Eur J Heart Fail 2009;11(2):130–9.
12. Oldenburg O, Bitter T, Lehmann R, et al. Adaptive servoventilation improves cardiac function and respiratory stability. Clin Res Cardiol 2011;100(2): 107–15.
13. Borghi-Silva A, Carrascosa C, Oliveira CC, et al. Effects of respiratory muscle unloading on leg muscle oxygenation and blood volume during high-intensity exercise in chronic heart failure. Am J Physiol Heart Circ Physiol 2008;294: H2465–72.
14. Ukkonen H, Burwash IG, Dafoe W, et al. Is ventilatory efficiency (VE/VCO$_2$ slope) associated with right ventricular oxidative metabolism in patients with congestive heart failure? Eur J Heart Fail 2008;10(11):1117–22.
15. Laveneziana P, O'Donnell DE, Ofir D, et al. Effect of biventricular pacing on ventilatory and perceptual responses to exercise in patients with stable chronic heart failure. J Appl Physiol (1985) 2009; 106:1574–83.
16. Dhakal BP, Murphy RM, Lewis GD. Exercise oscillatory ventilation in heart failure. Trends Cardiovasc Med 2012;22:185–91.
17. Meyer FJ, Borst MM, Zugck C, et al. Respiratory muscle dysfunction in congestive heart failure—clinical correlation and prognostic significance. Circulation 2001;103:2153–8.
18. Daganou M, Dimopoulou I, Alivizatos PA, et al. Pulmonary function and respiratory muscle strength in

chronic heart failure: comparison between ischae-mic and idiopathic dilated cardiomyopathy. Heart 1999;81(6):618–20.

19. Lavietes MH, Gerula CM, Fless KG, et al. Inspiratory muscle weakness in diastolic dysfunction. Chest 2004;126(3):838–44.

20. van der Palen J, Rea TD, Manolio TA, et al. Respiratory muscle strength and the risk of incident cardiovascular events. Thorax 2004;59(12):1063–7.

21. Filusch A, Ewert R, Altesellmeier M, et al. Respiratory muscle dysfunction in congestive heart failure – the role of pulmonary hypertension. Int J Cardiol 2011; 150:182–5.

22. Richter MJ, Tiede H, Morty RE, et al. The prognostic significance of inspiratory capacity in pulmonary arterial hypertension. Respiration 2014;88(1): 24–30.

23. Tikunov B, Levine S, Mancini D. Chronic congestive heart failure elicits adaptations of endurance exercise in diaphragmatic muscle. Circulation 1997;95(4):910–6.

24. Ramirez-Sarmiento A, Orozco-Levi M, Guell R, et al. Inspiratory muscle training in patients with chronic obstructive pulmonary disease: structural adaptation and physiologic outcomes. Am J Respir Crit Care Med 2002;166:1491–7.

25. Hart N, Kearney MT, Pride NB, et al. Inspiratory muscle load and capacity in chronic heart failure. Thorax 2004;59(6):477–82.

26. Bernardi L, Spadacini G, Bellwon J, et al. Effect of breathing rate on oxygen saturation and exercise performance in chronic heart failure. Lancet 1998; 351(9112):1308–11.

27. Bernardi L, Porta C, Spicuzza L, et al. Slow breathing increases arterial baroreflex sensitivity in patients with chronic heart failure. Circulation 2002; 105(2):143–5.

28. Parati G, Malfatto G, Boarin S, et al. Device-guided paced breathing in the home setting: effects on exercise capacity, pulmonary and ventricular function in patients with chronic heart failure: a pilot study. Circ Heart Fail 2008;1(3):178–83.

29. Ekman I, Kjellström B, Falk K, et al. Impact of device-guided slow breathing on symptoms of chronic heart failure: a randomized, controlled feasibility study. Eur J Heart Fail 2011;13(9):1000–5.

30. Seals DR, Suwarno NO, Dempsey JA. Influence of lung volume on sympathetic nerve discharge in normal humans. Circ Res 1990;67(1):130–41.

31. Mancini DM, Henson D, LaManca J, et al. Evidence of reduced respiratory muscle endurance in patients with heart failure. J Am Coll Cardiol 1994;24(4):972–81.

32. Suzuki S, Suzuki J, Ishii T, et al. Relationship of respiratory effort sensation to expiratory muscle fatigue during expiratory threshold loading. Am Rev Respir Dis 1992;145:461–6.

33. Suzuki S, Sato M, Okubo T. Expiratory muscle training and sensation of respiratory effort during exercise in normal subjects. Thorax 1995;50(4):366–70.

34. Sugiura H, Sako S, Oshida Y. Effect of expiratory muscle fatigue on the respiratory response during exercise. J Phys Ther Sci 2013;25:1491–5.

35. Derchak PA, Sheel AW, Morgan BJ, et al. Effects of expiratory muscle work on muscle sympathetic nerve activity. J Appl Physiol (1985) 2002;92(4):1539–52.

36. van Dixhoorn J, Duivenvoorden HJ, Staal JA, et al. Cardiac events after myocardial infarction: possible effect of relaxation therapy. Eur Heart J 1987;8(11):1210–4.

37. Mancini DM, Henson D, La Manca J, et al. Benefit of selective respiratory muscle training on exercise capacity in patients with chronic congestive heart failure. Circulation 1995;91:320–9.

38. Cahalin LP, Semigran MJ, Dec GW. Inspiratory muscle training in patients with chronic heart failure awaiting cardiac transplantation: results of a pilot clinical trial. Phys Ther 1997;77:830–6.

39. Johnson PH, Cowley AJ, Kinnear WJM. A randomized controlled trial of inspiratory muscle training in stable chronic heart failure. Eur Heart J 1998;19:1249–54.

40. Darnley GM, Gray AC, McClure SJ, et al. Effects of resistive breathing on exercise capacity and diaphragm function in patients with ischaemic heart disease. Eur J Heart Fail 1999;1(3):297–300.

41. Weiner P, Waizman J, Magadle R, et al. The effect of specific inspiratory muscle training on the sensation of dyspnea and exercise tolerance in patients with congestive heart failure. Clin Cardiol 1999;22:727–34.

42. Martinez A, Lisboa C, Jalil J, et al. Selective training of respiratory muscles in patients with chronic heart failure. Rev Med Chil 2001;129(2):133–8.

43. Cahalin L, Wagenaar R, Dec GW, et al. Endurance training in heart failure—a pilot study of the effects of cycle versus ventilatory muscle training. Circulation 2001;104(17):II-453.

44. Laoutaris I, Dritsas A, Brown MD, et al. Inspiratory muscle training using an incremental endurance test alleviates dyspnea and improves functional status in patients with chronic heart failure. Eur J Cardiovasc Prev Rehabil 2004;11(6):489–96.

45. Hulzebos EH, Helders PJM, Favie NJ, et al. Preoperative intensive inspiratory muscle training to prevent postoperative pulmonary complications in high-risk patients undergoing CABG surgery. JAMA 2006;296:1851–7.

46. Dall'Ago P, Chiappa GR, Guths H, et al. Inspiratory muscle training in patients with heart failure and inspiratory muscle weakness: a randomized trial. J Am Coll Cardiol 2006;47(4):757–63.

47. Laoutaris ID, Dritsas A, Brown MD, et al. Immune response to inspiratory muscle training in patients

with chronic heart failure. Eur J Cardiovasc Prev Rehabil 2007;14(5):679–85.

48. Laoutaris ID, Dritsas A, Brown MD, et al. Effects of inspiratory muscle training on autonomic activity, endothelial vasodilator function, and N-terminal pro-brain · natriuretic peptide levels in chronic heart failure. J Cardiopulm Rehabil Prev 2008; 28(2):99–106.

49. Chiappa GR, Roseguini BT, Vieira PJ, et al. Inspiratory muscle training improves blood flow to resting and exercising limbs in patients with chronic heart failure. J Am Coll Cardiol 2008;51(17):1663–71.

50. Padula CA, Yeaw E, Mistry S. A home-based nurse-coached inspiratory muscle training intervention in heart failure. Appl Nurs Res 2009;22(1):18–25.

51. Kulur AB, Haleagrahara N, Adhikary P, et al. Effect of diaphragmatic breathing on heart rate variability in ischemic heart disease with diabetes. Arq Bras Cardiol 2009;92(6):423–9.

52. Stein R, Chiappa GR, Güths H, et al. Inspiratory muscle training improves oxygen uptake efficiency slope in patients with chronic heart failure. J Cardiopulm Rehabil Prev 2009;29(6):392–5.

53. Winklemann ER, Chiappa GR, Lima CO, et al. Addition of inspiratory muscle training to aerobic training improves cardiorespiratory responses to exercise in patients with heart failure and inspiratory muscle weakness. Am Heart J 2009;158(5): 768–75.

54. Bosnak-Guclu M, Arikan H, Savci S, et al. Effects of inspiratory muscle training in patients with heart failure. Respir Med 2011;105(11):1671–81.

55. Mello PR, Guerra GM, Borile S, et al. Inspiratory muscle training reduces sympathetic nervous activity and improves inspiratory muscle weakness and quality of life in patients with chronic heart failure. J Cardiopulm Rehabil Prev 2012;32:255–61.

56. Laoutaris ID, Adamopoulos S, Manginas A, et al. Benefits of combined aerobic/resistance/inspiratory training in patients with chronic heart failure. A complete exercise model? A prospective randomized study. Int J Cardiol 2013;167(5):1967–72.

57. Palau P, Domínguez E, Núñez E, et al. Effects of inspiratory muscle training in patients with heart failure with preserved ejection fraction. Eur J Prev Cardiol 2013. [Epub ahead of print].

58. Marco E, Ramírez-Sarmiento AL, Coloma A, et al. High-intensity vs. sham inspiratory muscle training in patients with chronic heart failure: a prospective randomized trial. Eur J Heart Fail 2013; 15(8):892–901.

59. Adamopoulos S, Schmid JP, Dendale P, et al. Combined aerobic/inspiratory muscle training vs. aerobic training in patients with chronic heart failure: the Vent-HeFT trial: a European prospective multi-centre randomized trial. Eur J Heart Fail 2014; 16(5):574–82.

60. Mereles D, Ehlken N, Kreuscher S, et al. Exercise and respiratory training improve exercise capacity and quality of life in patients with severe chronic pulmonary hypertension. Circulation 2006;114: 1482–9.

61. Grunig E, Ehlken N, Ghofrani A, et al. Effect of exercise and respiratory training on clinical progression and survival in patients with severe chronic pulmonary hypertension. Respiration 2011;81: 394–401.

62. Kabitz HJ, Bremer HC, Schwoerer A, et al. The combination of exercise and respiratory training improves respiratory muscle function in pulmonary hypertension. Lung 2014;192:321–8.

63. Plentz RD, Sbruzzi G, Ribeiro RA, et al. Inspiratory muscle training in patients with heart failure: meta-analysis of randomized trials. Arq Bras Cardiol 2012;99(2):762–71.

64. Sbruzzi G, Dal Lago P, Ribeiro RA, et al. Inspiratory muscle training and quality of life in patients with heart failure: systematic review of randomized trials. Int J Cardiol 2012;156(1):120–1.

65. Lin SJ, McElfresh J, Hall B, et al. Inspiratory muscle training in patients with heart failure: a systematic review. Cardiopulm Phys Ther J 2012; 23(3):29–36.

66. Smart NA, Giallauria F, Dieberg G. Efficacy of inspiratory muscle training in chronic heart failure patients: a systematic review and meta-analysis. Int J Cardiol 2013;167(4):1502–7.

67. Montemezzo D, Fregonezi GA, Pereira DA, et al. Influence of inspiratory muscle weakness on inspiratory muscle training responses in chronic heart failure patients: a systematic review and meta-analysis. Arch Phys Med Rehabil 2014; 95(7):1398–407.

68. Hewitt J. The yoga of breathing posture and meditation. London: Random House; 1983. p. 89–91.

69. Stanescu DC, Nemery B, Veritier C, et al. Pattern of breathing and ventilatory response to CO_2 in subjects practising hata-yoga. J Appl Physiol (1985) 1981;51:1625–9.

70. Cross TJ, Sabapathy S, Beck KC, et al. The resistive and elastic work of breathing during exercise in patients with chronic heart failure. Eur Respir J 2012;39(6):1449–57.

71. Bertini P, Ferro B, Baldassarri R, et al. Beta-adrenergic antagonists improve oxygen saturation in acute pulmonary edema: a case series in the prehospital setting. Prehosp Emerg Care 2013; 17(3):421–3.

72. Azarbar S, Dupuis J. Lung capillary injury and repair in left heart disease: a new target for therapy? Clin Sci (Lond) 2014;127(2):65–76.

73. Cahalin LP, Forman DE, Manning K, et al. Inspiratory muscle testing and training in a patient with heart failure preserved ejection fraction and acute

cardiovascular decompensation. Am J Respir Crit Care Med 2014;189:A6453.

74. Available at: http://www.cms.gov/Medicare/Medicare-Fee-for-Service-Payment/AcuteInpatient PPS/Readmissions-Reduction-Program.html. Accessed October 2, 2014.

75. Goso Y, Asanoi H, Ishise H, et al. Respiratory modulation of muscle sympathetic nerve activity in patients with chronic heart failure. Circulation 2001;104(4): 418–23.

76. Harada D, Asanoi H, Takagawa J, et al. Slow and deep respiration suppresses steady-state sympathetic nerve activity in patients with chronic heart failure: from modeling to clinical application. Am J Physiol Heart Circ Physiol 2014. pii:ajpheart.00109.2014.

77. Black LF, Hyatt RE. Maximal respiratory pressures: normal values and relationship to age and sex. Am Rev Respir Dis 1969;99:696–702.

78. American College of Sports Medicine guidelines for exercise testing and prescription. 9th edition. Philadelphia: Lippincott Williams & Wilkins; 2014.

79. Bellemare F, Grassino A. Effect of pressure and timing of contraction on human diaphragm fatigue. J Appl Physiol (1985) 1982;53:1190–5.

80. Tomori Z, Donic V, Benacka R, et al. Resuscitation and auto resuscitation by airway reflexes in animals. Cough 2013;9(21):1–12.

Technology to Promote and Increase Physical Activity in Heart Failure

Nina C. Franklin, PhD, MS, LMT

KEYWORDS

- Heart failure • Self-management • Physical activity • Exercise adherence • Internet technology
- Social media • Telemedicine • Exercise promotion

KEY POINTS

- Heart failure is an important cause of cardiovascular disease–related morbidity and mortality and is closely linked to physical inactivity, obesity, and other unhealthy lifestyle behaviors.
- Habitual physical activity is firmly recommended for heart failure self-management but current levels among patients remain low, independent of age, ethnicity and race, gender, and socioeconomic status.
- Technology-based interventions are accessible, affordable, and have been proved effective in increasing physical activity levels but specific benefits among individuals with heart failure are undetermined.
- Health education, improved health literacy, and social support networks are associated with higher levels of self-efficacy, treatment adherence, and self-care engagement in heart failure patients.
- Technology-driven physical activity promotion tactics may foster greater patient engagement, adherence, and self-efficacy by enhancing health education, improving health literacy, and building social support systems.

INTRODUCTION

Cardiovascular disease (CVD) is the leading cause of death in the United States and abroad with severe heart-related morbidities affecting men and women across all ages and ethnic and racial groups.[1] Among the different CVDs, heart failure (HF) is a primary health concern, with a current US incidence, prevalence, and total cost of more than $800,000, $5 million, and $30 billion, respectively.[2] The development of HF is closely linked to common comorbidities of CVD, such as hyperlipidemia, hypertension, and diabetes.[3] In addition, controllable factors (ie, obesity and unhealthy lifestyle behaviors) also contribute greatly to HF risk, among which includes a sedentary lifestyle characterized by physical inactivity.[2,3] Among some populations, physical inactivity may increase the risk of HF by more than 50%.[4]

Habitual physical activity in the forms of structured exercise training and spontaneous physical activity (ie, walking, stair climbing, and performing household chores) is commonly recommended for the management of HF.[5,6] However, patients are less likely to engage in such activities often because of dyspnea, function-limiting comorbidities, and/or an utter lack of motivation.[7,8] Social networks and social support can enhance intrinsic and extrinsic motivation,[9] thereby fostering greater treatment adherence and self-care activities among HF patients, which influence disease

Disclosure Statement: The author declares that there are no conflicts of interest, financial or otherwise.
Integrative Physiology Laboratory, Department of Physical Therapy, College of Applied Health Sciences, University of Illinois at Chicago, 1919 West Taylor Street, M/C 898, Chicago, IL 60612, USA
E-mail address: njohns6@uic.edu

Heart Failure Clin 11 (2015) 173–182
http://dx.doi.org/10.1016/j.hfc.2014.08.006
1551-7136/15/$ – see front matter © 2015 Elsevier Inc. All rights reserved.

outcomes.[10,11] Furthermore, the widespread use of information and communication technology tools and resources (ie, computer networks, mobile applications, and wearable activity trackers) offers a potentially beneficial avenue for increasing physical activity levels and positive self-management behaviors primarily through improvements in intrinsic motivation.[12–14] In light of these facts, an effective strategy for encouraging exercise and other forms of physical activity in HF patients is one that capitalizes on the integral role of social support systems and the potential role of information and communication technology in facilitating self-management of HF.

Recent advances in social media and other Internet- and mobile-based information and communication technologies offer a unique approach to health promotion, disease prevention, and disease management. According to a recent report published by the Pew Research Center's Internet and American Life Project, nearly 90% of Americans use the Internet by way of a computer and/or mobile technology.[15] Among Internet users, social networking and health-specific Web sites are the most popular, used by approximately 70% of men and women including whites, African Americans, and Hispanics.[16,17] Moreover, the Deloitte 2010 Survey of Healthcare Consumers reports that people with chronic conditions are among the most likely to participate in online wellness programs and other World Wide Web–based interventions.[18] In addition, many interventions incorporate the use of wearable devices, such as pedometers, accelerometers, and heart rate monitors, allowing individuals to track their progress, set goals, and even share their activities and successes with people within their social networks,[17,19] which can further boost motivation and improve adherence.[20,21]

Given that approximately half of people with HF are expected to die within 5 years of being diagnosed,[2] innovative approaches to promoting exercise and physical activity in this population is of major clinical importance. Although engaging in such behaviors does not necessarily reverse HF, such practices can significantly improve the overall quality of life of patients by supporting healthy weight management, attenuating associated breathlessness, and improving other signs and general manifestations of the disease.[7,22,23] This article presents the ways in which technological advances in Internet- and mobile-based communication, social media, and self-monitoring devices can serve as a means to broadly promote increasing levels of physical activity to improve health outcomes in the HF population.

EXERCISE INTOLERANCE AND NONCOMPLIANCE IN HEART FAILURE

Regular physical activity in the form of exercise training is firmly recommended as a lifestyle measure for HF.[7,23] Unfortunately, although studies show that nearly 80% of people with HF admit to understanding the importance of exercise, only a mere 39% have actually adhered to a structured training regimen.[24] Exercise generally involves the performance of dynamic contractions of large muscle groups, which is usually not well tolerated by HF patients because of breathlessness, weakness, and extreme fatigue.[7,8]

Although such exercise intolerance is a classic symptom of HF, those patients who initiate and consistently adhere to an exercise training regimen are known to reap substantially beneficial results. The benefits of exercise training in HF include improved myocardial function, functional capacity, and peak oxygen consumption (Vo_2); reduced hospitalization rates; and ultimately increased probability of survival.[7,8,25] In light of such benefits, noncompliance of HF patients to exercise presents a major barrier to sound treatment.

Ineffective exercise promotion tactics may greatly contribute to a lack of compliance among HF patients. According to the World Health Organization, patient adherence in general is a multifactorial issue largely influenced by the health care team, specific disease characteristics, and patient-related factors including one's economical and environmental circumstances.[26] Adherence also largely depends on social influence; numerous studies show that social support is by far one of the most important factors affecting health behaviors and outcomes within the context of chronic conditions.[8,26,27] Given the critical role of social influences in health behaviors in the presence of disease, strategies that foster opportunities for social networking and participation may serve as a means to educate, empower, and motivate individuals to engage in healthier lifestyle choices.

Internet-based communication, coined under Web 2.0, has been shown to significantly enable unique social interactions among individuals with various chronic conditions, their supporters (ie, friends and family), and health care providers.[28,29] In addition, increasingly sophisticated mobile technologies have taken social computing beyond Web 2.0, as the widespread adoption and use of smartphones, tablet computers, and applications have introduced new and innovative ways to improve health and health care delivery.[30,31] Within the context of HF, such technologies provide a readily accessible, cost-effective, and easy-to-use medium that enables efficient delivery of time-unlimited support to patients. Such interactions by way of the World Wide Web may greatly promote exercise compliance and adherence to recommended self-care thereby supporting positive health outcomes among patients. Indeed, research pertaining to Internet- and mobile-based interventions for weight management and physical activity were among the first to identify positive results.[32–34]

EMBRACING TECHNOLOGY TO EDUCATE AND EMPOWER PATIENTS

Internet- and mobile-based information and communication technology tools and resources are becoming increasingly important methods for disseminating educational health information, which can improve health literacy in HF patients.[17,35] In the presence of disease, patient education is generally associated with increased treatment adherence, improved clinical outcomes, health care cost savings, and an overall enhanced quality of life.[35–37] A primary strategy of using technology to promote and increase physical activity in HF involves empowering patients through World Wide Web–based education and learning. Numerous studies show that patients feel empowered to make proactive decisions about their health and self-care regimens through World Wide Web–based education.[38–40] With added knowledge, patients also tend to exhibit higher levels of confidence in asking questions of health care providers to obtain more information when it comes to managing their conditions.[40,41]

Internet-based content should be innovatively customized, tailored, and presented in ways that meet the needs and preferences of HF patients.[42–44] Adapting and repurposing research-backed content through cross-platform communication strategies is critical and such content can be expanded by way of multiple channels.[28,45] Initiatives can specifically address the unique physical health needs of patients through expert articles and blogs, electronic books, simplified how-to videos, game-based learning, podcasts, and clinician-supervised patient forums. Such endeavors can continually make patients aware of the importance of implementing exercise and other forms of physical activity into their lifestyles for disease management and sustained good health.

To enhance self-efficacy among patients, while also optimizing health outcomes, World Wide Web–based educational information should address practical strategies for effective goal setting with realistic and feasible exercise regimens that are flexible and not overly complicated. This is especially important because HF patients generally find it difficult to include structured exercise in their everyday lifestyles.[8] Patients need to understand that even small amounts of exercise and physical activity can improve their condition and overall quality of life. Those who continually engage in activities viewed as useful or fun (ie, leisure walking, gardening, dancing, recreational sports, and mind-body exercise) tend to experience better outcomes.[8,46]

PROMOTING EXERCISE AND ADHERENCE THROUGH TECHNOLOGY

World Wide Web–based technologies can be used for exercise promotion in the HF population through the delivery of exercise prescription-related resources, physical activity monitoring devices (ie, pedometers, accelerometers, and heart rate and blood pressure monitoring), and virtual expert advice and coaching. These technologies are especially important for patients who otherwise would not have access to such services because of limited economic resources and geographic location. World Wide Web–based information and communication technology is highly contingent on patient resources, access, and general familiarity with the Internet.[47,48] However, recent advances in mobile technology offer an easily achievable solution for transcending this so-called "digital divide." Indeed, mobile use and smartphone penetration have increased exponentially in recent years, largely because of adoption among populations with lower incomes.[28,47]

By leveraging information and communication technology by way of Internet- and mobile-based tools and resources, HF patients can continually be encouraged and empowered to make exercise a top priority for disease management. Furthermore, incorporating persuasive elements, such as goal setting, physical activity tracking and monitoring, mobile notifications and alerts, and progress visualization, may produce promising results in the way of behavioral change and continued adherence among people with HF.[49–51]

The data collected via these tools also supports the health care team in routine patient management, because they are able to collect and share meaningful physiologic information from patients while maintaining essential patient-provider relationships, especially in cases when individuals are not in close proximity to their provider.[52–54] Results from numerous studies incorporating Internet- and mobile-based interactive communications in health care (telemedicine), such as the

Mobile Telemonitoring in Heart Failure Patients Study and Telemedical Interventional Monitoring in Heart Failure, indicate that home-based monitoring of vital signs and related-parameters (ie, heart rate, blood pressure, and body weight) substantially improves health outcomes in HF patients while also reducing the frequency and duration of related hospitalizations.[52,54] Incorporating such technologies to help facilitate physical activity monitoring and patient self-management by way of pedometers, accelerometers, and similar tracking devices would likely improve exercise compliance among this population. This holds true even among underserved and socially disadvantaged groups with limited access to information and communication technologies.[55–57]

USING TECHNOLOGY AS A MEANS OF SOCIAL SUPPORT AND ENGAGEMENT

Adequate social support is critical for promoting positive self-care behaviors among individuals with CVD including HF.[10,11,58] Social support essentially involves active communicative exchanges (verbal and nonverbal) between patients and their providers, family, and friends, which can greatly improve patient engagement in healthier behaviors, increase levels of coping self-efficacy, and foster effective disease-management.[11,26] Smaller social networks and a general lack of social support have been associated with increased CVD risk factors and higher incidences of myocardial infarction, stroke, and other related mortalities.[59,60] This is particularly evident among low-income and socially disadvantaged populations.[26,61] Internet- and mobile-based technologies are simple and highly effective means of enhancing active communications and interactions between patients and their social networks, especially among the economically disadvantaged.

The latest research trends suggest that health-related use of the World Wide Web and social media is much higher among socially disadvantaged populations when compared with more affluent groups, which makes this approach especially advantageous.[15,28] Social media encompasses various forms of technology including online forums, blogs (ie, WordPress and Tumblr), micro-blogs (ie, Facebook, Google+, Twitter, Instagram, and Pinterest), video blogs (ie, YouTube and Vine), and podcasting. Engaging in Internet- and mobile-based communication provides a means by which patients can encourage and motivate each other through shared experiences, and increased use of social media allows patients to connect with other patients. Such communication

technologies can also help foster stronger social collaborations between patients, their families, and their friends.

The effectiveness of communication technologies has been well studied in populations with diabetes and cancer.[62–64] Among individuals with diabetes, research shows that family members and friends tend to use social media as a means of sharing personal clinical information, requesting disease-specific guidance and feedback, and receiving emotional support. Such medium also provide a forum for reporting personal experiences, asking questions, and receiving direct feedback for people living with diabetes, all of which are effective strategies for enhancing patient engagement.[62,63] In relation to cancer, video-sharing Web sites, such as YouTube, have enabled innovative and effective exchanges of personal stories and testimonials (ie, sharing of cancer experiences between current patients and survivors, caregivers, and activists).[64]

Because most HF patients generally depend on the support of spouses and other family members, friends, and fellow patients,[65] technology-driven support may encourage increased compliance with physical activity behaviors for effective self-care. Specifically, communication technologies and social media create a means by which patients' social networks can fully support their efforts to exercise more. Effective strategies that can enhance patient accountability, commitment, engagement, and extrinsic and intrinsic motivation include establishment of an electronic exercise contract or agreement; an exercise buddy program between patients; and/or walking groups among family, friends, and neighbors with virtual sharing (ie, images and videos) of activity data (ie, pedometer steps and calorie-expenditure tracking) and health-related progress monitoring.[51,63]

Interestingly, videogame technology (ie, Nintendo Wii and Xbox active games) requiring motor activity (ie, exergames) within a social context has been shown to effectively promote healthy weight management and physical activity among the youth, older adults, and individuals with chronic disease.[47,66,67] In relation to CVD, telemedicine systems incorporating videogame-based technologies have also been proved successful in optimizing the health care of patients with HF.[68] Such systems may also serve as effective medium for enhancing social support and patient engagement in physical activity. Although structured exercise tends to be monotonous and, in some ways, unachievable for patients, exergames offer a range of familiar and fun fitness activities and sports (ie, tennis, bowling, and boxing) that can easily be varied and tailored to meet the individual needs and preferences of patients.

COST AND COMPARATIVE EFFECTIVENESS OF TECHNOLOGY IN HEART FAILURE

CVD in general is one of the most expensive chronic conditions to treat, accounting for total health care costs of more than $440 billion each year in the United States alone.[69] Using Internet- and mobile-based tools and resources to promote and increase physical activity and other self-care behaviors can significantly offset the burgeoning health care costs associated with HF, although specific evidence related to definite costs is needed. A large proportion of CVD-related costs can be attributed to the treatment of HF with estimated direct and indirect costs of $31 billion in 2012.[70] With forecasts of a steady rise in the incidence and prevalence of CVD over the next 10 to 20 years, the annual costs of HF are projected to experience a two-fold increase to $70 billion by 2030.[70] Unfortunately, posthospitalization transitions to patient self-care activities continue to constitute a sizable majority of annual costs associated with HF.[70,71] Nearly 25% of hospitalized patients are readmitted within 30 days of discharge and this number increases to 50% by 6 months.[71]

Rehospitalizations are largely caused by potentially preventable adverse outcomes often resulting from poor adherence to recommended treatment regimens (ie, improper medication usage, inadequate dietary practices, and noncompliance to physical activity or exercise recommendations).[71] Given that physical activity itself is a chief component of a comprehensive approach aimed at treating and managing HF,[7,8] information and communication technology offers an integrated and innovative approach to patient self-management by way of exercise. Harnessing such technology is also highly cost-effective for physicians, hospitals, health systems, allied health providers, and patients.[47,52,54]

Incorporating information and communication technologies into routine health care by way of telemedicine has continuously been shown to reduce avoidable hospitalizations, thereby generating substantial cost savings among individuals with HF in addition to other forms of CVD and related morbidities (hypertension and diabetes).[54,72] In fact, home-based telemonitoring and telemanagement programs for HF patients have been shown to result in substantially lowered health care costs with reductions in hospital readmissions of up to 36%.[16,73] Although data specifically pertaining to Internet- and mobile-based interventions for physical activity are limited, these technologies show great promise in helping patients maintain or increase their daily levels of exercise during and after cardiac rehabilitation in home- and community-based settings.[47,74,75] When coupled with routine, periodic health care, these interventions may ultimately lead to reduced hospitalizations, lower health care costs, and reduced out-of-pocket expenses for patients (ie, copays, travel to and from treatment, lost wages).

MAXIMIZING TECHNOLOGY ADOPTION AMONG HEART FAILURE PATIENTS

Based on the evidence presented so far, interventions incorporating information and communication technology clearly have the potential to significantly improve patient health outcomes, access to quality health care, and continuity in and among health services while also containing health care expenditures. Internet- and mobile-based technologies are uniquely beneficial in that these capabilities greatly enable self-management behaviors among patients by providing a means for rapid dissemination and sharing of health information; broader health outreach; tailored, targeted, and personalized health messaging; and patient interaction and engagement. Despite the many potential benefits, it is still unclear as to which types of technology patients prefer and whether or not they are viewed as useful, useable, and acceptable for their specific needs.[76,77]

The impact of information and communication technology-based interventions is highly contingent on patients' general understanding of the tools and resources provided by physicians and allied health providers and their decision to actually adopt and use them.[78,79] A lack of such information may present a challenge among certain patient populations including novice and nontechnology users; older adults; individuals with low income, education, or health literacy; and non-English speaking groups.

Fortunately, studies show that many individuals in these populations do have access to mobile devices, which enables adoption of numerous telemedicine-based interventions.[47,52,75] Moreover, with smartphone penetration continuing to increase on a global scale,[28,47] World Wide Web–based technological interventions will likely become a chief target for delivering health care in a user-friendly format to improve outreach and access to health care regardless of a patient's age, socioeconomic status, race and ethnicity, or geographic location.

There is limited evidence on effective technology interventions that specifically promote and increase physical activity among individuals with HF and other chronic diseases. However, a wide range of evidence suggests that World Wide Web–based information and interventions are adoptable and effective among individuals focused on losing weight and improving their health status.[28,47,80] Still, as with most interventions, engagement and retention are major barriers associated with World Wide Web–based tools and resources primarily because preferences and use tend to differ by age, gender, race and ethnicity, socioeconomic status, and education levels.[15,28,47]

To reduce such barriers, which may limit successful delivery of health care and health-promotion tactics by way of information and communication technologies, some investigators encourage the use of established analytical frameworks for evaluating World Wide Web–based interventions.[81–83] One framework that has gained widespread popularity for specifically addressing the strengths and weaknesses of chronic disease interventions is a multilevel model classified as RE-AIM.[81] This framework is based on a central premise that the "ultimate

impact of an intervention is due to its combined effects on 5 evaluative dimensions": (1) reach, (2) efficacy, (3) adoption, (4) implementation, and (5) maintenance.[84]

In accordance with its premise, the RE-AIM framework has been used to evaluate a range of interventions (ie, individual and group counseling, interactive computer-based, mail- and telephone-based) based on the following: (1) their ability to "reach" the target population; (2) their "efficacy" and effectiveness; (3) the extent to which they are pervasively "adopted" by target settings, institutions, and staff; (4) their successful "implementation" primarily in terms of deliverability and overall practicality in real-world settings; and (5) their maintainability and sustainability among individuals and in settings over time.[81]

Although evaluative methods of World Wide Web–based health promotion are undoubtedly in infancy stages and warrant extensive investigation, based on key tenets, the RE-AIM framework does offer a promising tool for maximizing technology adoption among HF patients for self-management of their condition. This holds true

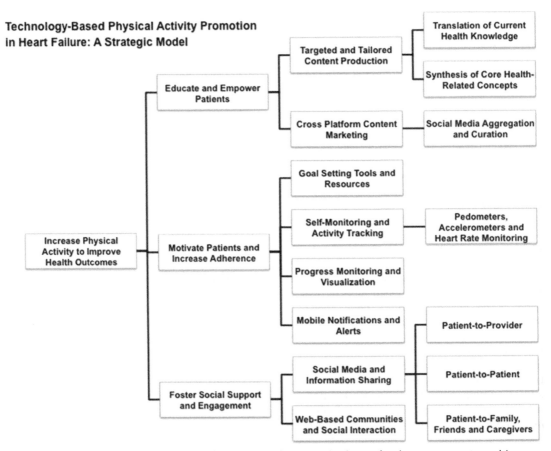

Fig. 1. A strategic model for harnessing information and communication technology to promote and increase physical activity in the HF population.

especially for World Wide Web–based interventions aimed to promote increased physical activity behaviors in this population, because their lack of follow through and adherence to treatment recommendations are major hurdles to improved health outcomes.[7,8] Internet- and mobile-based interventions that fail to effectively reach the diversity of HF patients are unlikely to be adopted, implemented, and maintained in real-world settings.[42,83] In light of these facts, incorporating analytical models like RE-AIM into the design and evaluation of World Wide Web–based interventions is a critical step for the overall success of technological approaches to HF management.

SUMMARY

Physical activity, weight control, and other self-management strategies are critical components of HF treatment. A sedentary lifestyle greatly contributes to obesity, worsens signs and symptoms, and increases the likelihood of CVD-related mortality yet most HF patients do not adhere to the recommended amounts of daily physical activity.[7,8] Given the extent of noncompliance to physical activity and exercise among patients and the multiplicity of factors that can influence engagement and, ultimately, health outcomes (ie, age, gender, race and ethnicity, disease comorbidities, socioeconomic status, and geographic location) more needs to be done to promote varying levels and types of exercise that are accessible, approachable, and affordable.

The continued growth and expansion of social networking sites and other adaptations of Internet- and mobile-based technologies offer great promise in beneficially impacting the delivery of specific interventions geared toward promoting and sustaining physical activity and exercise participation in the HF population. Additionally, incorporating the use of self-monitoring devices may further enhance the general impact of information and communication technology-related interventions. A strategic model for collectively implementing various technological approaches to promote and increase physical activity among individuals with HF is summarized in **Fig. 1**. Although the potential advantages are apparent in relation to improving health-related outcomes, these novel approaches definitely warrant further investigation to evaluate their overall efficacy, cost-effectiveness, and long-term maintainability.

REFERENCES

1. Pagidipati NJ, Gaziano TA. Estimating deaths from cardiovascular disease: a review of global methodologies of mortality measurement. Circulation 2013;127(6):749–56.
2. Go AS, Mozaffarian D, Roger VL, et al. Heart disease and stroke statistics–2014 update: a report from the American Heart Association. Circulation 2014;129(3):e28–292.
3. Grundy SM, Cleeman JI, Daniels SR, et al. Diagnosis and management of the metabolic syndrome: an American Heart Association/National Heart, Lung, and Blood Institute Scientific Statement. Circulation 2005;112(17):2735–52.
4. Young DR, Reynolds K, Sidell M, et al. Effects of physical activity and sedentary time on the risk of heart failure. Circ Heart Fail 2014;7(1):21–7.
5. Dontje ML, van der Wal MH, Stolk RP, et al. Daily physical activity in stable heart failure patients. J Cardiovasc Nurs 2014;29(3):218–26.
6. Tung HH, Jan MS, Lin CY, et al. Mediating role of daily physical activity on quality of life in patients with heart failure. J Cardiovasc Nurs 2012;27(1):16–23.
7. Pina IL, Apstein CS, Balady GJ, et al. Exercise and heart failure: a statement from the American Heart Association Committee on exercise, rehabilitation, and prevention. Circulation 2003;107(8):1210–25.
8. Conraads VM, Deaton C, Piotrowicz E, et al. Adherence of heart failure patients to exercise: barriers and possible solutions: a position statement of the study group on exercise training in Heart Failure of the Heart Failure Association of the European Society of Cardiology. Eur Heart J 2012;14(5):451–8.
9. King AC, Friedman R, Marcus B, et al. Harnessing motivational forces in the promotion of physical activity: the community health advice by telephone (CHAT) project. Health Educ Res 2002; 17(5):627–36.
10. Gallagher R, Luttik ML, Jaarsma T. Social support and self-care in heart failure. J Cardiovasc Nurs 2011;26(6):439–45.
11. Graven LJ, Grant JS. Social support and self-care behaviors in individuals with heart failure: an integrative review. Int J Nurs Stud 2014;51(2):320–33.
12. Jarvis-Selinger S, Bates J, Araki Y, et al. Internet-based support for cardiovascular disease management. Int J Telemed Appl 2011;2011:342582.
13. Stellefson M, Chaney B, Barry AE, et al. Web 2.0 chronic disease self-management for older adults: a systematic review. J Med Internet Res 2013; 15(2):e35.
14. Aneni EC, Roberson LL, Maziak W, et al. A systematic review of internet-based worksite wellness approaches for cardiovascular disease risk management: outcomes, challenges & opportunities. PLoS One 2014;9(1):e83594.
15. Fox S, Rainie L. The web at 25 in the U.S. Pew Research Center's Internet and American Life Project Website, 2014. Available at: http://www.

pewinternet.org/2014/02/27/the-web-at-25-in-the-u-s/Published. Accessed June 18, 2014.

16. Social Networking Fact Sheet. Pew Research Center's Internet and American Life Project Website. 2013. Available at: http://www.pewinternet.org/fact-sheets/social-networking-fact-sheet/Published. Accessed June 18, 2014.

17. Health Fact Sheet. Pew Research Center's Internet and American Life Project Website. 2013. Available at: http://www.pewinternet.org/fact-sheets/health-fact-sheet/Published. Accessed June 7, 2014.

18. Deloitte Survey. 2010 Survey of Health Care Consumers: Key Findings, Strategic Implications. Deloitte Website. 2010. Available at: http://www.deloitte.com/assets/Dcom-UnitedStates/Local%20Assets/Documents/US_CHS_2010SurveyofHealthCareConsumers_050610.pdf. Accessed June 8, 2014.

19. Lee JM, Kim Y, Welk GJ. Validity of consumer-based physical activity monitors. Med Sci Sports Exerc 2014;46(9):1840–8.

20. Snyder A, Colvin B, Gammack JK. Pedometer use increases daily steps and functional status in older adults. J Am Med Dir Assoc 2011;12(8):590–4.

21. Wijsman CA, Westendorp RG, Verhagen EA, et al. Effects of a web-based intervention on physical activity and metabolism in older adults: randomized controlled trial. J Med Internet Res 2013;15(11):e233.

22. Bartlo P. Evidence-based application of aerobic and resistance training in patients with congestive heart failure. J Cardiopulm Rehabil Prev 2007;27(6):368–75.

23. Piepoli MF, Conraads V, Corra U, et al. Exercise training in heart failure: from theory to practice. A consensus document of the Heart Failure Association and the European Association for Cardiovascular Prevention and Rehabilitation. Eur J Heart Fail 2011;13(4):347–57.

24. van der Wal MH, Jaarsma T, Moser DK, et al. Compliance in heart failure patients: the importance of knowledge and beliefs. Eur Heart J 2006;27(4):434–40.

25. Ismail H, McFarlane JR, Nojoumian AH, et al. Clinical outcomes and cardiovascular responses to different exercise training intensities in patients with heart failure: a systematic review and meta-analysis. JACC Heart Fail 2013;1(6):514–22.

26. Adherence to long-term therapies: evidence for action. World Health Organization Website. 2003. Available at: http://www.who.int/chp/knowledge/publications/adherence_introduction.pdf. Accessed June 8, 2014.

27. Maeda U, Shen BJ, Schwarz ER, et al. Self-efficacy mediates the associations of social support and depression with treatment adherence in heart failure patients. Int J Behav Med 2013;20(1):88–96.

28. Korda H, Itani Z. Harnessing social media for health promotion and behavior change. Health Promot Pract 2013;14(1):15–23.

29. Kolt GS, Rosenkranz RR, Savage TN, et al. WALK 2.0-using web 2.0 applications to promote health-related physical activity: a randomised controlled trial protocol. BMC Public Health 2013;13:436.

30. Cho MJ, Sim JL, Hwang SY. Development of smartphone educational application for patients with coronary artery disease. Healthc Inform Res 2014;20(2):117–24.

31. Yehle KS, Chen AM, Plake KS, et al. A qualitative analysis of coronary heart disease patient views of dietary adherence and web-based and mobile-based nutrition tools. J Cardiopulm Rehabil Prev 2012;32(4):203–9.

32. Khaylis A, Yiaslas T, Bergstrom J, et al. A review of efficacious technology-based weight-loss interventions: five key components. Telemed J E Health 2010;16(9):931–8.

33. Napolitano MA, Fotheringham M, Tate D, et al. Evaluation of an internet-based physical activity intervention: a preliminary investigation. Ann Behav Med 2003;25(2):92–9.

34. Hansen AW, Gronbaek M, Helge JW, et al. Effect of a web-based intervention to promote physical activity and improve health among physically inactive adults: a population-based randomized controlled trial. J Med Internet Res 2012;14(5):e145.

35. Evangelista LS, Rasmusson KD, Laramee AS, et al. Health literacy and the patient with heart failure–implications for patient care and research: a consensus statement of the Heart Failure Society of America. J Card Fail 2010;16(1):9–16.

36. Safeer RS, Cooke CE, Keenan J. The impact of health literacy on cardiovascular disease. Vasc Health Risk Manag 2006;2(4):457–64.

37. Parker RM, Ratzan SC, Lurie N. Health literacy: a policy challenge for advancing high-quality health care. Health Aff (Millwood) 2003;22(4):147–53.

38. Kuijpers W, Groen WG, Aaronson NK, et al. A systematic review of web-based interventions for patient empowerment and physical activity in chronic diseases: relevance for cancer survivors. J Med Internet Res 2013;15(2):e37.

39. Samoocha D, Bruinvels DJ, Elbers NA, et al. Effectiveness of web-based interventions on patient empowerment: a systematic review and meta-analysis. J Med Internet Res 2010;12(2):e23.

40. Steinwachs DM, Roter DL, Skinner EA, et al. A web-based program to empower patients who have schizophrenia to discuss quality of care with mental health providers. Psychiatr Serv 2011;62(11):1296–302.

41. Fleisher L, Bass S, Ruzek SB, et al. Relationships among internet health information use, patient behavior and self efficacy in newly diagnosed

cancer patients who contact the National Cancer Institute's NCI Atlantic Region Cancer Information Service (CIS). Proc AMIA Symp 2002;260–4.

42. Spittaels H, De Bourdeaudhuij I, Brug J, et al. Effectiveness of an online computer-tailored physical activity intervention in a real-life setting. Health Educ Res 2007;22(3):385–96.

43. Krebs P, Prochaska JO, Rossi JS. A meta-analysis of computer-tailored interventions for health behavior change. Prev Med 2010;51(3–4):214–21.

44. de Vries H, Brug J. Computer-tailored interventions motivating people to adopt health promoting behaviours: introduction to a new approach. Patient Educ Couns 1999;36(2):99–105.

45. Neiger BL, Thackeray R, Van Wagenen SA, et al. Use of social media in health promotion: purposes, key performance indicators, and evaluation metrics. Health Promot Pract 2012;13(2):159–64.

46. Yeh GY, McCarthy EP, Wayne PM, et al. Tai chi exercise in patients with chronic heart failure: a randomized clinical trial. Arch Intern Med 2011; 171(8):750–7.

47. Pratt M, Sarmiento OL, Montes F, et al. The implications of megatrends in information and communication technology and transportation for changes in global physical activity. Lancet 2012;380(9838): 282–93.

48. Kerr C, Murray E, Noble L, et al. The potential of web-based interventions for heart disease self-management: a mixed methods investigation. J Med Internet Res 2010;12(4):e56.

49. Wells S, Whittaker R, Dorey E, et al. Harnessing health IT for improved cardiovascular risk management. PLoS Med 2010;7(8):e1000313.

50. Kuhl EA, Sears SF, Conti JB. Internet-based behavioral change and psychosocial care for patients with cardiovascular disease: a review of cardiac disease-specific applications. Heart Lung 2006; 35(6):374–82.

51. Murtagh EM, Murphy MH, Boone-Heinonen J. Walking: the first steps in cardiovascular disease prevention. Curr Opin Cardiol 2010;25(5):490–6.

52. Scherr D, Kastner P, Kollmann A, et al. Effect of home-based telemonitoring using mobile phone technology on the outcome of heart failure patients after an episode of acute decompensation: randomized controlled trial. J Med Internet Res 2009; 11(3):e34.

53. Shah BR, Adams M, Peterson ED, et al. Secondary prevention risk interventions via telemedicine and tailored patient education (SPRITE): a randomized trial to improve postmyocardial infarction management. Circ Cardiovasc Qual Outcomes 2011;4(2): 235–42.

54. Koehler F, Winkler S, Schieber M, et al. Telemedical interventional monitoring in heart failure (TIM-HF), a randomized, controlled intervention trial investigating the impact of telemedicine on mortality in ambulatory patients with heart failure: study design. Eur J Heart Fail 2010;12(12):1354–62.

55. Pekmezi D, Dunsiger S, Gaskins R, et al. Feasibility and acceptability of using pedometers as an intervention tool for Latinas. J Phys Act Health 2013; 10(3):451–7.

56. Bennett GG, Wolin KY, Puleo E, et al. Pedometer-determined physical activity among multiethnic low-income housing residents. Med Sci Sports Exerc 2006;38(4):768–73.

57. Clarke KK, Freeland-Graves J, Klohe-Lehman DM, et al. Promotion of physical activity in low-income mothers using pedometers. J Am Diet Assoc 2007;107(6):962–7.

58. Shaya FT, Yan X, Farshid M, et al. Social networks in cardiovascular disease management. Expert Rev Pharmacoecon Outcomes Res 2010;10(6): 701–5.

59. Gafarov VV, Panov DO, Gromova EA, et al. The influence of social support on risk of acute cardiovascular diseases in female population aged 25-64 in Russia. Int J Circumpolar Health 2013;72. http://dx.doi.org/10.3402/ijch.v72i0.21210.

60. Vogt TM, Mullooly JP, Ernst D, et al. Social networks as predictors of ischemic heart disease, cancer, stroke and hypertension: incidence, survival and mortality. J Clin Epidemiol 1992;45(6):659–66.

61. Wilkinson RG, Marmot MG. Social determinants of health: the solid facts. 2nd edition. Denmark: World Health Organization; 2003.

62. Greene JA, Choudhry NK, Kilabuk E, et al. Online social networking by patients with diabetes: a qualitative evaluation of communication with Facebook. J Gen Intern Med 2011;26(3):287–92.

63. Chomutare T, Tatara N, Arsand E, et al. Designing a diabetes mobile application with social network support. Stud Health Technol Inform 2013;188: 58–64.

64. Chou WY, Hunt Y, Folkers A, et al. Cancer survivorship in the age of Youtube and social media: a narrative analysis. J Med Internet Res 2011;13(1):e7.

65. Clark AM, Spaling M, Harkness K, et al. Determinants of effective heart failure self-care: a systematic review of patients' and caregivers' perceptions. Heart 2014;100(9):716–21.

66. Taylor MJ, McCormick D, Shawis T, et al. Activity-promoting gaming systems in exercise and rehabilitation. J Rehabil R D 2011;48(10):1171–86.

67. Lamoth CJ, Alingh R, Caljouw SR. Exergaming for elderly: effects of different types of game feedback on performance of a balance task. Stud Health Technol Inform 2012;181:103–7.

68. Finkelstein J, Wood J, Cha E, et al. Feasibility of congestive heart failure telemanagement using a Wii-based telecare platform. Conf Proc IEEE Eng Med Biol Soc 2010;2010:2211–4.

69. Heidenreich PA, Trogdon JG, Khavjou OA, et al. Forecasting the future of cardiovascular disease in the United States: a policy statement from the American Heart Association. Circulation 2011; 123(8):933–44.

70. Heidenreich PA, Albert NM, Allen LA, et al. Forecasting the impact of heart failure in the United States: a policy statement from the American Heart Association. Circ Heart Fail 2013;6(3):606–19.

71. Desai AS. Home monitoring heart failure care does not improve patient outcomes: looking beyond telephone-based disease management. Circulation 2012;125(6):828–36.

72. Wakefield BJ, Holman JE, Ray A, et al. Effectiveness of home telehealth in comorbid diabetes and hypertension: a randomized, controlled trial. Telemed J E Health 2011;17(4):254–61.

73. Giordano A, Scalvini S, Zanelli E, et al. Multicenter randomised trial on home-based telemanagement to prevent hospital readmission of patients with chronic heart failure. Int J Cardiol 2009;131(2):192–9.

74. Antypas K, Wangberg SC. An Internet- and mobile-based tailored intervention to enhance maintenance of physical activity after cardiac rehabilitation: short-term results of a randomized controlled trial. J Med Internet Res 2014;16(3):e77.

75. Maddison R, Pfaeffli L, Stewart R, et al. The HEART mobile phone trial: the partial mediating effects of self-efficacy on physical activity among cardiac patients. Front Public Health 2014;2:56.

76. Danner M, Hummel JM, Volz F, et al. Integrating patients' views into health technology assessment: analytic hierarchy process (AHP) as a method to elicit patient preferences. Int J Technol Assess Health Care 2011;27(4):369–75.

77. Hill JH, Burge S, Haring A, et al. Communication technology access, use, and preferences among primary care patients: from the Residency Research Network of Texas (RRNeT). J Am Board Fam Med 2012;25(5):625–34.

78. Xie B, Wang M, Feldman R, et al. Internet use frequency and patient-centered care: measuring patient preferences for participation using the health information wants questionnaire. J Med Internet Res 2013;15(7):e132.

79. Hsu J, Huang J, Fung V, et al. Health information technology and physician-patient interactions: impact of computers on communication during outpatient primary care visits. J Am Med Inform Assoc 2005;12(4):474–80.

80. Hageman PA, Pullen CH, Hertzog M, et al. Web-based interventions for weight loss and weight maintenance among rural midlife and older women: protocol for a randomized controlled trial. BMC Public Health 2011;11:521.

81. Glasgow RE, Askew S, Purcell P, et al. Use of RE-AIM to address health inequities: application in a low-income community health center based weight loss and hypertension self-management program. Transl Behav Med 2013;3(2):200–10.

82. Ancker JS, Miller MC, Patel V, et al. Sociotechnical challenges to developing technologies for patient access to health information exchange data. J Am Med Inform Assoc 2014;21(4):664–70.

83. Blackman KC, Zoellner J, Berrey LM, et al. Assessing the internal and external validity of mobile health physical activity promotion interventions: a systematic literature review using the RE-AIM framework. J Med Internet Res 2013;15(10):e224.

84. Glasgow RE, Vogt TM, Boles SM. Evaluating the public health impact of health promotion interventions: the RE-AIM framework. Am J Public Health 1999;89(9):1322–7.

Printed and bound by CPI Group (UK) Ltd, Croydon, CR0 4YY

03/10/2024

01040377-0019